Problem Solving for Better Health

A Global Perspective

Barry H. Smith, MD (Cornell '72), **PhD** (MIT '68), is director of The Rogosin Institute, of which the Dreyfus Health Foundation is a division. He is professor of Clinical Surgery at Weill–Cornell Medical College and attending physician at the NewYork–Presbyterian Weill–Cornell Medical Center. He has been directly involved in international health for more than 35 years, as well as medical research and patient care, administration, and health policy.

Joyce J. Fitzpatrick, PhD (New York University '75), **MBA** (Case Western Reserve University '92), **BSN** (Georgetown '66), **RN, FAAN,** has been an International Nursing Program consultant to the Dreyfus Health Foundation of The Rogosin Institute since 2004. She is the Elizabeth Brooks Ford Professor of Nursing at the Frances Payne Bolton School of Nursing at Case Western Reserve University, where she was previously dean for 15 years. She has served as a consultant to nursing leaders, educators, and clinicians throughout the world.

Pamela Hoyt-Hudson, BSN (Georgetown '86), **RN,** has directed the International Nursing Program at the Dreyfus Health Foundation of The Rogosin Institute for the past eight years. She has dedicated herself to sharing the Dreyfus Health Foundation's problem-solving methodologies with communities and healthcare professionals to develop more nurse leaders who are committed to improving health and healthcare around the world.

Problem Solving for Better Health

A Global Perspective

Barry H. Smith, MD, PhD
Joyce J. Fitzpatrick, PhD, MBA, BSN, RN, FAAN
Pamela Hoyt-Hudson, BSN, RN
Editors

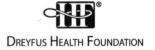

DREYFUS HEALTH FOUNDATION

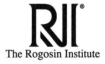

The Rogosin Institute

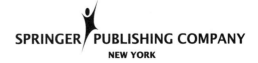

SPRINGER PUBLISHING COMPANY
NEW YORK

Springer Publishing Company, LLC
11 West 42nd Street
New York, NY 10036
www.springerpub.com

Acquisitions Editor: Allan Graubard
Production Editor: Gayle Lee
Cover Design: Steven Pisano
Project Manager: Ashita Shah
Composition: Newgen Imaging Systems

ISBN (Hardcover): 978-0-8261-0468-7
ISBN (Paperback): 978-0-8261-2867-6
E-book ISBN: 978-0-8261-0469-4

10 11 12 13/ 5 4 3 2 1

The author and the publisher of this work have made every effort to use sources believed to be reliable to provide information that is accurate and compatible with the standards generally accepted at the time of publication. Because medical science is continually advancing, our knowledge base continues to expand. Therefore, as new information becomes available, changes in procedures become necessary. We recommend that the reader always consult current research and specific institutional policies before performing any clinical procedure. The author and publisher shall not be liable for any special, consequential, or exemplary damages resulting, in whole or in part, from the readers' use of, or reliance on, the information contained in this book. The publisher has no responsibility for the persistence or accuracy of URLs for external or third-party Internet Web sites referred to in this publication and does not guarantee that any content on such Web sites is, or will remain, accurate or appropriate.

Library of Congress Cataloging-in-Publication Data

Problem solving for better health : a global perspective / Barry H. Smith, Joyce J. Fitzpatrick, Pamela Hoyt-Hudson, editors.
    p. ; cm.
 Includes bibliographical references.
 ISBN 978-0-8261-0468-7
1. Health promotion. 2. World health. 3. Public health. 4. Dreyfus
Health Foundation. 5. Problem solving. I. Smith, Barry H. II. Fitzpatrick, Joyce J., 1944-
III. Hoyt-Hudson, Pamela
 [DNLM: 1. Dreyfus Health Foundation. 2. World Health. 3. Evidence-Based
Practice. 4. Models, Organizational. WA 530.1 P962 2009]
 RA427.8.P755 2009
 613–dc22   2009043425

Printed in the United States of America by Bang Printing

This book is dedicated to the memory of Jack J. Dreyfus, Jr. Jack's "inability to copy what others have done," vision, concern for his fellow human beings, and unflagging, noncompromising commitment to a better world have made so much possible and set the highest standards for us all to follow.

Contents

Note: The countries listed in Section II "Problem Solving for Better Health: Perspectives From Around the World" illustrate case stories from many of the Dreyfus Health Foundation program locations around the globe. Although we extended the invitation to contribute to all program leaders, not all were able to submit chapters in time for this publication.

Contributors

Stephanie Ahmed, DNP, FNP, RN, Director, Clinical Operations, Dovetail Health, Needham, MA

Roy Ahn, MPH, ScD, Associate Director, Policy and Research, Division of Global Health and Human Rights, Department of Emergency Medicine, Massachusetts General Hospital; Instructor in Surgery, Harvard Medical School, Boston, MA

Mahmoud M. Alkam, BSc, Dip PH, Dip Ophth, MSc, PSBH and CBH National Coordinator, Jordan, Amman, Jordan

Frank C. Andolino, DDS, Executive Director and Cofounder, Kageno Worldwide, Inc., New York, NY

Lauren P. Babich, MPH, former Deputy Director, Lesotho–Boston Health Alliance; Instructor, Department of Family Medicine, Boston University, Boston, MA

Darwish Badran, MD, PhD, Director, Center for Educational Development, University of Jordan, Amman, Jordan

Daniel Becker, MD, Chairman of the Board, Center for Health Promotion (Centro de Promoção da Saúde), Rio de Janeiro, Brazil; PSBH National Coordinator, Brazil, and Regional Coordinator, Latin America

William J. Bicknell, MD, MPH, Director, Lesotho–Boston Health Alliance; Professor, Departments of International Health and Family Medicine, Schools of Public Health and Medicine, Boston University, Boston, MA

David E. Bloom, PhD, Chairman and Clarence James Gamble Professor of Economics and Demography, Department of Global Health and Population, School of Public Health, Harvard University, Boston, MA

Daniella Bonatto, MD, Project Coordinator, Center for Health Promotion (Centro de Promoção da Saúde); Urban and Regional Planning Research Institute—Federal University of Rio de Janeiro, Rio de Janeiro, Brazil

Katarzyna Broczek, MD, PhD, Assistant Professor, Department of Geriatrics, Medical University of Warsaw, Warsaw, Poland

Elizabeth Cafiero, MS, Research Assistant, Department of Global Health and Population, School of Public Health, Harvard University, Boston, MA

Jianmei Cai, RN, First Affiliated Hospital of Guangxi Medical University, Nanning, People's Republic of China

Yongqiang Cai, MD, Professor, Inner Mongolia Medical College, Hohhot, People's Republic of China

Kathleen Leask Capitulo, DNSc, RN, FAAN, Executive Director, Transcultural Nursing Leadership Institute, New York, NY

Ignacio Paniagua Castro, MD, President, Salvadoran Physicians for Social Responsibility (Médicos Salvadoreños para la Responsabilidad Social), San Salvador, El Salvador; PSBH National Coordinator, El Salvador

Yunchao Chen, RN, First Affiliated Hospital of Guangxi Medical University, Nanning, People's Republic of China

Ruth Chikasa, International President, Girls' Brigade International Council; Director, Foundation for Better Health, Ndola, Zambia; PSBH National Coordinator, Zambia, and Regional Coordinator, Africa

Maureen L. Chirwa, PhD, RNM, Managing Director, Prime Health Consulting and Services; Director, Health Management Unit, University of Malawi College of Medicine, Zomba; Director, Local Initiative for Better Health, Lilongwe; PSBH National Coordinator, Malawi

Marsha Johnson Copeland, PSBH National Coordinator, United States, Dreyfus Health Foundation, New York, NY

Inge B. Corless, PhD, RN, FAAN, Professor, School of Nursing, Institute of Health Professions, Massachusetts General Hospital, Boston, MA

Arthur G. Cosby, PhD, William L. Giles Distinguished Professor and Director, Social Science Research Center, Mississippi State University, Starkville, MS

Xia Dai, RN, First Affiliated Hospital of Guangxi Medical University, Nanning, People's Republic of China

Sheila M. Davis, DNP, RN, ANP, FAAN, Clinical Assistant Professor, School of Nursing, Institute of Health Professions, Massachusetts General Hospital, Boston, MA

Carlyla Dawson, Director of Operations, Kageno Worldwide, Inc., New York, NY

Jill B. Derstine, EdD, RN, FAAN, Clinical Associate Professor, College of Nursing and Health Professions, Drexel University; Professor Emeritus, Department of Nursing, College of Health Professions, Temple University, Philadelphia, PA

Evgenia Dimitrova, PhD, RN, Senior Lecturer in Nursing, Medical University–Pleven, Bulgaria

Giedre Donauskaite-Tang, PSBH National Coordinator, Lithuania, Vilnius, Lithuania

Kátia Edmundo, PhD, Director, Center for Health Promotion (Centro de Promoção da Saúde), Rio de Janeiro, Brazil

Carolyn L. Engelhard, MPA, Assistant Professor and Health Policy Analyst, Department of Public Health Sciences, School of Medicine, University of Virginia, Charlottesville, VA

Ana Florea, President, Andrea Foundation, Bucharest, Romania

Paul Florea, Vice President, Andrea Foundation, Bucharest, Romania; PSBH and CBH National Coordinator, Romania

Arthur Garson, Jr., MD, MPH, Executive Vice President and Provost, University of Virginia, Charlottesville, VA

John J. Green, PhD, Director, Institute for Community-Based Research and Associate Professor of Sociology and Community Development, Delta State University, Cleveland, MS

Wanda Guimarães, General Coordinator, Center for Health Promotion (Centro de Promoção da Saúde), Rio de Janeiro, Brazil

Le Thi Luc Ha, MD, Lecturer, Faculty of Nursing, Hue University College of Medicine and Pharmacy, Hue, Vietnam

Wenxing Han, BS, Inner Mongolia Medical College, Hohhot, People's Republic of China

Ying Han, MD, Inner Mongolia Medical College, Hohhot, People's Republic of China

Xiaohong He, RN, First Affiliated Hospital of Guangxi Medical University, Nanning, People's Republic of China

Frances C. Henderson, EdD, RN, Nursing Consultant, Dreyfus Health Foundation's Partners Investing in Nursing's Future Project and PSBHN Initiatives, Cleveland, MS

Ian R. Holzman, MD, FAAP, Chief, Division of Newborn Medicine, Mount Sinai Medical Center, New York, NY

Muhong Huang, RN, First Affiliated Hospital of Guangxi Medical University, Nanning, People's Republic of China

Yihua Huang, RN, First Affiliated Hospital of Guangxi Medical University, Nanning, People's Republic of China

Yuzhu Huang, RN, First Affiliated Hospital of Guangxi Medical University, Nanning, People's Republic of China

Valerie D. Jackson, PSBH Program Director, Solutions for Better Living, Houston, TX

Wesley N. Jenkins, MHS, Executive Director, Babyland Family Services, Inc., Newark, NJ; PSBH Program Coordinator, Newark, NJ

Kui Jia, RN, First Affiliated Hospital of Guangxi Medical University, Nanning, People's Republic of China

Shuang Kang, BS, Inner Mongolia Medical College, Hohhot, People's Republic of China

V. Raman Kutty, MD, MPH, MPhil, Professor, Achutha Menon Centre for Health Science Studies, Sree Chitra Tirunal Institute for Medical Sciences and Technology; Chairman, Health Action by People, Trivandrum, India; PSBH National Coordinator, India

Hong Lee, RN, Vice President, Fujian Provincial Hospital, Fuzhou, People's Republic of China

Sarah J. Leonard, MSCD, Assistant Director, The College Board Advanced Placement Program, New York, NY

Daniel M. Levine, PhD, Chief Information Officer, Director, Clinical Research Laboratory, and Co-Director, Lipid Research Laboratory, The Rogosin Institute; Associate Professor of Biochemistry, Weill Medical College of Cornell University, New York, NY; Director, Children's Help Net Foundation, Briarcliff Manor, NY

Malgorzata Leznicka, MSc, Assistant Lecturer, Department of Healthcare Organization and Management, Ludwik Rydygier Collegium Medicum in Bydgoszcz, Nicolaus Copernicus University, Torun, Poland

Jianmei Li, RN, First Affiliated Hospital of Guangxi Medical University, Nanning, People's Republic of China

Weiwei Li, First Affiliated Hospital of Guangxi Medical University, Nanning, People's Republic of China

Xiaohe Li, MD, Lecturer, Inner Mongolia Medical College, Hohhot, People's Republic of China

Zhijun Li, MD, Professor, Inner Mongolia Medical College, Hohhot, People's Republic of China

Guixian Liang, RN, Director of Nursing, First Affiliated Hospital of Kunming Medical College, Kunming, People's Republic of China

Rong Liang, RN, First Affiliated Hospital of Guangxi Medical University, Nanning, People's Republic of China

Xiaokun Liang, PhD, RN, Associate Professor, School of Nursing, Peking Union Medical College, Beijing, People's Republic of China

Socorro Lima, Director, Center for Health Promotion (Centro de Promoção da Saúde), Rio de Janeiro, Brazil

Jing Lin, MD, Assistant Professor, Mount Sinai School of Medicine; Attending Faculty, Neonatal ICU, Kravis Children's Hospital, Mount Sinai Medical Center, New York, NY

Juan Lin, RN, Deputy Director of Nursing, Fujian Provincial Hospital, Fuzhou, People's Republic of China

Zhanghua Lin, RN, First Affiliated Hospital of Guangxi Medical University, Nanning, People's Republic of China

Hengli Ling, RN, First Affiliated Hospital of Guangxi Medical University, Nanning, People's Republic of China

Guimei Liu, RN, First Affiliated Hospital of Guangxi Medical University, Nanning, People's Republic of China

Huaping Liu, PhD, RN, FAAN, Dean and Professor, School of Nursing, Peking Union Medical College, Beijing, People's Republic of China

Jianfen Liu, MSN, RN, Associate Professor, School of Nursing, Peking Union Medical College, Beijing, People's Republic of China

Wanling Liu, MD, Professor, Inner Mongolia Medical College, Hohhot, People's Republic of China

Mauricio Lozano, MD, Vice President and Coordinator of Research on Social Violence, Salvadoran Physicians for Social Responsibility (Médicos Salvadoreños para la Responsabilidad Social), San Salvador, El Salvador; CBH National Coordinator, El Salvador

Andrew Leung Luk, PhD, RN, Professor of Nursing, Kiang Wu Nursing College, Macau Special Administrative Region, People's Republic of China

Ruxiang Luo, RN, First Affiliated Hospital of Guangxi Medical University, Nanning, People's Republic of China

Aisyah Maulina, MSc, Senior Staff, Indonesian Foundation for Better Health, Jakarta Selatan, Indonesia

Jing Meng, MD, Inner Mongolia Medical College, Hohhot, People's Republic of China

Sebastian J. Milardo, MS, Director of Operations, Dreyfus Health Foundation, New York, NY

Julian D. Miller, AB, PSBH Program Coordinator, Mississippi Delta, Winstonville, MS

Shelagh Murphy, RN, RM, International Nursing Program Consultant, UK; Dreyfus Health Foundation, New York, NY

Joyce P. Murray, EdD, RN, FAAN, Professor, Nell Hodgson Woodruff School of Nursing, Emory University; Director, Ethiopia Public Health Training Initiative, The Carter Center, Atlanta, GA

Mary Muyoka, RN, RM, RPHN, RFP, Founder and Director, Nekeki, Kitale, Kenya; PSBH National Coordinator, Kenya

Geisa Nascimento, Project Advisor, Center for Health Promotion (Centro de Promoção da Saúde), Rio de Janeiro, Brazil

Tonya T. Neaves, MPPA, Research Fellow and Project Coordinator, Social Science Research Center, Mississippi State University, Starkville, MS

Njoki Ng'ang'a, MSc, RNC, Donna A. Sanzari Women's Hospital, Hackensack University Medical Center, Hackensack, NJ; Director of Nursing, International Organization for Women and Development, New York, NY

Patrice K. Nicholas, DNSc, MPH, RN, ANP, FAAN, Director, Global Health and Academic Partnerships, Division of Global Health Equity and the Center for Nursing Excellence, Brigham and Women's Hospital; Professor, Institute of Health Professions, Massachusetts General Hospital, Boston, MA

Thomas P. Nicholas, BSBA, Product Delivery Analyst, Bank of America; Department of Patient Care Services, Brigham and Williams Hospital, Boston, MA

Adelaida Oreste, MD, MPH, President, Center for Integral Health and Development (CISADE); Director, Human Resources of the Ministry of Public Health and Social Assistance; Professor of Health Science, Autonomous University of Santo Domingo, Dominican Republic; PSBH National Coordinator, Dominican Republic

Alex Papilaya, MD, DTPH, Director, Indonesian Foundation for Better Health, Jakarta Selatan, Indonesia; PSBH National Coordinator, Indonesia

Taufik Pramudja, Senior Staff, Indonesian Foundation for Better Health, Jakarta Selatan, Indonesia

Tiesheng Que, BS, Professor, First Affiliated Hospital of Guangxi Medical University, Nanning, People's Republic of China

Dame Sheila Quinn, DBE, DSc (hon), BSc, RGN, International Nursing Program Consultant, UK; Dreyfus Health Foundation, New York, NY

Egidia Rugwizangoga, BSN, RN, Registered Nurse, Surgical Unit, Brigham and Women's Hospital, Boston, MA

Héctor Marroquín Segura, MD, Professor, Escuela de Ciencias de la Salud, Universidad del Valle de México, San Luis Potosí, Mexico; PSBH National Coordinator, Mexico

Jin Shen, MD, Professor, First Affiliated Hospital of Kunming Medical College, Kunming, People's Republic of China

Ye Shen, Teacher, Shanghai Minhang District Qiying School, Shanghai, People's Republic of China

Oleksandra Sluzhynska, MD, PhD, President, SALUS Charitable Foundation, Lviv, Ukraine; PSBH and CBH National Coordinator, Ukraine

Jan Sobotka, PhD, Assistant Professor, Department of Preventive Medicine and Hygiene, Institute of Social Medicine, Medical University of Warsaw, Warsaw, Poland; PSBH National Coordinator, Poland, and Regional Coordinator, Eastern Europe, the Middle East, and Central Asia

Aptie Sookoo, BAS, ASc, Public Health Inspector, Hastings & Prince Edward Counties Health Unit, Belleville, Ontario, Canada

Diane Stanton, MA, RNC, NE-BC, Clinical Nurse Manager, Neonatal Intensive Care Unit, Kravis Children's Hospital, Mount Sinai Medical Center, New York, NY

Gongliang Tao, Shanghai, People's Republic of China

Tai-zhen Tao, Professor, Shanghai Medical Workers College, Shanghai, People's Republic of China

Shelly B. Terrazas, MBA, MS, Assistant Director, Ethiopia Public Health Training Initiative and Mental Health Liberia Program, The Carter Center, Atlanta, GA

Tran Duc Thai, MD, former Dean, Faculty of Nursing, Hue University College of Medicine and Pharmacy, Director, Gamma Knife Center and Neurosurgery Unit, Hue University Hospital, Hue, Vietnam; PSBH National Coordinator, Vietnam

Eric Tribut, Masters in Political Science, Associate Member of Grupo GEA, Lima, Peru

Lynda Tyer-Viola, PhD, RNC, Assistant Professor, School of Nursing, Institute of Health Professions, and Senior Advisor, Division of Global Health and Human Rights, Department of Emergency Medicine, Massachusetts General Hospital, Boston

Yanka Tzvetanova, MA, MPsych, Senior Lecturer of English, Department of Foreign Languages, Medical University–Pleven; Director, Association for Better Health; PSBH and CBH National Coordinator, Bulgaria

Alysa N. Veidis, MSN, RN, FNP, Director of Nursing Programs, Lesotho—Boston Health Alliance, Department of Family Medicine, Boston University Medical Center, Boston, MA

Ana Viamonte-Ros, MD, MPH, Secretary of Health and State Surgeon General, Department of Health, State of Florida, Tallahassee, FL

K. Vijayakumar, MD, DPH, Dip NB, Professor, Department of Community Medicine, Medical College, Trivandrum, Kerala, India, and Secretary, Health Action by People, Trivandrum, Kerala, India

Guoqiang Wang, MD, Lecturer, Inner Mongolia Medical College, Hohhot, People's Republic of China

Jianwei Wang, MD, Professor, Inner Mongolia Medical College, Hohhot, People's Republic of China

Mingjun Wang, Assistant Professor, First Affiliated Hospital of Guangxi Medical University, Nanning, People's Republic of China

Weirong Wang, Professor, Shanghai Medical Workers College, Shanghai, People's Republic of China

Zhenfeng Wang, MD, Professor, Inner Mongolia Medical College, Hohhot, People's Republic of China

Na Wei, BS, Inner Mongolia Medical College, Hohhot, People's Republic of China

Ruili Wei, RN, First Affiliated Hospital of Guangxi Medical University, Nanning, People's Republic of China

Yongfeng Wei, RN, First Affiliated Hospital of Guangxi Medical University, Nanning, People's Republic of China

Hanchun Wen, Assistant Professor, First Affiliated Hospital of Guangxi Medical University, Nanning, People's Republic of China

Judith Woodruff, JD, Program Director, Health Workforce, Northwest Health Foundation, and Program Director, Partners Investing in Nursing's Future, Portland, OR

Zengming Xiao, MD, Director of Orthopedic Surgery, First Affiliated Hospital of Guangxi Medical University, Nanning, People's Republic of China

Wenhua Xin, MD, Lecturer, Inner Mongolia Medical College, Hohhot, People's Republic of China

Youhua Yao, MS, Linfen Community Health Service Center, Zhabei District, Shanghai, People's Republic of China

Ningxian Yu, RN, First Affiliated Hospital of Guangxi Medical University, Nanning, People's Republic of China

Weiping Yu, MD, Deputy Director, Caojiadu Community Health Center, Jing'an District, Shanghai, People's Republic of China

Sheryl M. Zang, EdD, RN, FNP, CNS, Clinical Associate Professor of Nursing, SUNY Downstate Medical Center, Brooklyn, NY

Jin Zeng, RN, First Affiliated Hospital of Guangxi Medical University, Nanning, People's Republic of China

Weihua Zeng, Linfen Community Health Service Center, Zhabei District, Shanghai, People's Republic of China

Xiaofen Zeng, RN, First Affiliated Hospital of Guangxi Medical University, Nanning, People's Republic of China

Hua Zhang, BS, Linfen Community Health Service Center, Zhabei District, Shanghai, People's Republic of China

Huaping Zhang, RN, First Affiliated Hospital of Guangxi Medical University, Nanning, People's Republic of China

Lidong Zhang, MD, Inner Mongolia Medical College, Hohhot, People's Republic of China

Man Zhang, BS, Inner Mongolia Medical College, Hohhot, People's Republic of China

Weibo Zhang, MD, Shanghai Mental Health Center, Xuhui District, Shanghai, People's Republic of China

Xiaoxia Zhang, RN, Nurse in Charge, Wuyi Mountain Municipal Hospital, Wuyishan, People's Republic of China

Yan Zhao, MD, Inner Mongolia Medical College, Hohhot, People's Republic of China

Jincai Zhong, MS, Professor, First Affiliated Hospital of Guangxi Medical University, Nanning, People's Republic of China

Yuxia Zhong, MD, Inner Mongolia Medical College, Hohhot, People's Republic of China

Aimin Zhou, RN, First Affiliated Hospital of Guangxi Medical University, Nanning, People's Republic of China

Xiaomin Zhou, BS, Assistant Professor, First Affiliated Hospital of Guangxi Medical University, Nanning, People's Republic of China

Jinge Zhu, RN, First Affiliated Hospital of Guangxi Medical University, Nanning, People's Republic of China

Shitai Zhu, Shanghai, People's Republic of China

Na Zhuo, BS, Inner Mongolia Medical College, Hohhot, People's Republic of China

Anna Zucchetti, MSc, MPhil, Founder and Executive Director, Grupo GEA, Lima, Peru; PSBH National Coordinator, Peru

Jacek Zyrkowski, MD, Internal Medicine, TORMED, Torun, Poland

Preface

Barry H. Smith

This book is about human potential and possibilities for change. It is an exciting story because it describes not only what has already been accomplished but also what remains to be done to achieve better health and better quality of life for all the world's people. The book, then, is both a progress report and a call to further action.

Section I opens with an introductory chapter, "Stating the Problem and Finding Solutions." This chapter on problem solving for a better world lays the groundwork necessary for understanding the stories that follow, and provides a broad definition of health, which is absolutely crucial to our efforts. The following chapter describes the history of the Dreyfus Health Foundation (DHF), the Problem Solving for Better Health® (PSBH®) program, and the principles on which its methodology is based.

Section II, "PSBH: Perspectives From Around the World," contains the stories that bring PSBH to life. The chapters here include only a portion of what has been achieved over the past 22 years since the inception of the program. The section begins with stories from Africa: Ghana, Kenya, Lesotho, Malawi, Niger, and Zambia. These chapters illustrate the wonderful warmth, beauty, challenges, and enormous promise of this great continent. The focus then shifts to Asia, with accounts of the program and projects in

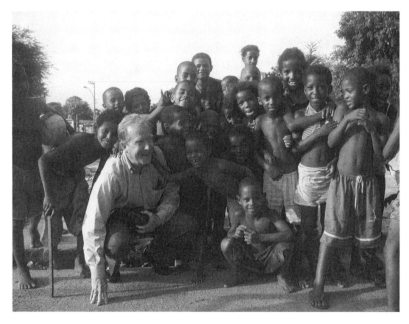

Barry H. Smith with "the future of Brazil" in the *favela* Vila Paciência, Rio de Janeiro, Brazil.

China, India, Indonesia, Kyrgyzstan, and Vietnam. Comprising more than two-fifths of the world's population, this region has a long, dramatic history forged by cultural and economic tidal waves from war, ideology, economic dynamism, and the stark contrasts between urban and rural well-being. Following Asia is Eastern Europe, where changes in government, economy, and social organization during the past 30 years have been equally dramatic. The people of Bulgaria, Lithuania, Poland, Romania, and Ukraine have striking stories to tell about what they have achieved, sometimes despite the negative forces that their history has presented to them. Latin America and the Caribbean is the next region of focus. From Brazil, the Dominican Republic, El Salvador, Guyana, Mexico, and Peru come messages of hope that transcend class and ethnicity and speak of the richness and challenges faced by these countries' many cultures. There is also a report from Jordan, representing the Middle East, with yet another story of hope and transformation that involves a countrywide effort to change lives and health. Finally, there is the United States, represented by three areas: Houston, Texas; Newark, New Jersey; and the Mississippi Delta. As often occurs, many partnerships have developed in Mississippi as a result of the collective work being done in the region. Views from some of these DHF partners are included in the chapter on the Mississippi Delta.

Section III broadens our horizons by describing other approaches to global health, illustrating how different models can be compatible, and not compete, with each other. Here, Garson and Engelhard present an innovative approach to expanding the health workforce by utilizing senior citizens, thereby engaging the aging population to solve health problems. Nicholas and colleagues follow with their examination of global health partnerships, and the chapter on The Carter Center's Ethiopia Public Health Training Initiative addresses the shortage of healthcare providers, an exemplar of what can be done on a broad scale. Bloom and Cafiero follow with their views on the need for improved implementation of public health interventions, and the final chapter of the section, "Corporate Social Responsibility and Global Health," presents the link between economic activity as it exists in the corporate world, and the health and quality of life of the communities involved.

Clearly, we must develop more programs to leverage the power of each individual approach in a way that accelerates progress toward better health. Hence, Section IV is about the future. PSBH, as well as all other approaches to improving health and quality of life for more people, ultimately must come face to face with the demand to scale up. This is a crucial effort, and Garson's chapter in this section, on connecting individual problem solving with evidence-based policy for achieving a healthier world, is a strong start in this direction. Finally, "The Call to Action" addresses the points discussed in the preceding chapters while laying out a set of specific tasks and goals that must and can be accomplished. If you finish this book with a renewed sense of hope and confidence that we can and will make the necessary change, and you are motivated to actively participate in the effort to do so, then this book will have served its purpose.

A Note From the Editors

This book would not have been possible without the efforts of Carley E. Smith. Carley worked tirelessly, volunteering her time and editorial expertise for this project. As the former Director of Operations for the Dreyfus Health Foundation (DHF), Carley continues to cultivate relationships with DHF coordinators and teams around the world. We are deeply grateful to Carley, our DHF ambassador.

Acknowledgments

We would like to acknowledge the involvement of thousands of committed people around the world who have contributed to the global work illustrated in this book. We are indebted to those who have organized and participated in Problem Solving for Better Health® workshops and projects in their countries—for all they have given to their communities, for all they have taught us, and for all their passion for creating a better world. We could not include descriptions of all the projects and the people who implemented them—that would require many, many volumes. Instead, this book is a snapshot of the good work that is being done throughout the world. As such, it should be a stimulus and encouragement to us all.

We extend special thanks to the book's contributors and to the national coordinators and local teams of the Dreyfus Health Foundation (DHF) programs. We also wish to recognize the monumental efforts of New York–based DHF staff members, present and past, who spent countless hours identifying key contributors, researching relevant data, and preparing the final product for publication. We thank Carol Slotkin and Valerie Ciliento, whose editorial, translation, and organizational skills assured that the book got off to a strong start. We also thank Sebastian J. Milardo, Karen Meerabux, and Marsha Johnson Copeland for their keen eyes and for keeping us organized and on schedule. We thank Ana Maria Cruz for her translation assistance, and we thank, anonymously by request, a colleague who was enormously instrumental in many aspects of the book's preparation. In addition we thank Dr. Arthur Garson, Jr., who willingly read the entire manuscript several times with a critical eye. We are especially indebted to Springer Publishing for its expert advice and unending patience. In particular we thank Allan Graubard, our editor, who advised and supported us along the way, and Joanne Jay, Gayle Lee, Jason Roth, Pascal Schwarzer, Elizabeth Stump, and Ashita Shah of Newgen Imaging. We are extremely grateful to *all* the people who have contributed their time and expertise on behalf of this book.

—*Barry H. Smith, Joyce J. Fitzpatrick, and Pamela Hoyt-Hudson*

Problem Solving for Better Health

A Global Perspective

I

Introduction

1

Stating the Problem and Finding Solutions

Barry H. Smith

Our world is broken. Grinding poverty, injustice, inequality, violence and warfare, hatred, racism, urban decay, global warming, worldwide recession, corruption at all levels, declining seas, eroding soil, growing deserts, the emergence of new diseases, and the persistence, even increased prevalence, of old diseases affect hundreds of millions of people. Despite many attempts to fix existing problems, we seem to be drifting sideways and losing ground rather than moving on an upward track. We have achieved some successes, such as the elimination of smallpox, the provision of sanitation to 1 billion people, the emergence of new middle classes in countries like China and India, and the South African "miracle;" however, we have not succeeded nearly as well as we should have.

Economists have estimated that, since the 1960s, developed countries have provided more than 2.6 trillion USD to less fortunate countries. Given the investment made, far less has been accomplished than should have been (Burnside & Dollar, 2000; Easterly, 2003, 2006). There are many different points of view on the value, and even necessity, of foreign aid, but the bottom line is that policies to date have not resulted in the kind or quality of improvements expected. As Easterly (2003) wrote, "The goal of having the high-income people make some kind of transfer to very poor people remains a worthy one, despite the disappointments of the past. But the appropriate goal of foreign aid is neither to move as much money as politically possible, nor to foster society-wide transformation from poverty to wealth. The goal is simply to benefit some poor people some of the time."

There are different levels that must be considered in relation to aid and what it should mean and accomplish. There is the macroeconomic level and questions such as whether or not foreign aid can stimulate or achieve the growth of a country's economy (Sachs, 2005). Data such as those provided by Easterly (2006) shed doubt on any simple relationship here (Figure 1.1).

At the microeconomic level, there is much more opportunity to see the benefits of foreign aid. The provision of a new well or a pipe system to bring water directly to villagers, who previously had to walk long distances to obtain it, is a clear benefit. However, many benefits at the microeconomic level are short lived or unsustainable.

Turning more specifically to health issues, what is the situation? It parallels what has been described earlier for a wide range of global issues. There is a relationship among economics, health, and life expectancy. Such a relationship is not surprising, nor is it necessarily simple. The World Health Organization's (WHO) Commission on Social

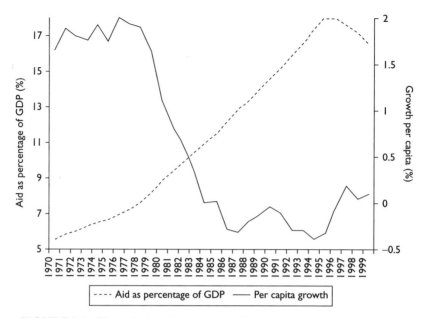

FIGURE 1.1   The relationship between aid as a percentage of gross domestic product (GDP) and per capita growth for Africa. The rise of foreign aid would appear to correlate with a marked fall in per capita growth. Of course, it is not as simple as that. The fact remains, however, that foreign aid did not help per capita economic growth in Africa from 1970 to 2000 in any significant degree (Easterly, 2006).

Determinants of Health (2008d) summarized this well: "Wealth alone does not have to determine the health of a nation's population. Some low-income countries such as Cuba, Costa Rica, China, [the] state of Kerala in India and Sri Lanka have achieved levels of good health despite relatively low levels of national incomes." For example, life expectancy at birth is 75.14 years (2009 estimate) in Sri Lanka with a per capita income of 4,300 USD, as compared with 78.11 years in the United States, where per capita income is 47,000 USD. The small difference in life expectancy is hard to understand, given the more than 10-fold difference in per capita income. In the People's Republic of China, life expectancy is 73.47 years with a per capita income of 6,000 USD. Once again, compared with the United States, which has a per capita income almost eight times that of the Chinese figure, the difference in life expectancy is less than 5 years.

The situation is even more complicated than that. National figures hide inequities within a country. This is well known, but just how big the differences can be in developed and undeveloped, as well as in "rich" and "poor," countries, is surprising. Some facts from the WHO Commission on Social Determinants of Health show this clearly:

■ A child born in a Glasgow, Scotland, suburb can expect a life 28 years shorter than another living only 13 km away. A girl in Lesotho is likely to live 42 years less than another in Japan. In Sweden, the risk of a woman dying during pregnancy and childbirth is 1 in 17,400; in Afghanistan, the odds are 1 in 8.

■ Life expectancy for Indigenous Australian males is shorter by 17 years than all other Australian males.

- Maternal mortality is 3 [to] 4 times higher among the poor compared with the rich in Indonesia. The difference in adult mortality between least and most deprived neighborhoods in the United Kingdom is more than 2.5 times.
- Child mortality in the slums of Nairobi is 2.5 times higher than that in other parts of the city. A baby born to a Bolivian mother with no education has a 10% chance of dying, while one born to a woman with at least secondary education has a 0.4% chance.
- In the United States, 886,202 deaths could have been averted between 1991 and 2000 if mortality rates between Whites and African Americans were equalized. (This contrasts to 176,633 lives saved in the United States by medical advances in the same period.)
- In Uganda, the death rate of children younger than 5 years in the richest fifth of households is 106 per 1,000 live births, but in the poorest fifth of households it is even worse—192 deaths per 1,000 live births—that is, nearly a fifth of all babies born alive to the poorest households are destined to die before they reach their fifth birthday. Set this against an average death rate for children younger than age 5 in high-income countries of 7 deaths per 1,000 (WHO, 2008d).

Another way to examine the problem from the point of view of health involves the leading causes of disability-adjusted life years (DALYs) and mortality. Table 1.1 lists the leading causes of disability and Table 1.2 lists the leading causes of mortality.

The tables present a large amount of data, but they do not tell the whole story. For example, there is no way to know that 99% of the women who died in pregnancy and childbirth were from developing countries. Similarly, it is not obvious that tobacco use is a risk factor for six of the eight leading causes of death, with 8.3 million tobacco-related deaths projected for 2030 and more than 80% of these deaths occurring in developing countries.

It is also apparent that a surprisingly large proportion of the DALYs and causes of death are dependent on human behavior. Of course, there are problems that do not directly relate to human behavior, such as purely genetic diseases or some bacterial or viral diseases, but these are relatively few. For much of these lists human behavior plays an important role. Moreover, many of the problems listed are found in both the developed and the developing world.

In the early years of the 21st century, it is clear that health is a global issue, with the health of one region dependent on the health of all the others. Since many emerging diseases, as well as noncommunicable diseases, do not honor nation-state boundaries, the interdependence of all humanity is evident. The obvious question then is, "Who is going to do what needs to be done to improve health?" The most common answers to this question are cautionary. There are very few health professionals. Fiscal resources are strained for all governments, especially with the recent global economic downturn. We need new and better programs. We need new technology. Can we really hope to change the situation, or is it simply too big and complex to achieve better health for many, let alone Health for All (which was a goal set by WHO for the year 2000 but is not yet close to being achieved)?

Whether support comes from governments, international agencies, or private foundations, none of the efforts to date have succeeded to the extent that we would wish them to. The Bill & Melinda Gates Foundation (http://www.gatesfoundation.org/global-health), for example, has made an enormous and broad-based commitment to global health. The

TABLE 1.1   *Leading Causes of Burden of Disease (DALYs), Countries Grouped by Income, 2004*

Disease or Injury	DALYs (millions)	Percent of Total DALYs	Disease or Injury	DALYs (millions)	Percent of Total DALYs
World			*Low-Income Countries*		
1. Lower respiratory infections	94.5	6.2	1. Lower respiratory infections	76.9	9.3
2. Diarrheal diseases	72.8	4.8	2. Diarrheal diseases	59.2	7.2
3. Unipolar depressive disorders	65.5	4.3	3. HIV/AIDS	42.9	5.2
4. Ischemic heart diseases	62.6	4.1	4. Malaria	32.8	4.0
5. HIV/AIDS	58.5	3.8	5. Prematurity and low birth weight	32.1	3.9
6. Cerebrovascular disease	46.6	3.1	6. Neonatal infections and other*	31.4	3.8
7. Prematurity and low birth weight	44.3	2.9	7. Birth asphyxia and birth trauma	29.8	3.6
8. Birth asphyxia and birth trauma	41.7	2.7	8. Unipolar depressive disorders	26.5	3.2
9. Road traffic accidents	41.2	2.7	9. Ischemic heart disease	26.0	3.1
10. Neonatal infections and other*	40.4	2.7	10. Tuberculosis	22.4	2.7
Middle-Income Countries			*High-Income Countries*		
1. Unipolar depressive disorders	29.0	5.1	1. Unipolar depressive disorders	10.0	8.2
2. Ischemic heart disease	28.9	5.0	2. Ischemic heart disease	7.7	6.3
3. Cerebrovascular disease	27.5	4.8	3. Cerebrovascular disease	4.8	3.9
4. Road traffic accidents	21.4	3.7	4. Alzheimer's and other dementias	4.4	3.6
5. Lower respiratory infections	16.3	2.8	5. Alcohol use disorders	4.2	3.4
6. COPD	16.1	2.8	6. Hearing loss, adult onset	4.2	3.4
7. HIV/AIDS	15.0	2.6	7. COPD	3.7	3.0
8. Alcohol use disorders	14.9	2.3	8. Diabetes mellitus	3.6	3.0
9. Refractive errors	13.7	2.4	9. Trachea, bronchus, lung cancers	3.6	3.0
10. Diarrheal diseases	13.1	2.3	10. Road traffic accidents	3.1	2.6

*This category also includes other noninfectious causes arising in the perinatal period apart from prematurity, low birth weight, birth trauma, and asphyxia. These noninfectious causes are responsible for about 20% of DALYs shown in this category.
COPD: chronic obstructive pulmonary disease; DALYS: disability-adjusted life years.
Source: WHO, (2008c).

TABLE 1.2   *The 10 Leading Causes of Death by Broad Income Group, 2004*

Disease or Injury	Deaths in Millions	Percentage of Deaths
Low-Income Countries		
Lower respiratory infections	2.94	11.20
Coronary heart disease	2.47	9.40
Diarrheal diseases	1.81	6.90
HIV/AIDS	1.51	5.70
Stroke and other cerebrovascular diseases	1.48	5.60
COPDs	0.94	3.60
Tuberculosis	0.91	3.50
Neonatal infections	0.90	3.40
Malaria	0.86	3.30
Prematurity and low birth weight	0.84	3.20
Middle-Income Countries		
Stroke and other cerebrovascular diseases	3.47	14.20
Coronary heart disease	3.40	13.90
COPD	1.80	7.40
Lower respiratory infections	0.92	3.80
Trachea, bronchus, lung cancers	0.69	2.90
Road traffic accidents	0.67	2.80
Hypertensive disease	0.62	2.50
Stomach cancer	0.55	2.20
Tuberculosis	0.54	2.20
Diabetes mellitus	0.52	2.10
High-Income Countries		
Coronary heart disease	1.33	16.30
Stroke and other cerebrovascular diseases	0.76	9.30
Trachea, bronchus, lung cancers	0.48	5.90
Lower respiratory infections	0.31	3.80
COPD	0.29	3.50
Alzheimer's and other dementias	0.28	3.40
Colon and rectum cancers	0.27	3.30
Diabetes mellitus	0.22	2.80
Breast cancer	0.16	2.00
Stomach cancer	0.14	1.80
World		
Coronary heart disease	7.20	12.20
Stroke and other cerebrovascular diseases	5.71	9.70
Lower respiratory infections	4.18	7.10
COPD	3.02	5.10
Diarrheal diseases	2.16	3.70

Continued

TABLE 1.2   *Continued*

Disease or Injury	Deaths in Millions	Percentage of Deaths
HIV/AIDS	2.04	3.50
Tuberculosis	1.46	2.50
Trachea, bronchus, lung cancers	1.32	2.30
Road traffic accidents	1.27	2.20
Prematurity and low birth weight	1.18	2.00

COPD: chronic obstructive pulmonary disease.
Source: World Health Organization (2008b).

foundation's Global Health Program emphasizes the importance of scientific innovation and discovery. Priority areas include (1) discovery of new insights to fight serious diseases and other problems affecting developing countries; (2) development of effective and affordable vaccines, medicines, and other health tools; and (3) delivery of proven health solutions to those who need them most (Bill & Melinda Gates Foundation, 2009). Undergirding these efforts is a strong foundation of technology. However, this tremendous effort has not achieved all that it could. Even with good new solutions and technology, how are these to be delivered to the people?

The answer given by the chapters in this book is that it is possible to achieve better health for millions and that it is practical to do so. In fact, we have to do it. There can be no excuses. There is simply too much at stake, not only for the present but also, even more important, for a future that will not be very attractive if we do not act now to make a big difference. To examine how this can be done, let us take a step back and talk about health more generally. What exactly do we mean by health?

Definition of Health

The Constitution of WHO defines health as "… a state of complete physical, mental and social well-being and not merely the absence of disease or infirmity" (WHO, 2006). Moving beyond the confining parameters of what has been mainstream Western and scientific medicine, the field of population health, for example, has led us to see health as a product of many factors including both the biological and social. The social determinants of health are defined by WHO (2008a; see also Taylor, 2008) as "the circumstances in which people are born, grow up, live, work and age, and the systems put in place to deal with illness. These circumstances are in turn shaped by a wider set of forces: economics, social policies, and politics." Specific factors that are determinants of health include the following: income and social status, social support networks, education and literacy, employment working conditions, social environments, physical environments, life skills, personal health practices and coping skills, healthy childhood development, biology and genetic endowment, health services, gender, and culture. A more strictly "social" list drawn up in Canada includes aboriginal status, early life, education, employment and working conditions, food security, gender, healthcare services, housing, income and its distribution, social safety net, social exclusion, and unemployment and employment security (Raphael, 2008).

From the nature of the aforementioned lists it is easy to see how these parameters or variables shape the health inequities that exist, whether within a given country or between countries. Recognizing this, WHO established the Commission on Social Determinants of Health in 2005 to propose ways to reduce health inequities by working through social determinants. Although there have been vast changes in medical care since 1900, McKinlay, McKinlay, and Beaglehole (1989) estimated that only 10%–15% of the increase in longevity since the turn of the century is due to improved healthcare, at least in the developed nations. Similarly, it was not improvements in individual behavior that produced these results. It was much more the improvements in daily life that were responsible. Key elements, consistent with the aforementioned lists, included education, early childhood conditions, food processing and availability, health and social services, and employment security and conditions—all social determinants of health. The bottom line is that health, in its broadest sense, is a product of society and the degree to which that society is functioning well or poorly.

The Challenge

Taking this broadened approach to health would seem to make the problem of improving health for hundreds of millions of people around the world much worse. The implication of this is that all sectors of society—economics, transportation, education, agriculture, and distribution—must be improved before health will improve. Beyond that, the numbers of people who must be reached are staggering. United Nations projections indicate that the world population will grow from 6.1 billion in 2000 to 8.9 billion in 2050, a 47% increase, or the addition of 57 million people a year on average (United Nations Department of Economic and Social Affairs [UN DESA] Population Division, 2004). The same source notes that the 50-year increase will be more than twice the current population of China and more than double that of the combined current population of all the developed regions of the world. Added to this is the fact that most of the demographic increase will take place in the less developed regions of the world. These regions will increase their population by 58%, while the developed regions increase by only 2%, according to the projections (UN DESA Population Division, 2004). Africa is projected to add 1 billion to its population, with the continent's share of the global population rising from 13% to 20% (UN DESA Population Division, 2004). In other words, 99% of the population increase will occur in regions where public health systems are weakest or nonexistent. Beyond that, there is the dramatic shift of people from rural areas to densely packed urban centers with an associated shift in disease patterns and the opportunity for emerging diseases to spread rapidly.

Further unsettling facts come from the World Bank, United Nations International Children's Emergency Fund, and Joint United Nations Program on HIV/AIDS. Approximately 3 billion people live on less than 2 USD a day, adjusted for purchasing power (Chen & Ravaillion, 2004); 840 million people do not have enough to eat; 1 billion people do not have access to clean water or adequate sanitation; 1 billion cannot read or write; 10 million children die every year from preventable diseases; and new epidemic or pandemic diseases, from AIDS to SARS and H1N1 influenza, are global problems threatening the entire world population.

The population problem has yet another important aspect: changing global demographics, with aging being the most prominent of these. Projections indicate that the percentage growth of the population over 65 worldwide will increase by 84.8% from 2000 to 2050, but by 344% in less developed regions over this same period; the percentage of the total population over 65 will rise from 5.2% in 1950 to 15.9% by 2050 (UN DESA Population Division,

2004). The point of listing all these figures is to emphasize the size of the problem. The chronic illnesses of the aging population are far more complex and expensive to manage than communicable diseases. Noncommunicable diseases are projected to account for more than 75% of all deaths by 2030 (WHO, 2008c), and an increasing percentage of these problems will be in the over-65 population. With the struggles the world already has meeting the needs of the present population burden, the difficulties will only grow. The resources needed to meet the challenges are unlikely to grow at the pace required to even keep up with the problems. Many aspects of the disease burden are far outpacing the systems designed to control them. All the other societal sectors are strained as well.

Does this mean the situation is hopeless? Should we just continue to improve immunization and the detection and treatment of tuberculosis, build more clinics, educate the public about health and disease, and fix broken health systems? Although there has been some success with these approaches and there is no shortage of plans, the realization of the plans to date has fallen far short of the goals that have been set (Easterly, 2006). Can we meet the challenge and, if so, how? As I have already stated, the answer given in this book is that it is not only possible to achieve better health for millions but also practical to do so. In fact, we must do it. There can be no excuses.

Responding to the Challenge

Recognizing the multiplicity of factors on which good health relies and the numbers presented earlier, it is clear that there will never be sufficient medical personnel, public health professionals, or financial resources to meet the challenges. The sheer size and continuing yearly growth of the global human population, including a large portion of that population surpassing 65 years of age, appear to be highly discouraging. How can we possibly cope with such numbers and the issues associated with them?

The answer is that we need to radically change our thinking. Yes, such numbers represent a burden to the system, but they also present us a solution. People are not the problem; they are a major part of the solution. "The people" whom our health systems are designed to serve must be integrated as active participants and not simply passive recipients or objects of the programs that are planned.

How is this integration to be achieved? Traditional thinking about people as passive recipients of the knowledge held by medical and public health experts must be changed. I emphasize this point because biases from within these fields are deep and subtle, and ultimately limiting and harmful. As an example, I recount a conversation I had with a Ministry of Health official. When asked for her evaluation of the status of health programs in her country, she responded that the country had excellent health programs. After I replied that was good to hear, the official continued, "But they don't work." Puzzled, I asked, "How can that be? The programs are excellent, but they don't work?" Her reply was quick. "That's easy. The people don't follow our instructions. They are lazy. They are stupid. You can't trust them." Perhaps this is an extreme example, but it is also an honest one—and it is a widespread view. We need to change the dominant way of thinking.

In his book, *Development as Freedom*, Amartya Sen (1999) points out that poverty is not really the problem for poor people. The problem is the denial of opportunities for poor people to exercise their innate abilities to solve problems using local knowledge and skills bred of experience in a particular environment and with a set of challenges.

This does not mean that the people have all the knowledge, answers, or tools required to promote their own health or prevent disease, but it does mean that they can be the ones to turn the knowledge they do have into action, belief, behavioral change, and practice within their communities. How do we engage the people in the process of improving health and quality of life? It is crucial for them to take ownership of the problems they face and make a commitment to be actively involved in the solutions they need. They must see a given issue as a priority for them and not for someone else.

One approach here, developed by the Dreyfus Health Foundation (DHF), is Problem Solving for Better Health® (PSBH®; DHF, 2009; Hoyt, 2007; Smith et al., 1994). The PSBH process involves asking people to think about the two or three most important problems in their community or region, from their point of view. These should be problems that they believe they can do something about as individuals or in small groups, implementing solutions that they have created and are possible for them to accomplish. The solutions may be informed by knowledge that has come from an external source, but they must ultimately belong to the individuals who have made a commitment to solving the problems and have detailed the implementation of the solutions.

PSBH is a tool for individual use. It consists of the scientific method adapted to community-level needs and issues. It includes a series of steps, which begin with (1) defining the problem precisely (nature, size, causes, and contributing factors); (2) prioritizing the problem from the point of view of the community and asking if it can be addressed by an individual (at least initially); (3) identifying and sorting out possible solutions, choosing one solution and asking a "Good Question" ("Will doing *what*, with *whom*, and *where*, for *how long*, achieve the *desired objective*?"); (4) developing an action plan (including background and rationale, "Good Question," hypothesis, methods, and evaluation); and (5) taking action (DHF, 2009). As a tool, PSBH must be met with a strong commitment to making a positive change. It requires a blend of intellect and passion. It involves community organization, with optimism about the ability to achieve change and a strong sense that it is realistic to expect it (Hoyt, 2007; Smith et al., 1994).

PSBH is a way to help organize a community. It has its own intrinsic strength and applicability, but it is also intended to sow the seeds of a transformative process. It is about creating change through a self-sustaining, dynamic, and forward-looking approach to continuous community improvement, with a strong emphasis on improving quality of life for individuals and families. PSBH is certainly not the only approach to community organization and short- and long-term transformation, but it is a time-tested and proven means of achieving such goals. It serves to illustrate what 21st-century health promotion and healthcare must do if they are to make a much larger impact. The public must take active ownership of the solutions, ensuring their implementation, effectiveness, and sustainability.

Effective organization of communities at the grassroots level is not simple. It requires hard work and a consistent, forward-looking plan that has at its heart local individuals and teams. These people must incorporate the transformative process into the fabric of their communities. The better-health process shares much in common with political process and should incorporate lessons from this discipline into its own planning. Examples of effective community organization can be found in post-1949 China, as well as Barack Obama's recent presidential campaign in the United States, and Dr. Thomas Frieden's campaigns for tobacco control and trans-fat reduction in New York City, among others. Obama, with a skillful use of the Internet, built a 13-million-member grassroots network. He indicated that this network would play a critical role as the "Organizing for America" group in achieving the goals of his agenda, once he was in the White House. Efforts to achieve better health must build similar grassroots-led networks and find ways to become self-sustaining and self-replicating.

Health professionals should also recognize that they may be part of the problem. Although it is not particularly palatable, and some of his terminology bears the stamp of the 1970s, Paulo Freire's *Pedagogy of the Oppressed* makes the point clearly (Freire, 2000). Freire described the oppressed (the "poor") as living in an existential duality: at once themselves, they also live with their image as projected by their "oppressors"—as ignorant, incapable, being good for nothing. It is not surprising, then, that poor individuals suffer fatalistic and self-deprecatory attitudes about their situation. Freire (2000, pp. 61–63) quoted poor individuals who say:

> The peasant begins to get courage to overcome his dependence when he realizes that he is dependent. Until then, he goes along with the boss and says, "What can I do? I am only a peasant." … The peasant feels inferior to the boss because the boss seems to be the only one who knows things and is able to run things.

Freire (2000, pp. 60–66) also adds an admonishment to those who seek to help the oppressed:

> Those who authentically commit themselves to the people must re-examine themselves constantly. The conversion [to a true humanist] is so radical as to not allow … ambiguous behavior. To affirm this commitment but to consider oneself the proprietor of revolutionary wisdom—which must then be given to (or imposed on) the people—is to retain the old ways. The man or woman who proclaims devotion to the cause of liberation yet is unable to enter into communion with the people, whom he or she continues to regard as totally ignorant, is grievously self-deceived. The convert who approaches the people but feels alarm at each step they take, each doubt they express, and each suggestion they offer, and attempts to impose his "status," remains nostalgic towards his origins. … At all stages of liberation, the oppressed must see themselves as women and men engaged in the ontological and historical vocation of becoming more fully human … action on the side of the oppressed … must be action with the oppressed. Those who work for liberation must not take advantage of the emotional dependence of the oppressed…. Using their dependence to create still greater dependence is an oppressor tactic.

Unfortunately, often with the best intentions, many health professionals' efforts have been beset and greatly diminished by the sense that they are the experts bringing knowledge and enlightenment to those who have none of their own. Young professionals entering the health education field must be taught that the new reality they face, and may help to create, and the techniques they use in doing so should be different from those of the past.

Problem-solving education of the kind I have described earlier is essential for both health professionals and the people themselves. In such education, as Freire (2000, p. 83) explained, "People develop their power to perceive critically the way they exist in the world with which and in which they find themselves; they come to see the world not as a static reality, but as a reality in process, in transformation." For the health professional, the conversion is a radical one in the direction of humility and listening. For the poor individual, such education is liberation. Both the professional and the oppressed are beings in the "process of becoming—as unfinished, uncompleted beings in and with a likewise unfinished reality" (Freire, 2000, p. 84). Mutual transformation in space and time is the common theme.

If better health for millions more people is to be realized, an enhanced ability to deal with the complex interactions among various sectors of society that affect health must be developed. Health is a product of society. A well-functioning community or society will produce better health than one that is marginally functional or dysfunctional. Public health and medicine, for understandable and practical reasons, have often focused on particular habits, diseases, or conditions such as tobacco, adverse lipid profiles, the obesity epidemic, or type 2 diabetes and their accompanying knowledge, attitudes, beliefs, and practices. Twenty-first century health planning and action efforts should focus more rigorously on the multiple factors in a society that predict health outcomes. These factors include economics, housing, nutrition, education, spirituality, family structure, gender relations, childcare, and transportation. A chart of the multiple influences that ultimately define the level of health and quality of life for one community in the Mississippi Delta, a DHF PSBH program site, makes these multiple influences and resources clear (Figure 1.2).

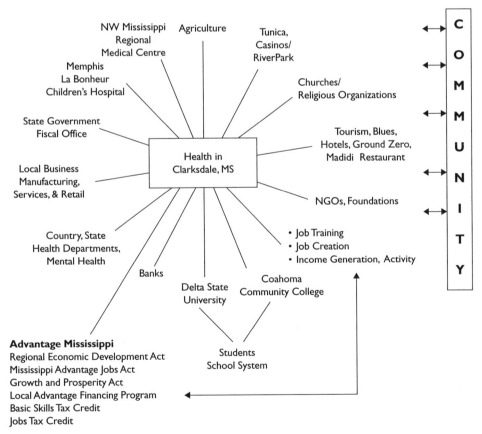

FIGURE 1.2 Health, in its broadest sense, as a product of multiple facets of a community or society. NGO = nongovernmental organization.

The fact is that people cannot be described by a disease label such as diabetes, HIV/AIDS, tuberculosis, peripheral vascular disease, or other diagnoses medicine provides. The complete human being is much more than one or more medical diagnoses or behavioral habits and practices. A more effective public health discipline can bring the multiple factors contributing to people's total well-being, health, and quality of life together to predict outcomes both qualitatively and quantitatively. As a result, it can plan interventions that are more likely to be successful in promoting health and preventing disease. It will also draw in multiple resources, many of which do not seem to have a direct relationship to health, to achieve the health goals that have been set. Achieving this analytical and predictive power will require new mathematical approaches, perhaps with elements taken from chaos theory (Resnicow & Page, 2008) and the sophisticated GPS-based data collection and analysis programs that have already been developed (Scotch, Parmanto, Gadd, & Sharma, 2006). Further developing and embracing these techniques must be a priority. Without such techniques, our plans will not achieve meaningful change.

The 21st-century challenges for achieving better health and quality of life for hundreds of millions of people are tremendous and so are the opportunities. To meet the challenges, all concerned with the improvement of health on the local, national, and global scales must work collectively rather than in isolation. Health is a product of the multiple aspects of society and requires a multifaceted approach to health promotion, the prevention and treatment of disease, and the improvement of quality of life for all people. A revolutionary change in our concept of the workforce for health is necessary. It is the people themselves who must be mobilized and encouraged to do what needs to be done. Energized and motivated, they can do it.

A Call to Action

There is no excuse for the continuation of the current level of suffering and untapped human potential. If we do not succeed in our efforts to change the situation, then the future will be very bleak. When the statistics, current plans, and planning processes are put into proper perspective, it is clear that what is required is a revolution in our approach. As indicated in the Preface, that is what this book is about—a global revolution by, and for, the people. It is a revolution that is ongoing. The people who tell their stories in this book are at the front lines of this revolution that is taking place around the world today. They are the heroes. They are making a difference. We invite you, too, to answer the call to action and become part of the revolution for better health and quality of life worldwide.

References

Bill & Melinda Gates Foundation (2009). Retrieved August 12, 2009, from http://www.gatesfoundation.org/global-health

Burnside, C., & Dollar, D. (2000). Aid, policies and growth. *American Economic Review, 90*(4), 847–868.

Chen, S., & Ravaillion, M. (2004, June). *How have the world's poor fared since the early 1980s?* Development Research Group. (World Bank Policy Working Paper No. 3341.) Retrieved August 12, 2009, from http://www.worldbank.org/research/povmonitor/MartinPapers/How_have_the_poorest_fared_since_the_early_1980.pdf

Dreyfus Health Foundation. (2009). *Problem solving for better health handbook*. Retrieved August 12, 2009, from http://www.dhfglobal.org

Easterly, W. (2003). Can foreign aid buy growth? *Journal of Economic Perspectives, 17*(3), 23–48.

Easterly, W. (2006). *The white man's burden*. New York: Penguin Press.

Freire, P. (2000). *Pedagogy of the oppressed* (30th anniv. ed.). New York: Continuum.

Hoyt, P. (2007). An international approach to Problem Solving for Better Health-Nursing™ (PSBHN). *International Nursing Review, 54*, 100–106.

McKinlay, J., McKinlay, S. M., & Beaglehole, R. (1989). A review of the evidence concerning the impact of medical measures on recent mortality and morbidity in the United States. *International Journal of Health Services, 19*(2), 181–208.

Raphael, D. (2008). *Social determinants of health: Canadian perspectives* (2nd ed.) Toronto: Canadian Scholars' Press Inc.

Resnicow, K., & Page, S. E. (2008). Embracing chaos and complexity: A quantum change for public health. *American Journal of Public Health, 98*(8), 1382–1389.

Sachs, J. (2005). *The end of poverty: Economic possibilities for our time*. New York: Penguin Press.

Scotch, M., Parmanto, B., Gadd, C. S., & Sharma, R. K. (2006). Exploring the role of GIS during community health assessment problem solving: Experiences of public health professionals. *International Journal of Health Geographics, 5*, 39–49.

Sen, A. (1999). *Development as freedom*. New York: Anchor Books, Random House.

Smith, B., Barnett, S., Collado, D., Conner, M., DePasquale, J., Gross, L., et al. (1994). Problem- solving for better health. *World Health Forum, 15*(1), 9–15.

Taylor, H. (2008). *Introduction to public health practice*. Retrieved November 30, 2009, from http://ocw.jhsph.edu/courses/publichealthpractice101/lectureNotes.cfm

United Nations Department of Economic and Social Affairs/Population Division. (2004). *World population to 2300*. Retrieved August 12, 2009, from http://www.un.org/esa/population/publications/longrange2/WorldPop2300final.pdf

World Health Organization. (2006, October). *Constitution of the World Health Organization* (45th ed.). Retrieved August 12, 2009, from http://www.who.int/governance/eb.constitution/en/index.html

World Health Organization. (2008a). *Commission on social determinants of health—Final report*. Retrieved August 12, 2009, from http://www.who.int/social_determinants/thecommission/finalreport/en/index.html

World Health Organization. (2008b). *Global burden of disease*. Fact sheet No. 310: Top 10 causes of death. Retrieved May 26, 2009, from http://who.int/mediacentre/factsheets/fs310/en/print.html

World Health Organization. (2008c). *The global burden of disease, 2004 update*. Retrieved on August 12, 2009, from http://www.who.int/healthinfo/global_burden_disease/GBD_report_2004update_full.pdf

World Health Organization. (2008d). *Inequities are killing people on a grand scale, reports WHO's Commission*. Retrieved August 12, 2009, from http://www.who.int/mediacentre/news/releases/2008/pr29/en/index.html

2

The Dreyfus Health Foundation and Problem Solving for Better Health

Introduction

Barry H. Smith

The Dreyfus Health Foundation (DHF) began over 35 years ago as the Dreyfus Medical Foundation. Jack Dreyfus, founder of Dreyfus & Co. and the Dreyfus Fund, established the Foundation after treatment with phenytoin (PHT), also known as Dilantin, led to his recovery from an endogenous depression. Finding that the uses of PHT were not widely known, he started the foundation to study, collect, and disseminate information and sponsor collaborative, clinical, and basic health research on the drug's benefits.

PHT was introduced into clinical practice in the United States in 1937 as the first nonsedative treatment for epilepsy. Since then, PHT has been reported useful for a wide range of symptoms and disorders, including depression, anxiety, mania, repetitive thinking, various types of pain, cardiac arrhythmias, neuromuscular disorders, impulsive aggression, cocaine abuse, Alzheimer's disease, burns, and wound and skin ulcer healing.

Experience with PHT around the world made it clear that the drug was an example of an inexpensive and readily available medical resource that was greatly underutilized. At DHF, we believed that lessons learned from this experience could be applied to the broader arena of healthcare. Many approaches to improving health globally were falling short of their intended goals because the problems being addressed were often poorly defined. As a result, proposed solutions were inadequate, as were the action plans for implementing them. Readily available resources to assist in the solutions were largely overlooked. Instead, everyone waited for external help that seemed to contain all the answers, but generally did not. Paralysis by analysis—overanalyzing a situation with little effort directed toward actions—played an additional role in slowing progress. The widespread belief that nothing can be done without large amounts of funding added to inaction. Collecting data often seemed more important than doing something about the problems. Problem-solving skills were not what they should or could have been.

History of Problem Solving for Better Health

Our commitment to making a difference in global health led us to develop the Problem Solving for Better Health® (PSBH®) methodology in 1988. This was at the same time that

DHF joined The Rogosin Institute, a major U.S. medical research and healthcare facility affiliated with Weill Cornell Medical College and NewYork–Presbyterian Hospital.

The first PSBH program was launched in August 1989 at West China University of Medical Sciences (WCUMS; now part of Sichuan University) in Chengdu, Sichuan Province, China. I created the program with the Director of Medical Education at the University of Texas Medical Branch at Galveston, Texas, Dr. Abdul Sajid (who died in a tragic accident shortly thereafter). The two of us shared a frustration with the lack of impact of the standard approaches to better-health projects around the world. They saw a clear need for a program that encouraged people to:

1. Think more critically about the problems they face;
2. Take more responsibility for solving those problems to create better health and a better quality of life;
3. Develop confidence in their abilities to solve the problems without waiting for someone else, from within or outside the country, to do it;
4. Make use of available resources to solve the problem. (Instead of saying "Give us some money and we'll solve the problem," the PSBH approach teaches "Let us solve the problem first and then see what is really needed to implement the solution proposed.")

The first program at WCUMS was implemented over a 10-day period and involved approximately 60 physicians from all over China. The program, which included stages of project development and implementation, was a great success, and results were disseminated nationally. Because WCUMS was one of the Chinese medical schools linked to the China Medical Board (CMB) in New York City, a 4-year collaboration between DHF and CMB developed. This led to the expansion of PSBH to a number of other cities in Asia where a broad range of programs evolved. A nationwide program for librarians on the use of medical literature resulted from a close working relationship with the Institute for Medical Information of the Chinese Academy of Medical Sciences. In another example, the presidents of 11 Chinese medical schools participated in a PSBH workshop at China Medical University in Shenyang centered on the multiple administrative and educational issues facing the medical schools.

The emphasis on medical schools and physicians, in one sense, was a departure from the PSBH goal of working with communities. However, starting in this way was most appropriate, given the existing relationships. Many of the early workshops in China also included nurses and nursing students. Their enthusiasm led to a special emphasis on PSBH for nurses, a program that later came to be known in China and elsewhere as Problem Solving for Better Health-Nursing™ (PSBHN™).

The Problem Solving for Better Health Process

The PSBH methodology emphasizes using available resources to solve health problems, rather than waiting for solutions from the outside. PSBH was designed to give people, perhaps the most important available resource, the confidence to unleash their innate abilities to solve problems. The methodology integrates the No Excuses™ approach in which, rather than making excuses for not achieving better health for more people, the people concerned determine what positive actions can be initiated. Active participation and commitment is encouraged from all concerned. The responsibility for change is placed on the individual, enabling him or her to identify local solutions to local problems. The process begins with a training workshop (usually 1–3 days) that helps the participants move through the five steps of the PSBH process. Country and regional facilitators, who have been trained to facilitate the workshops, serve as resource persons to lead the small group discussions that are integral to the PSBH process.

The steps of the PSBH process are as follows:

1. Defining the problem, including the *nature, size, cause,* and *contributing factors;*
2. Prioritizing the problem (identifying a piece of the problem that one can realistically solve);
3. Defining a solution (asking a "Good Question");
4. Creating an action plan, including the *why, what, how,* and plans for *evaluation;*
5. Taking action.

Asking the "Good Question" is an important component of the process. The "Good Question" includes the following dimensions: Will doing *what,* with *whom, where,* and for *how long,* achieve the *desired objective?*

Participants are encouraged to use available resources, including information and funding, to address the problems they have identified. Each participant leaves the workshop with a clearly defined problem, a "Good Question," and a practical action plan. Most important, participants return to their communities with a renewed commitment to making a difference.

After a period of 3–6 months, the participants reconvene at a follow-up workshop to present their projects to a local team comprising workshop facilitators and organizers. Site visits and small group meetings with local facilitators are additional means of support for the participants. These gatherings provide fora where the project leaders can share lessons learned and develop solutions to obstacles they encountered. The local facilitators are key to the success of the model. Country and regional coordinators, volunteers who provide a liaison to the DHF staff, also provide support to the local volunteer facilitators. Evaluation, sustainability, and replication are important factors in the overall PSBH program success.

Problem Solving for Better Health Initiative

The Problem Solving for Better Health Initiative™ (PSBHI™) program emphasizes building broad coalitions and partnerships to impact health and quality of life within a given community or region. It aims to solve health problems by utilizing multisectoral collaborations and community-wide participation. The invited participants include representatives from government and nongovernmental organizations, educational institutions, cultural organizations, private enterprises, sports clubs, and the community itself.

The PSBHI program generally takes place after the PSBH program has been well established in a location and many better-health projects have been successfully implemented there. At a PSBHI workshop the following questions are asked: "How can we help even more people achieve better health and quality of life for themselves and their communities? How can the successful PSBH ideas be linked together in a coordinated fashion to serve people even more effectively? Through such coordinated efforts, can broader, community-wide problems or issues be addressed?" At the workshop each participant is taken through a process that helps him or her plan a project designed to solve a series of linked problems identified.

Communications for Better Health

The Communications for Better Health® (CBH®) program, developed in 1990, creates innovative, dynamic, and interactive centers that disseminate local and international health information. The program also functions to collect, organize, and exchange relevant experiences and solutions to health problems through locally prepared digests. Other means of communication, such as radio, video, and the Internet, are also used. In regions where communication is difficult, it is especially important to increase the availability and use of information to solve health problems.

The CBH program is implemented within a hospital, university, medical library, or nongovernmental organization. After evaluating the community's health needs, the CBH team selects current, relevant health information from local and international medical sources, as well as PSBH project data, and repackages it into a digest, which is distributed within the region and abroad. In certain countries, readers can request full-text articles on specific topics of health and medical interest through an order form in the digest. Recipients of the digests include health workers, hospital staff, students, educators, nongovernmental organizations, community members, and PSBH project leaders.

Formalization of Problem Solving for Better Health-Nursing

Barry H. Smith and Joyce J. Fitzpatrick

In 2002, PSBHN was officially launched in recognition of the need for even greater involvement of nurses. Nurse Pamela Hoyt-Hudson joined DHF as International Nursing Program Coordinator and since that time has provided leadership for both U.S.-based and global PSBHN initiatives. PSBHN is now active in 15 countries, and the successful results of the model have been published (Hoyt, 2006, 2007). As a result of the program, thousands of nurses and nursing students have been mobilized to assume a more active role in their communities and work environments.

Problem Solving for Better Health-Nursing

Pamela Hoyt-Hudson

Shortly after launching the PSBH program, Dr. Smith recognized that nurses were a key resource in changing healthcare, so he invited Dame Sheila Quinn and Shelagh Murphy, both well-recognized nurses from the United Kingdom, to join the DHF team. Through the years they have served as consultants, workshop facilitators, and advisers, participating in implementation and evaluation of many projects in many countries.

Dame Sheila Quinn began her work with DHF in 1995 as the first International Nursing Program Consultant. Her notable professional accomplishments include several prestigious appointments and recognitions, including President of the Royal College of Nursing in the United Kingdom and recipient of the Christiane Reimann Prize from the International Council of Nurses. Dame Sheila is especially gifted with a keen sensitivity to nursing needs and issues in various cultures. Throughout her career, she has proposed many successful strategies to help nurses cope with and improve their work environments throughout her career. Dr. Smith and Dame Sheila envisioned the creation of a PSBH program specifically designed for nurses, and in 2002 the PSBHN program was officially launched. Dr. Smith and Dame Sheila believed that bringing nurses together in a workshop setting (separate from participants from other disciplines and/or community members) would provide an opportunity for nurses to assert their voices and assume leadership roles.

Dame Sheila then introduced DHF to another esteemed nursing expert, Shelagh Murphy. Both she and Dame Sheila have covered the globe as International Nursing Program consultants for DHF, helping to launch PSBHN programs in countries such as Bulgaria and China. They are admired not only for their expertise but also for their passion and human spirit. It is not possible to adequately measure their impact on nurses and nursing throughout their involvement with the program, nor their positive influence on so many members of the extended DHF network over the past 15 years. They have touched the lives of countless people.

A Nursing Perspective

Shelagh Murphy and Dame Sheila Quinn

The best thing about the PSBH methodology is its simplicity. We have had the privilege of being involved in many PSBH workshops held all over the world, and in each workshop participants have grasped the idea quite quickly. As facilitators and international nursing consultants, our role is to help workshop participants progress through the practical problem-solving steps so that each person comes away from the workshop with his or her own project action plan in hand, ready for implementation. Additionally, we work closely with the DHF country facilitators to help participants identify existing local resources to support the implementation phase of their projects. Nurses relate to the PSBH process easily because they are already trained to assess, plan, implement, and evaluate. Problem solving and critical thinking are universally important nursing skills. The PSBH methodology provides an innovative approach to problem solving and can be applied in a variety of settings, including hospitals, academic institutions, and communities.

There are many examples of such applications of PSBHN in this book. Several examples include small local projects that eventually evolved into regional, and sometimes national, initiatives. The projects are diverse in theme, and yet they all have one thing in common: They make a real difference in the lives of their target audiences. Just as important, they

---

Shelagh Murphy and Dame Sheila Quinn, both based in the UK, are Dreyfus Health Foundation International Nursing Program Consultants.

make a real difference in the lives of those who complete the projects. Documenting transformational change among the project leaders is not easy. We, as facilitators, see the personal transformation and hear the participants' testimonials, but measuring such change remains a challenge. Preliminary reports from PSBHN pilot programs show that the process positively influences nurses' attitudes toward the profession, increases their job satisfaction, and helps to develop leadership skills.

The DHF, under the leadership of Dr. Smith and his team, has made a real contribution to improving the health and quality of life of people around the world. DHF national coordinators, who set up the programs in their countries, select the participants, and make all the necessary arrangements for the workshops and follow-up programs, must be commended. The national coordinators and local DHF team members work on a volunteer basis, devoting much time and energy to making the workshops and follow-up monitoring process successful. It has been a privilege to be a part of this global mission to improve health.

Conclusion

Since its origin in 1988, the PSBH program in its various forms has been implemented in more than 30 countries around the world. New PSBH programs often evolve as a result of serendipity or word of mouth among colleagues also working in the field of global health. Approximately 60,000 people from all walks of life have participated in PSBH activities, and almost 40,000 large and small PSBH projects have been developed. The smallest project involved helping one person; some have reached millions. But PSBH is about much more than the projects it has generated. At its core, it is about transformation—transforming people's attitudes and confidence to create a culture of change and achieve better health worldwide.

References

Hoyt, P. (2006). Problem solving for better health-nursing: A working approach to the development and dissemination of applied research in developing countries. *Applied Nursing Research, 19*(2), 110–112.

Hoyt, P. (2007). An international approach to Problem Solving for Better Health-Nursing™ (PSBHN). *International Nursing Review, 54,* 101–106.

II

Problem Solving for Better Health: Perspectives From Around the World

3

Ghana

Barry H. Smith

Ghana is located in sub-Saharan West Africa and borders Cote d'Ivoire, Burkina Faso, Togo, and the Atlantic Ocean's Gulf of Guinea. Home to approximately 24 million people, it is the beating heart of West Africa, full of life and energy. Ghanaians are a diverse people, including Akan, Mole-Dagbon, Ewe, and Ga-Dangme, among other ethnic groups. They are, however, united as a people known for their artistic talent and exuberance throughout Africa and around the world. The Ghanaians are among the early shapers of the Problem Solving for Better Health program.

The Problem Solving for Better Health® (PSBH®) program in Ghana was inspired by a taxi ride from New York City to John F. Kennedy Airport in 1984. As often happens during taxi rides, the driver and I began to talk. He told me that he had been the Minister of Foreign Affairs in Liberia until a coup had ousted the government from power. With threats against his life in Liberia, he came to the United States and now made his living as a taxi driver. He asked me what I did for a living, and I explained that I was a physician and medical director of a New York foundation (now called the Dreyfus Health Foundation [DHF]), a charitable entity working to improve the quality of health and life around the world. The driver asked if we might consider developing a program in Ghana, his home country. (Although he had served in the Liberian government, he was actually Ghanaian.) He was interested in anything he could do to help his people. He suggested that I contact Dr. Kenneth Mills-Robertson, his cousin, a young Ghanaian physician.

Coincidentally, Ghana was one of the countries we had already been considering for possible program development. A United States Agency for International Development official had suggested that we stay out of West Africa because of what he considered the great difficulties of establishing a useful program there. But I found this caution intriguing and had been considering Ghana as a starting point. However, I did not know how or where to begin making contacts in Ghana until that taxi ride to the airport. Dr. Mills-Robertson confirmed his interest, and we agreed that the first step would be an exploratory trip to Ghana. Accordingly, Dr. Douglas Clark, a surgeon who was working with the DHF, and I set off for West Africa, where Dr. Mills-Robertson was to be our guide and mentor in Ghana.

We arrived in Accra, the capital, at about 5 a.m. The Accra airport was quite small, and the arrival of a large jet taxed all of its services. With credit cards not functional in Ghana at the time, one prominent "service" was a currency check. Each passenger was escorted into a small, curtained booth, the door to which was guarded by a soldier with an automatic weapon. Here, an official checked the accuracy of each passenger's currency declaration. When my turn came, I was informed that I had 60 USD more than I had declared. This, I was told, was a very serious offense. After a lengthy discussion that included an invitation to central police headquarters in Accra, I suggested that the 60 USD be split between the official and the guard, a suggestion that was readily accepted. I was assured that there was no longer any offense.

Relieved, I met Dr. Clark and Dr. Mills-Robertson at the baggage area only to learn that our luggage had not arrived. When we explained that we had no luggage, and therefore nothing to declare, the customs official informed us that there was a 100 USD fee for lost luggage. We paid the fee, despite being uncertain how or when we would be able to retrieve our bags; we were headed to a hospital in Sekondi-Takoradi, a city on the western coast of Ghana, a good 5 hours by road.

Then fortune began to smile on us. A very distinguished man with regal bearing was nearby, waiting for his daughter who was returning from London. Seeing our confusion and distress, he asked if he could help us. He introduced himself as Lawton Ackah-Yensu, from Accra and Cape Coast. Hearing why we had come, and learning that Dr. Mills-Robertson's wife had been a close school friend of his daughter's, he immediately took us to his home in Accra. He was amused by our lack of a plan for traveling to Sekondi-Takoradi. Ever polite and considerate, Lawton succeeded in finding a car and driver willing to take us to our destination but warned us that the roads were not in good shape. Adding to the discomfort of driving over countless potholes with no rear shock absorbers were the frequent roadblocks en route, manned by armed soldiers. At these, a check often began with the muzzle of a weapon stuck through the open car window. Flight Lieutenant Rawlins' second revolution was still fresh enough for everyone on the road to be a bit on edge.

We finally arrived in Sekondi-Takoradi and checked into the Atlantic Hotel, which had a beautiful view of the Atlantic Ocean but lacked basic utilities like running water and light fixtures. (As a note—beer can be used as a substitute for water for a number of personal hygiene functions, most notably brushing one's teeth. The taste is not fantastic with toothpaste, but it works.) Three days into our visit, we were shocked by the sight of Lawton Ackah-Yensu trudging up the hill to the hotel (cars could only get so far along the road). He was carrying our missing luggage! Surprisingly, we were not charged any further fees for lost luggage.

But none of the little problems mattered. What was important were the meetings that started the next morning at the Effia Nkwanta Regional Hospital in Takoradi with its Medical Director, Dr. Ebenezer Binder, and his colleagues. From these meetings onward, we developed a partnership that worked its way through some traditional grants for health projects to a full-fledged PSBH program in 1991. The partnership continues today.

Central to the development of the PSBH program was Lawton Ackah-Yensu. This marvelous man, whom we had met by chance at the airport in Accra, was, at various periods of his life, captain of the Ghanaian national soccer team; a national sports broadcaster;

head of the State Insurance Corporation; chief of some 100,000 people in the Cape Coast region; and the heart and soul of the PSBH program, which he oversaw from 1985 until his death in 1999, an event that was felt nationwide. The mention of Lawton's name in any village I visited throughout the country brought immediate warm welcomes and hospitality that always involved the offer of a bottle of Accra Brewery beer or a soft drink, no matter how humble the home.

The PSBH workshops in Ghana began officially in 1991, but these had been preceded by several workshops that pointed toward the problem-solving process. Thus, it is fair to say that many of the concepts and principles of PSBH were developed together with Ghanaian colleagues from many parts of the country, though they clearly began with colleagues in the western and central regions. The clear commitment of the DHF and the Ghanaian PSBH team was to help the people of Ghana help themselves to better health and a better quality of life. What we were doing was not about workshops and training processes, or even specific projects, so much as it was about instilling a transformative process in a broad cross section of citizenry, from villagers to Ministry of Health officials. This process has several crucial elements: hope for a better tomorrow, belief in the possibility of change, use of available resources, personal responsibility for change, and, most importantly, action.

Since PSBH was formally launched in 1991 in Ghana, 36 problem-solving workshops have been held, involving some 2,000 participants, from farmers, fishermen, and taxi drivers to government officials. Over 1,250 health projects implemented throughout the country have benefitted more than a million Ghanaians. Examples of specific accomplishments include a national program in cooperation with the government for the treatment of Buruli ulcers with topical phenytoin; a national nutrition education program in collaboration with the Ministry of Health, which includes a guidebook with instructions on how to use locally available materials, such as food tins, to measure appropriate amounts of nutritious foods; a teen pregnancy program in Oforikrom, Kumasi, that serves hundreds of young women and has been exported to the United States (to Philadelphia); Ghana's first breast cancer awareness center, Mammocare; a cerebral meningitis education campaign for the people of Zangu in the northern region, where many children die of the disease; a nationwide oral hygiene program, using chew sticks made from local trees to clean teeth; an adult tourism apprenticeship program in Cape Coast using an American Express training program; a health education radio program in Cape Coast, with participation by local chiefs; health seminars for skilled workers during meetings at the Business Advisory Centre in Cape Coast; a health education program on Radio Z in Koforidua; and trainings for taxi drivers in first aid techniques, enabling them to serve as emergency caregivers on the roads of Cape Coast. Accomplishing these programs and the more than 1,200 projects involved many individuals and institutions, including numerous Ghanaian hospitals and clinics, the Ghana Health Service, the Ghana Registered Midwives Association, and the Ghana Registered Nurses Association.

Along the way as PSBH developed in Ghana, we formed a council to guide the program, including Lawton Ackah-Yensu, Dr. Adrian Nii-Oddoye, Dr. Joana Nerquaye-Tetteh, Dr. Ebenezer Binder, Dr. David Oppong-Mensah, and Lynda Arthur. Ultimately, we established the Health Foundation of Ghana under Ghanaian law, directed by Lynda Arthur. This formalized and institutionalized the PSBH process in Ghana. Also, developing alongside PSBH was a special program for nurses called Problem Solving for Better Health-Nursing™. This program recognizes the importance of nurses for a truly transformative process for better health and quality of life, not only in Ghana but also in every country around the world.

Yet another component of the PSBH program in Ghana was the development of Communications for Better Health® (CBH®). Ghana was the pilot site for this program, which arose from DHF's conviction that information is a necessary part of any effective problem-solving process. We launched CBH in 1990 in cooperation with Daniel Addo, librarian of the University of Ghana Medical School, Korle Bu, Accra. When the program began, the digest, *Current Medical Literature, Ghana,* was sent to various individuals and institutions. In November 2000, the Health Foundation of Ghana adopted the CBH program. The digest was renamed *Ghana Health Digest* and distributed to doctors, nurses, pharmacists, libraries, members of Parliament, business organizations, embassies, banks, district health management teams, and the public. Requests for the digest are frequently made via the Health Foundation's website.

In addition to print format, content is also disseminated via radio, video, and the Internet. The Ghana Broadcasting Corporation reads sections from the publication on the health segment of its national morning *Breakfast Show.* Articles are regularly printed under the health section of the *Daily Graphic,* a national newspaper. Health messages, in local dialects, are captured on video and used to educate those living in isolated, rural communities throughout the country. The editorial board of the *Digest* comprises faculty from the University of Ghana Medical School and Ghanaian doctors, and the publication attracts many advertisers. Ghana was the first country where the government made a formal effort to incorporate CBH into its health programs. This success is indicative of the pervasiveness and effectiveness of the work of the Ghanaian PSBH team and the problem-solving process itself. It illustrates transformation on a national level. It is also transformation that involves the people at the grassroots level, as well as the vertical structure of Ghanaian society, including the government.

Ghana was clearly vital in the development of the concepts and principles of PSBH. As the second site of the launching of the PSBH program, after China in 1989, Ghana can well be said to be one of the program's "parents." For CBH, the country truly served as the birthplace of this element of the PSBH process. More important, however, is the degree of success of the country's programs—Ghana has been a true leader and standard setter. From the beginning of PSBH in the western region of Ghana to the national spread of many of its programs, and the broad utility of CBH, the level of achievement of the people of Ghana is something for all of us in other countries to study and emulate.

4

Kenya

Located in the heart of East Africa, Kenya shares borders with Somalia, Ethiopia, Sudan, Uganda, and Tanzania, with Lake Victoria, Africa's largest lake, in the southwest, and the Indian Ocean forming the country's coast on the east. Its location, multiple and diverse human roots, and history have earned it recognition as the "Cradle of Humanity." In Kenya's history, the Arab world of the coast met the great Masai and Kikuyu peoples of the interior to create, along with European influences, the Kenya of today. Led by an energetic local team, a Dreyfus Health Foundation partnership with Kageno has extended the Problem Solving for Better Health program to Rusinga Island in western Kenya.

Problem Solving for Better Health in Kenya

Mary Muyoka

From my perspective as a community nurse in rural Kenya, health is a precious commodity, fragile and complex. Health is influenced greatly by human behavior, environmental issues, genetics, and scientific research. In today's world, there is a great deal of suffering and poor health, despite the efforts of so many organizations with global health missions. It is critical that international development agencies work closely with local nongovernmental organizations (NGOs) and community-based organizations so that local needs can be addressed effectively. It takes a great deal of understanding and collaboration before change can occur in developing countries such as Kenya.

Dreyfus Health Foundation in Kitale

In 2001, I was introduced to Kelvin Mow, the Dreyfus Health Foundation (DHF) representative who was participating in a World Health Organization seminar that I was hosting in Kitale. After the seminar, he shared information about DHF's global programs, and we agreed that Nekeki, a local Kenyan NGO, and DHF should partner, given the organizations' similar missions and shared goals. Nekeki is a national organization founded in

---

Mary Muyoka is Founder and Director of Nekeki, the Dreyfus Health Foundation's implementing partner in Kitale, Kenya and Problem Solving for Better Health National Coordinator for Kenya.

1993 by women from the North Rift Valley and western Kenya and registered in 1994 by the Kenyan government. Nekeki's main goal is to enhance the health status of women and children. A member of the National Council of NGOs, Nekeki is based in Kitale, and has eight permanent staff members, seven board members, and 150 volunteers with diverse skills from different communities and institutions. The organization collaborates with Kenyan government ministries as well as with local and international agencies.

In October 2002, Nekeki hosted an initial DHF workshop to present the Problem Solving for Better Health® (PSBH®) tools and train new facilitators for a PSBH program in Kenya. Forty-five Kenyans were trained as workshop facilitators, and 15 became active volunteers. These volunteers included a district commissioner, a probation officer, two public health officers, six teachers, a nutritionist, a youth development officer, a laboratory technologist, a social worker, and a women's development officer.

The next year, Nekeki conducted a PSBH workshop with 45 farmers in Matunda, which is located in the Trans-Nzoia district, 400 km northwest of Nairobi and situated at the foot of Mount Elgon. The farmers sought advice on increasing their maize production. Workshop participants were trained in the PSBH process and mentored by members of the Ministry of Agriculture and Ministry of Livestock Development. After the workshop, each farmer prepared and planted one experimental acre of land employing farming skills learned during the workshop, including the application of soil nutrients to improve his or her yield. As a result, each acre produced 25–30 bags of maize, compared with only 2–5 bags in previous years. During the course of the project, agricultural extension officers from the Ministry of Agriculture visited the farmers once a month and held educational field days. Since 2004, the farmers have continued to utilize their acquired skills and maintain their increased yields. Project seed funding helped the farmers to start a village group cooperative (Matunda Farm), which enabled them to trade their crops for clothing, school fees, and healthcare. Food security has improved in Matunda, and the Co-Operative Bank of Kenya has provided microfinancing to assist with project sustainability.

In 2004, several participants from a second PSBH workshop in Matunda developed projects related to mosquito control and malaria prevention. The project leaders were able to leverage additional resources because of their success in using minimal seed funding to drain and bury stagnant water pools, clear overgrown bushes, and encourage proper sanitation practices in their community. Population Services International supplied the project with treated mosquito nets to ensure project sustainability. At the same workshop, another 15 participants developed projects focusing on clean water for Matunda. A minimal amount of seed funding was provided to buy necessary materials to drill and protect 89 boreholes and install pumps to retrieve fresh drinking water and prevent water-borne diseases. Because of these efforts, Matunda now enjoys clean water.

At a third PSBH workshop in Matunda, DHF and the German Foundation for World Population helped train 200 young adults to counsel their peers on sexually transmitted diseases (STDs) and HIV/AIDS. Those trained then visited 120 primary and 48 secondary schools in the Trans-Nzoia and Bungoma districts and provided education on peer pressure, STDs, HIV/AIDS, and survival skills. As a result of their projects, the young adults were able to decrease the number of teen pregnancies and STDs and increase the number of youth seeking voluntary counseling and testing (VCT) services.

Another workshop was held in Miendo in the Bungoma district, 460 km northwest of Nairobi. A total of 115 participants developed projects to address malaria (50), malnutrition (40), and HIV/AIDS (25). Each participant chose five neighbors to work closely with during the implementation of his or her project. This program was jointly supported by DHF (PSBH training and project seed funding), the Monsanto Fund (training in nutrition and organic farming), the Bungoma Family Helper Project (training in HIV/AIDS mentoring and VCT referral), the microfinance institution Faulu Kenya (training in capacity building and sustainability), and Friends Lugulu Mission Hospital (training in proper nutrition for people living with AIDS, children, and others). With Nekeki, the German Foundation for World Population trained youth in VCT services in the Western and North Rift provinces, and Friends Lugulu Mission Hospital started a mobile program to deliver antiretroviral therapy (ART) and provide home care in surrounding villages.

In Begeng'i, a village in the Busia district approximately 500 km northwest of Nairobi, Peris Wandera, a retired nurse, developed two projects, one to address HIV/AIDS and the second to address malnutrition. The HIV/AIDS project received support from DHF and the government of Kenya, while DHF and the Monsanto Fund supported the nutrition project. In the latter project, agricultural, livestock, and trade extension officers trained 40 farmers in cereal, dairy, and poultry farming; pig keeping; horticulture; tree husbandry; and microfinancing. A local radio station assisted the farmers in obtaining markets for their produce. The nutrition project was replicated, ultimately involving an additional 200 trainees. The National Council of NGOs and the Kenyan government reviewed the project and determined it to be a practicable solution to reducing poverty.

In another development, DHF initiated a collaboration with TechnoServe, which was supporting a project with Nyala dairy farmers in the Nyandarua and Laikipia districts focused on the collection, storage, and marketing of dairy products. The farmers requested aid with health problems affecting their communities. With TechnoServe's support, DHF and Nekeki held a workshop to train 50 Nyala dairy farmers in the PSBH process. The farmers developed projects to address HIV/AIDS, plastic recycling, environmental health, malnutrition, dairy and poultry farming, horticulture, children's health, and family planning. Their projects received seed funding from DHF and the Monsanto Fund. In addition, TechnoServe assisted with microfinance and in identifying potential donors. One significant result of these collective efforts was that the farmers acquired a milk-cooling system to maintain milk at proper temperatures for transportation.

Following the farmers' workshop, members of their communities expressed interest in addressing health problems on a wider scale. In March 2004, a Problem Solving for Better Health Initiative™ workshop was held in Kimilili, a town in the Bungoma district at the foot of Mount Elgon with a high prevalence of HIV/AIDS (20%–30% in 2003) and high mortality. Fifty-five people (government officials and other local leaders) were trained in the PSBH process and implemented projects to address HIV/AIDS, including the opening of four pharmacies, the distribution of condoms, and the training of VCT counselors. The German Foundation for World Population provided information, education, and communication (IEC) materials to further support this effort. Representatives from AMKENI—a project funded by the United States Agency for International Development—trained mentors and provided ART rehabilitation. With the support of the Ministry of Health, the Kimilili subdistrict hospital continues to accept referrals from the village for testing and treatment. The project is ongoing and has secured additional funds from the National AIDS/STD Control Program to ensure sustainability.

Also in 2004, the head teacher at the Misemia Primary School in Bikeke, a poverty-stricken village in the Trans-Nzoia district, requested that the PSBH program be launched in the school district. The primary school had 25 teachers for 1,500 pupils, and 350 of these children were orphaned by the HIV/AIDS epidemic. Bikeki's main source of income was the brewing and selling of alcohol. There were many cases of child labor, abuse, and rape in the community, and approximately 40–80 teen girls dropped out of school annually due to pregnancy. The academic performance in the district was so poor that the children could not qualify for further education in the national schools.

As a result of the primary school teacher's request, Nekeki organized a PSBH workshop for the district that year. Fifty-five teachers were trained in the PSBH methodology and implemented projects in their respective schools. DHF provided seed funding for the projects, and Nekeki connected the trained teachers to the German Foundation for World Population, which provided sex education, IEC materials, and information on microfinance. The Elton John AIDS Foundation supplied uniforms and books and provided funds for microfinance. The Kenyan government, through the Community Development Trust Fund, built four classrooms at the Misemia Primary School, and the German Foundation for World Population built four more. Through this collective effort, the school has improved its performance in the national examinations, ranking second in the district in 2005.

In addition, projects focusing on HIV/AIDS and sex education have helped to reduce the number of STDs and teen pregnancies in the district. The Kenyan government now permits HIV/AIDS and adolescent health education to be incorporated into the school curriculum. Nekeki has received requests for the PSBH program from other schools and churches, which have set aside space for the counseling of students.

Problem Solving for Better Health-Nursing™ (PSBHN™) has also been successfully introduced in Kenya. While visiting relatives in the United States, Dr. Mary MaduMadu attended a PSBHN informational presentation in Bridgeport, Connecticut. After the presentation, Dr. MaduMadu expressed interest in launching a nursing program in Kenya, specifically for retired nurses. She wanted to mobilize a network of retired nurses to take action and make a difference in health in the rural villages where they were born and raised. Pamela Hoyt-Hudson, DHF's International Nursing Program Coordinator, encouraged her to put her vision down on paper and submit it formally to DHF. Along with DHF's regional coordinator for Africa, Ruth Chikasa, I reviewed the proposal, and we agreed it was an important idea to pursue. Dr. MaduMadu's mother, a retired nurse in her home community, assumed responsibility for organizing this network of nurses, as they had been her friends and colleagues for many years. Nurses in Kenya often retire by 55, leaving an able workforce idle in the midst of a severe worldwide nursing shortage.

In 2004, 135 nurses from the Kilifi, Malindi, Kwale, and Mombasa districts trained at a PSBHN workshop. These nurses developed projects on HIV/AIDS, orphans, malaria, ART rehabilitation, horticulture, tree planting, and poultry and dairy farming. The projects were supported with seed funding from DHF and the Monsanto Fund. One project implemented at Malindi airport addressed pollution that led to an increase in birds nesting in the airport hangars. As a result of interference from the birds, several airplane accidents occurred. A retired nurse began a cleanup and sanitation program with support from the Municipal Council of Malindi and the government of Kenya. To date, there have been no further accidents as a result of bird interference.

Finally, DHF established a partnership with the NGO Kageno in July 2006, due to the efforts of a DHF volunteer, Ellen Schoninger. Ellen introduced Dr. Frank Andolino, founder of Kageno, to DHF, as she believed that the PSBH program would add value to the grassroots efforts of Kageno in Kenya. The following section discusses more about the partnership between DHF and Kageno.

The PSBH program in Kenya has been sustainable because of the involvement of international and local stakeholders. We have turned to the government of Kenya for partnership and have benefited from Kenyan's policies, expertise, and willingness to help us strengthen our grassroots efforts in Kenyan communities. We are also grateful to additional partners who have joined our collective mission, including TechnoServe, Kageno, Faulu Kenya, Friends Lugulu Mission Hospital, the German Foundation for World Population, and the Elton John AIDS Foundation, among others.

Kageno Partnership

Carlyla Dawson and Frank C. Andolino

The population of Kenya is currently estimated at around 39 million with over 70 tribal groups, giving the nation a rich cultural heritage. However, the population growth and diverse cultural heritage have created several development obstacles. Many perspectives need to be taken into consideration in devising strategies for solving these problems. For example, cultural traditions differ by region, so an approach to the prevention of HIV/AIDS may work in one region but not in another. Another obstacle is the dramatic difference between the urban and rural areas. Frequently, large development organizations devise universal solutions to local problems without taking into consideration diverse populations. This is one of the reasons why work at the community level is so crucial.

In Kenya, NGOs contribute significantly to overall healthcare. Over the past several years, the government in Kenya has worked to improve healthcare systems, and in 1994 the Kenya Health Policy Framework was approved as a blueprint for developing and managing health services in the country, with specific attention paid to collaborating with NGOs. The framework identifies long-term strategic goals, sets the agenda for Kenya's health sector, and recognizes the importance of NGOs in that process.

The policy initiatives in the framework deal with constraints limiting the government's ability to meet healthcare needs of the Kenyan people, including a decline in expenditure on the health sector, inefficient utilization of resources, centralized decision-making, inadequate management skills, worsening poverty levels, increasing burden of disease, and rapid population growth. These factors have contributed to a significant decline in the quality of health in Kenya over the past several years and have solidified the need for additional resources and help from NGOs.

NGOs from all over the world have collaborated with the Kenyan government to address some of these issues at both the national and local levels. Large international organizations such as the World Health Organization work best at the national level, helping with policy creation and general overall management of the healthcare sector. Organizations such as Kageno and the DHF work better at the local level, providing

Carlyla Dawson is Director of Operations and Frank C. Andolino is the Executive Director and Cofounder of Kageno Worldwide, Inc., a Dreyfus Health Foundation partner in Kenya.

insight into individual community problems and appropriate solutions, while leveraging local resources more efficiently than large organizations. The purpose of this chapter is to describe how Kageno and DHF have been working at the local level with the Kenyan government to help improve health in Kenyan communities.

Kageno Worldwide, Inc.

Kageno Worldwide, Inc., was founded in 2003 by Alphonce Okuku, a Kenyan, who is now the country director; Rob Place, a U.S. Peace Corps volunteer; and Frank Andolino, an orthodontist from the United States, who is currently the acting executive director. In 5 years, Kageno grew from a grassroots effort into a robust organization, implementing community development projects in two countries (Kenya and Rwanda) that have employed 600 people and mobilized nearly 1,000 volunteers.

Kageno's founding vision was one of sustainable solutions to global poverty achieved through a set of interdependent programs that would address the complex web of issues faced by impoverished people. As such, Kageno empowers communities toward diversified economies; more educated populations; and stronger infrastructures for community health, clean water, and healthy environments (through reforestation, preservation, and sanitation) to break cycles of poverty and allow healthier, more sustainable communities to emerge.

In addition, Kageno establishes sustainability for its nonprofit programs by combining the needs-based approach of the nonprofit sector with the entrepreneurship of successful for-profit business models. At the local level, microloans and well-designed small business ventures have moved individuals toward self-sufficiency. Kageno seeks partnerships with for-profit businesses that can help boost dormant revenue streams from the community's existing environmental, cultural, and human resources.

Partnering With Dreyfus Health Foundation

In early 2002, Kageno founders visited the village of Kolunga Beach on Rusinga Island, which was in the midst of a crisis. The unemployment rate was higher than 80%, with no jobs available except for the seasonal fishing industry. Women and girls regularly engaged in "fish for sex" (*jaboya* in the local dialect), avoiding starvation by prostituting themselves to migrant fishermen in exchange for fish. Rather than attending school, children spent their days scavenging for food in piles of trash strewn with human feces. More than 40% of the population had HIV/AIDS, and the village's main source of drinking water was Lake Victoria, which receives millions of liters (L) of untreated sewage each day. The village had only one latrine per 1,200 individuals and no means to safely deposit human waste. There was no formal trash removal program, and a population unable to afford any other form of cooking fuel had stripped the area of foliage.

To further the work in which it was already engaged on Rusinga Island, Kageno formed a partnership with the DHF in 2006. Kageno's executive director, Dr. Frank C. Andolino, met with DHF staff about the PSBH program and found that the grassroots approach of the PSBH methodology fit well with Kageno's vision and mission.

In July 2006, DHF and Kageno organized a 3-day workshop on Rusinga Island to train 28 community members to be PSBH problem solvers. Community members and trainees were happy to meet with Mary Muyoka, Ruth Chikasa, Pamela Hoyt-Hudson, and volunteer consultant Ellen Schoninger to discuss the problems in their community. Training sessions were interactive and included brainstorming; all participants were challenged to rethink their own roles and ways of solving the problems. All too often development organizations come into a community with a devised solution to a specific problem that they (the outsiders) have seen. This approach often fails due to a lack of understanding with regard to the origin of the problem, what resources are locally available, and what solutions already exist within the community. Through the PSBH program, Kageno and DHF sought to engage the community in the process.

Innovative Solutions

During the workshop, community members identified many problems. They also provided helpful insight into the issues and offered many viable solutions. One of the problems addressed was the rampant spread of HIV/AIDS—6 out of the 22 action plans submitted dealt with this issue. Other problems participants identified included typhoid, malaria, teen pregnancy, and lack of clean water. Descriptions of some of the projects developed to address these issues follow.

Reducing the Practice of "Fish for Sex" and the Rate of HIV/AIDS

One of the most alarming concerns raised at the workshop was an unusual and disturbing phenomenon occurring within the fishing community on Rusinga Island. The practice of "fish for sex" was identified as one of the leading causes of the rapid spread of HIV/AIDS along the shores of Lake Victoria. Alphonce Okuku suggested that if the women had capital to buy fish they would no longer need to exchange sex for the fish. Another aspect of this problem was the lack of HIV/AIDS awareness and education on methods of prevention.

Alphonce developed an action plan that he carried out from September 2006 to October 2007. His objectives were to use microlending to improve the living standards of poor women in Kolunga Beach by 40% within 1 year, provide condoms, and educate women on the dangers of HIV/AIDS. Project activities included visiting the Ministry of Health and the chief's *baraza* (a gathering to share information and raise awareness) to seek permission to carry out the project, recruiting project participants, providing condoms and education on their use, educating women about the risks of "fish for sex," and initiating a microlending program with 20 women.

Alphonce and a team of community health workers identified the women for the microlending program pilot through a process of group and individual meetings, keeping in mind the sensitive nature of the issue. After the identification process, each woman was given 1,500 Kenyan shillings (Kshs; 30 USD) and asked to attend weekly meetings to make loan payments, discuss health topics, and learn business and life skills. Through the microloan program, women created businesses selling fish, vegetables, fruits, soft drinks, and cereal, and also managed hotels and stores.

The program not only economically empowered the women but also addressed many of the social issues that contributed to their problems. The educational component is the most important part of the program. Kageno and DHF wanted to give the beneficiaries not only the skills needed to succeed in the microloan program but also the life skills needed to survive. They expanded the program to address all issues related to the health of the individuals and their families. During the weekly meetings, the women attended short educational talks on how to prevent HIV/AIDS, malaria, tuberculosis, and typhoid; how to provide their children with nutritious food; the importance of a clean living environment; and the need to use treated water for drinking.

The social impact of this program has been significant. Prior to its inception, many of the behavioral issues were not discussed in any public forum. Group meetings allow the issues to be voiced and have proved to be a powerful deterrent to unsafe practices. The meetings serve as counseling sessions where the women can support each other and discuss problems they face in their daily lives. Financial gains from the program were not significant in the beginning, but the social impact has been profound since day 1. Most striking, as a result of the joint effort by Kageno and DHF, the 20 women are no longer involved in prostitution.

Kageno's experience has illustrated that a small amount of money provided by a well-managed microlending program can result in a vigorous economic cycle. The benefits extend beyond individual beneficiaries because the jobs generated help to improve living standards in the entire community. The program has helped to stimulate the local economy by injecting capital and diversifying the market. The creation of diversified occupations has reduced the dependency on the fishing industry and decreased the oversaturation of specific trades.

In the first round of the microlending program, Kageno experienced a repayment rate of 100%. The success of the initiative led Kageno to expand the program to involve more individuals. As the program grew and more funding became available, the loans were increased and now range anywhere from 1,000–5,000 Kshs (20–100 USD). The success and significant impact of the program has continued to attract new donors from around the world. Currently, there are a total of 189 individual recipients involved in the microlending project, and that number will continue to increase. In order to make the program sustainable, Kageno introduced a small but important addition to the program. Each loan is to be paid back with a small amount of interest that goes into a fund to be used to provide additional loans. This allows the participants themselves to expand the program in a sustainable manner.

To address the sustainability of the individual borrowers' success and to ensure that they continue to benefit, Kageno introduced a "saving for the future" component to the design of the program. With no banking institutions on Rusinga Island, the possibility of saving never existed for these women. Now, in addition to the weekly payments and interest, they contribute whatever amount they can to savings. This mechanism is crucial to the success of the women in the program.

Kageno has worked hard to develop a financially sustainable institution by modeling the microlending program after the well-known and successful Grameen Bank or "Banking for the Poor" philosophy. The program empowers the recipients by giving them the tools needed to solve their problems, rather than solving their problems for them. The initial capital for the program comes from an external source, but the members run the program with the help of Kageno. They choose their members, elect officers, and establish bylaws. Kageno has provided the opportunity and the resources, but the community does the rest.

The future of the Microfinance and Empowerment Program, as the program is now called, is promising, as more funding becomes available. Since the initial program began, more than 75 women have been given an alternative to prostitution, and many more have seen firsthand that there are now other options available. Kageno hopes to see the elimination of the practice of "fish for sex" on Rusinga Island as the program continues to expand.

Reducing Typhoid Fever on Rusinga Island

Typhoid fever is a significant problem on Rusinga Island due to a lack of understanding about the transmission and prevention of the disease, along with the unavailability of tools for accurate diagnosis of typhoid. During the PSBH workshop, it became apparent to the community members that the spread of typhoid is an easily solvable problem. The main cause was contaminated water, because many people on Rusinga Island drink water directly from the lake, which is known to have high levels of fecal contamination.

Duncan Ouma carried out his PSBH project combating typhoid from July 2006 to July 2007. Its objectives were to reduce typhoid cases on Rusinga Island in 1 year, create awareness of the importance of using clean water, identify centrally located sites for and distribute seven 100-L clean water tanks around the island, and provide Water Guard (the locally available water treatment product) to community members. The project activities included holding community meetings to discuss the importance of clean water and using Water Guard, mobilizing women's groups to discuss the importance of clean water, purchasing Water Guard and the 100-L tanks, and conducting demonstration sessions on the proper use of Water Guard.

Duncan first conducted several small-scale meetings with community members to raise awareness of the connection between contaminated water and typhoid fever, including instruction on contamination-prevention methods. Then seven 100-L water tanks were purchased and distributed to seven homes, and several dozen bottles of Water Guard were distributed. Duncan conducted follow-up visits to make sure the tanks and the Water Guard were properly used.

With his program, Duncan reduced the cases of typhoid fever at the local clinic from 15% to 7% and increased awareness through 10 successful community meetings, reaching more than 200 individuals. The program's impact was even greater, as meeting participants discussed the issues at home with family, friends, and neighbors. By the conclusion of the program, there was a significant increase in the demand for water tanks and Water Guard, as well as community awareness of how to prevent the spread of the disease. The total cost of the program was 310 USD, half of which purchased seven 100-L tanks that served more than 100 individuals. As is the case with any health-related intervention, the economic impact of the program can be seen in the increased productivity of the community. In addition, the increased demand for water tanks and Water Guard boosted the local economy, as both products are bought and sold locally.

Reducing Malaria on Rusinga Island

Kenya suffers from a high incidence of malaria due to its location and climate, with Rusinga Island particularly affected. The majority of the population suffers from the disease more than five times a year, losing about 25 working days. One of the main contributing factors leading to the high incidence is the lack of education regarding prevention. In addition, the population does not have the capital to purchase the chemicals to treat mosquito nets, which would make the nets more effective. The solution was to educate the people on how to protect themselves from malaria by using treated mosquito nets and keeping their compounds free of debris and stagnant water. Locally available chemicals would be purchased to treat nets and to spray heavily affected areas around the island. These two simple solutions would work to reduce malaria on the island.

The objectives of the action plan submitted by Teresa Onono to reduce malaria on Rusinga Island included reducing cases by 5% within 1 year (from 90 to 80 per month), educating the community about malaria prevention, treating mosquito nets, and eliminating mosquito breeding grounds. Teresa carried out her action plan from July 2006 to February 2007. Activities included seeking permission for the project from the Ministry of Health, area chief, and local leaders; collecting data from local clinics; conducting community seminars; clearing bushes and filling holes; educating people on the use of mosquito nets; spraying mosquito nets and screens; collecting dirty tins and disposing of them; organizing peer education; and conducting a final evaluation.

With government permission, Teresa visited local clinics to collect data on the incidence rate of malaria and locations with the most outbreaks. Several community meetings were held to teach the participants how to treat mosquito nets, recognize signs and locations where mosquito breeding might take place, and prevent mosquitoes from breeding. They were taught how cleaning the compound and clearing the bushes around their homes would not only reduce the breeding ground for the mosquitoes but also improve the overall health of those who live in the compound. Chemicals were purchased, and key areas around the island were sprayed. Other activities included filling potholes on the roads and holes in the fields to prevent the collection of stagnant water during the rainy season.

As a result of this project, much of Rusinga Island is no longer considered a good breeding ground for this deadly disease. The total cost of the program was 198 USD. Fifty mosquito nets were treated for a cost of less than 2 USD each, providing protection for at least 200 people. Moreover, the population spends less money on malaria medication and other medicine, and productivity has increased because people no longer lose days of work due to illness.

Reducing the Schoolgirl Dropout Rate on Rusinga Island

The problem identified by Frederick Okumu was girls dropping out of school because of lack of exposure to family planning methods and lack of social empowerment tools. Early marriage, a common practice on Rusinga Island, is defined by the community as marrying before the age of 16. One major factor in the dropout rate is the cultural belief that girls hold less value than boys. A solution devised by Frederick was to teach girls at an early age that they have choices. He suggested that they receive this education as early as primary school, in order to increase the number of girls advancing to secondary school. Frederick also suggested a focus on changing parents' opinions about the need to educate their daughters. Because parents often encourage early marriage, they, themselves, needed to be educated on the benefits of secondary education for their daughters.

Frederick submitted an action plan and carried out his project from July to December 2006. The objective was to reduce early sex and marriage by 30% among a target group of 150 girls within a 6-month period. Activities included seeking permission from school administrators; organizing meetings with teachers, parents, administrators, counselors, and the Ministry of Education; educating girls on risks of early sex, how to protect themselves, and the disadvantages of early marriage; and empowering girls to make smart decisions regarding family planning and marriage.

The main activities took place at Uya Primary School, one of the largest primary schools on Rusinga Island. Having first informed teachers and parents about the program to obtain their support, Okumu held weekly meetings that included videos about pregnancy prevention, role-playing on how to avoid the pressure of early marriage, and family planning method discussions. The girls were told how and where they could find local reproductive health services. Also, monthly meetings were held with parents and teachers, illustrating the importance of girls completing secondary school.

As a result of this program, there has been an increase in the number of girls finishing secondary school and a change in attitude about the importance of girls finishing their secondary education. Parents showed great interest in the initiative, and teachers have started to incorporate some of the discussions into the general curriculum. In total, more than 200 girls and more than 50 parents attended regular meetings. The cost of the program can be calculated at about 0.70 USD per girl.

Clean Environment, Better Health

When Kageno first came to Kolunga Beach on Rusinga Island, the village had only one latrine per 1,200 individuals. The majority of the population was using the shores of Lake Victoria to eliminate body waste. Because the lake is also the main source of water for the village, this created many health problems, the worst being chronic diarrhea and dehydration, the leading causes of death among children on Rusinga Island and in Africa generally. Joyce Opala knew of a Care Kenya program that teaches people how to build slabs and blocks from local raw materials, which could be used to construct latrines.

Joyce submitted an action plan to help reduce the number of diarrhea cases on the island by building these pit latrines, and she carried out her project from August 2006 to January 2007. Her main objective was to educate residents on how to build the latrines. Activities included seeking permission from the chief, encouraging the local health officer to educate the community on the connection between diarrhea and the use of pit latrines, consulting the Beach Management Unit, constructing at least one pit latrine per home and three for Kolunga Beach, and teaching the community how to properly clean the latrines and the importance of maintaining them.

With Care Kenya's assistance, Joyce organized an educational program to teach the community how to build the slabs and blocks for the latrines, which resulted in the construction of pit latrines in three homes. All materials were purchased and made locally, and the three households provided the labor. Kageno then decided to take the project further by providing funds to construct 30 additional latrines. The community came together and donated the land and the labor.

This program shows how community materials and resources can be leveraged with the assistance of outside help. The community had the materials and was willing to provide the labor, but lacked the necessary capital and training to build the latrines. As a result of the project, awareness of the importance of latrines has risen, and along with it, the demand for the necessary materials. Local authorities have made it a priority to find more land to construct additional latrines. The cost for each latrine was approximately 65 USD, and each latrine services about 10 individuals.

Endangered Fish in Lake Victoria (Uta Beach)

Illegal fishing practices are detrimental to the fishing industry of Lake Victoria. These practices include the use of chemicals, nets with smaller than usual holes, and overfishing in general. The chemicals are used to tranquilize the fish to prevent escape from the net. Illegal nets are used to catch the largest number of fish possible. The main effect of using these two techniques is the reduction in the amount of fish in the lake as a whole. Illegal nets also catch immature fish that have not yet had a chance to lay their eggs, preventing reproduction of the species. The problem has grown due to the rising number of fishermen and the increased demand for fish, which are sold locally and internationally. Without action, this problem will only worsen.

Julious Kinanga's action plan to counter the practice of using illegal fishing nets in Lake Victoria was carried out from August to October 2006. His objectives were to protect the endangered fish by reducing the proportion of fishermen who use illegal nets and chemicals from 20% to 10% by the end of the year, sustain the general fish population, educate fishermen about the results of overfishing, and raise awareness of illegal fishing practices and their impact on the fishing industry of Lake Victoria. The project activities included visiting the fisheries department to seek permission, visiting the chief and his assistant in their respective *barazas* to create awareness, introducing and discussing the project with the Beach Management Unit at Uta Beach, organizing a peaceful demonstration against illegal nets and chemicals, organizing five workshops for fishermen, interviewing members of the community and the fishermen, and discouraging marketers from purchasing and selling immature fish.

Julious taught the community the importance of stopping all illegal fishing practices. Peaceful demonstrations created momentum behind the movement to counter illegal practices and demonstrate support. During a 2-month period, Julious toured the beach to identify fishermen making or repairing illegal fishing nets. He educated the fishermen about the harmful effects of using these nets and encouraged them to change their practices. In addition, he met with local marketers to discourage them from purchasing immature fish.

Of the 32 identified illegal nets, only 12 are still operational, and the use of chemicals has almost disappeared. Many fishermen are looking for alternatives, such as buying proper fishing gear and using other techniques to reduce the number of fish that escape. The fishermen now seem to realize that by overfishing, using illegal nets, and fishing with chemicals, they are destroying one of the only income-generating activities they have available to them. By changing the attitude toward illegal fishing methods, there is hope for the future of Lake Victoria's fishing community and an industry that is the main provider of jobs in the region.

Conclusion

Countless lives on Rusinga Island have been positively affected by the joint effort of Kageno and the DHF. The grassroots approach allowed community members to deal with issues affecting their future by giving them tools to find solutions. Engaging the community in the development process has proven to be a successful and sustainable strategy. The PSBH process has enabled the community to feel a sense of ownership of the programs, which has contributed to their success.

To date, Kageno's accomplishments on Kolunga Beach include initiating a Microfinance and Empowerment Program that has created approximately 600 new jobs for local people and lifted 76 women out of prostitution, constructing two nursery schools (one on Rusinga Island and one on Mfangano Island) where children learn in modern classrooms and receive a daily nutritious meal, opening a VCT center that provides HIV/AIDS services, building a dispensary, constructing a solar-powered clean-water pump that delivers an ample supply of safe water to the entire village, constructing 30 latrines, implementing a formal trash collection program, planting 50,000 new trees, developing innovative recycling programs, and introducing agroforestry techniques to improve soil quality. Kageno will continue assisting and empowering the people on Rusinga Island.

5

Lesotho

Lesotho, the "Mountain Kingdom," is home to 2 million Basotho people and their monarch, King Letsie David Mohato III. Lesotho is completely surrounded by South Africa, with 80% of its land at least 1,800 m above sea level and some peaks in the rugged Drakensberg range on the country's eastern border rising above 3,000 m. Interactions with European traders, Boer pioneers, French missionaries, the Zulu people, and the British have helped shape the Basotho people, who today are striving to build a modern nation on the proud foundation of their traditions and history of independence. A collaboration between Boston University and the Dreyfus Health Foundation has made Problem Solving for Better Health a truly national program here.

Problem Solving for Better Health in Lesotho

Lauren P. Babich and William J. Bicknell

Boston University (BU) has demonstrated its confidence in Problem Solving for Better Health® (PSBH®) since 2000, when the BU School of Public Health Summer Certificate Program started teaching PSBH to its students as a useful method for empowering communities to improve their own health. When the BU chancellor made an institutional commitment to work with Lesotho during the country's HIV/AIDS crisis in 2003, PSBH was immediately considered as a starting point. Initially, PSBH in Lesotho was seen as a way to address the HIV/AIDS crisis specifically (Figure 5.1). With help from PSBH program leaders from Indonesia and Zambia, the program soon expanded to address the overwhelming problems faced by Lesotho's hospitals. The program has been enormously successful in propelling the transformation of several hospitals in two

Lauren P. Babich, an instructor in the Department of Family Medicine, Boston University Medical Center, is the former Deputy Director of the Lesotho–Boston Health Alliance (LeBoHA). William J. Bicknell is Director of LeBoHA and a professor in the Departments of International Health and Family Medicine in the Schools of Public Health and Medicine, Boston University.

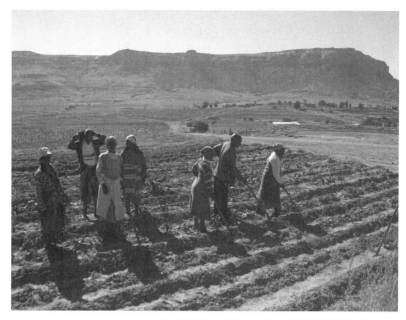

FIGURE 5.1 Problem Solving for Better Health participants cultivate a field donated by the local chief for a project that provides food to an orphanage for HIV/AIDS children near Maseru.

northern districts of Lesotho. The goal of PSBH in Lesotho is to energize and empower a self-perpetuating and growing cadre of educated and motivated persons who, on a daily basis, carry out efficient and quality improvement activities that directly relate to the practical and immediate improvement of day-to-day health services and ministry functioning in Lesotho.

From Indonesia to Boston: Problem Solving for Public Health Practitioners

PSBH in Lesotho began serendipitously. Dr. William (Bill) Bicknell, then Chairman of the Department of International Health at the BU School of Public Health and Associate Vice President for International Health at the university, heard an old African proverb from his wife: "If you think you are too small to make a difference, try sleeping in a closed room with a mosquito." At this time, Bill worked with a long-time colleague in Indonesia, Dr. Alex Papilaya. When Alex heard the proverb he smiled and said, "That's the motto of Problem Solving for Better Health; let me tell you about the program." A few months later, Alex was in Boston and a meeting was arranged between Bill and the director of the Dreyfus Health Foundation (DHF), Dr. Barry H. Smith, in New York. As a result of this meeting, PSBH became a component of BU's very successful 3-month Summer Certificate Program in International Health. The first 2½-day PSBH workshop was a huge success, and the summer was extraordinary, with international DHF facilitators from Indonesia, England, Romania, Brazil, Zambia, and New Jersey participating. The summer program has changed at BU, but to this day PSBH remains a vital component, taught as a valuable tool for community-based problem solving and development.

From Boston to Lesotho: Problem Solving for HIV/AIDS

When PSBH was introduced in Lesotho, the country was suffering the world's fourth highest prevalence of HIV, with an estimated 31% of adults (aged 15–49) infected with the virus (Lesotho Ministry of Health and Social Welfare [MOHSW], 2003). Lesotho reported its first case of AIDS in 1986, but due to a combination of denial and lack of capability, the government did not respond until the start of the 21st century (Kimaryo, Okpaku, Githuku-Shongwe, & Feeney, 2003). In 2000, the government of Lesotho declared HIV/AIDS a "national disaster," adopted a National AIDS Strategic Plan, and organized the Lesotho AIDS Program Coordinating Authority (LAPCA) to direct the implementation of the plan (Kimaryo et al., 2003). From that point, information, education, and communication strategies became the primary focus (Lesotho Planned Parenthood Association [LPPA], 2003).

In 2003, it was essential to increase the level of national response to HIV/AIDS. LAPCA had too much responsibility and not enough authority (Kimaryo et al., 2003); people were more knowledgeable about HIV/AIDS but were not changing their behavior (LPPA, 2003); HIV testing services had very limited availability (LPPA, 2003); and HIV prevalence was on the rise, particularly in rural areas (MOHSW, 2003).

Bill and BU had worked in Lesotho intermittently since the 1990s and knew an AIDS program in the country was achievable. Lesotho boasted excellent national leadership; low levels of corruption; good infrastructure, including hospitals and health centers; one ethnic and linguistic group who spoke Sesotho and English, with English as an official language; and high literacy. These factors convinced the BU president to support and fund BU-partnered projects in Lesotho (Babich, Bicknell, Culpepper, et al., 2008; Babich, Bicknell, Jack, & Culpepper, 2008).

In August 2003, shortly after BU had made a 10-year minimum commitment to work with the government of Lesotho on the HIV/AIDS epidemic, Bill and Arden O'Donnell, then deputy of BU's Lesotho program, visited Lesotho. The visit led to a list of priority areas mutually agreed upon by the Minister of Health and Social Welfare, Dr. Motloheloa Phooko, Bill, and Arden. The Ministry and BU agreed to focus on preserving the lives of Lesotho's citizens through building the capacity of the country's health workforce and maximizing the efficiency of Lesotho's existing health system and its use of resources. But there was a pervasive undercurrent to the issues. Lesotho was plagued by a national epidemic of inaction as well as by HIV/AIDS. Individuals and organizations alike waited for direction from above. There was too little initiative and not much experience with practical problem solving. Recognition of the overwhelming extent of HIV/AIDS failed to result in specific steps to begin to address it. It would take time for the government to develop and begin implementation of a national strategy, and even more time for this strategy, or strategies, to reach the community level. There was a great need to produce a critical mass of change agents who could not only act but also train others to act to create an ever-increasing cadre of committed individuals to combat the national scourge and personal threat on a daily basis.

As Bill flew home from this visit, he thought more and more about PSBH, and in early September of 2003 he called Barry. Lesotho was small enough for DHF and BU to make a difference. In January 2004, Barry made a trip to Lesotho with Bill, Arden, and the student interns who would organize the first workshop. Barry met with the Minister of Finance and Development Planning, the Minister of Health and Social Welfare, and the U.S. Ambassador to explain the PSBH process, and he quickly gained support from all of them. The ambassador was against workshops in general but was quickly convinced that PSBH was "a different kind of workshop."

With support from DHF, BU trained 157 people between April 2004 and March 2005 to adapt the principles of PSBH to focus exclusively on HIV/AIDS, thereby producing a cadre of people in and outside the government who (1) are knowledgeable about the prevention and treatment of HIV/AIDS, (2) understand the PSBH process and its value in everyday life, and (3) have the skills and commitment to apply the techniques of PSBH to the treatment of HIV/AIDS. Participants from all sectors were represented at the three PSBH HIV/AIDS workshops, including representatives from eight government ministries, several district public service departments, five institutions of higher education, eight district hospitals, and six nongovernmental organizations (NGOs). The goal was to get as many people as possible engaged in combating AIDS on a daily basis, in a variety of ways, based on good science and an understanding of cultural, social, and economic factors relevant to HIV/AIDS control.

The projects tackled a wide range of HIV/AIDS-related issues, including needs for the following: education to prevent HIV/AIDS through knowledge, attitude change, and behavior change strategies; increased availability and uptake of voluntary counseling and testing (VCT) services; development and expansion of services for people living with HIV/AIDS (PLWHA) and orphans and vulnerable children; improvement of clinical services for better diagnosis and referrals, management of opportunistic infections, and availability of postexposure prophylaxis for rape victims; development of workplace programs and policies to reduce stigma and increase uptake of VCT services, reduce stress among those caring for HIV/AIDS patients, and improve coordination to implement HIV/AIDS programs; increased availability and use of condoms; education to promote disclosure among PLWHA; addressing underlying contributors, such as unemployment, poverty, rape, and alcohol abuse; and development and promotion of positive alternatives to risky behaviors, including life skills and job training and HIV/AIDS activist clubs. Also, a small number of individuals opted to address problems unrelated to HIV/AIDS. Allowing people to address problems more relevant to their everyday work results in a greater chance of success and reinforces the PSBH process.

There are several success stories from this first series of workshops. One example is Nthabiseng Ramokhele-Mbole's project. Mrs. Ramokhele-Mbole, a prison officer in the rural district of Qacha's Nek, wanted to address the problem the prison faces with transmission of HIV/AIDS among inmates, due to the men having unprotected sex with their fellow inmates. She addressed this problem by teaching the inmates about HIV/AIDS in general, the risks of HIV infection associated with men having sex with men (MSM), and the proper use of condoms. She worked with rehabilitation officers to arrange visits to the prison by trained counselors from the nearby government hospital to provide education to the inmates. HIV awareness and health talks were conducted for the inmates once a week, and pastors integrated the education into their regular Sunday preaching. Occasionally, youth from a nearby center joined the sessions and shared their experiences and perceptions. Inmates participated actively during these talks, and many volunteered to be tested. Condoms were provided, despite denial of MSM activity, and the inmates frequently reported that their condoms were "missing." This project was to end in March 2006, but it is now a long-term program that reaches out to new prisoners.

Barry attended the first two PSBH HIV/AIDS workshops, along with international facilitators from the United States, South Africa, and Zambia. Over the course of these three workshops, and others that followed, members of the Zambian team provided invaluable help in guiding the development of PSBH in Lesotho. Ruth Chikasa, Dr. Dixon Tembo, Chilufya Mwaba, and the Rev. Kangwa Mabuluki contributed their knowledge of the PSBH process by training local participants as facilitators. In addition, Dr. Alex Papilaya came from Indonesia and was instrumental in laying a strong foundation for a hospital-based program, Problem Solving for Better Hospitals (PSBHospitals). Some of the most successful participants in the workshops were identified as cofacilitators and grew into the roles of facilitators and workshop leaders. These individuals benefited from the experience and mentorship of the skilled international facilitators, and now PSBH in Lesotho is entirely staffed from within.

Growth in Lesotho: Problem Solving for Better Hospitals

Over the past 10–12 years, providing health services in Lesotho, particularly hospital services, has become more difficult. Problems include staff shortages, unresponsive and cumbersome administrative practices, equipment maintenance problems, and limited budgets. In spite of this, facilities are, for the most part, new and in good condition; the drug supply is adequate; and laboratory services are available.

As advanced HIV disease/clinical AIDS increased in Lesotho, three things were certain: hospitals were overwhelmed with AIDS patients, all the non-AIDS patients' needs continued, and hospital staff members were dying of AIDS in large numbers. This terrifying reality made efficiency and doing the most with the least ever more important. PSBHospitals was one of the few immediate interventions with the potential to make a difference and make a difference fast.

Two PSBHospitals workshops, based on DHF's Indonesian model, were held, one in 2004 and one in 2006. The goal was to produce a cadre of motivated people from government and Christian Health Association of Lesotho (CHAL) hospitals, as well as from the central Ministry of Health and Social Welfare (MOHSW), with the skills and knowledge sufficient to identify and solve important problems affecting the efficiency and quality of hospital services. The two workshops involved 109 individuals from the central MOHSW, MOHSW hospitals, central CHAL, CHAL hospitals, Maseru Private Hospital, auxiliary services (e.g., the National Drug Service Organization), Lesotho Flying Doctors Services, and nursing schools.

Teboho McPhearson, a maintenance technician from Scott Hospital (CHAL), worked hard to implement his project addressing the frequent breakdowns of life-saving and biomedical equipment. He determined that the cost for a maintenance contract (R26,000, or 3,500 USD per year) was not available in the budget to service the machines. Yet he discovered that a one-time call for preventive maintenance cost only R4,500 (600 USD). By introducing semiannual preventive maintenance calls, Teboho found a way to keep the machines operating for only 35% of the cost of a service contract, an amount within the hospital's recurrent budget. When he started his project, 80% of the machines were broken. After the first preventive maintenance call, that number was reduced to 40%.

Shortly thereafter, many other CHAL hospitals adopted this problem-solving practice. More than 2 years later, Teboho reported that he had negotiated a maintenance service contract for the laboratory equipment. He also reported that PSBH helped him learn how to fix small problems that can lead to fixing bigger problems.

Sister Constancia 'Mele, hospital administrator at Mamohau Hospital (CHAL), took on the challenge of reducing unpaid hospital bills. Sister 'Mele put posters around the entire hospital explaining the fees, and made a list of all the people and families in each area who had not paid their bills. She met with the chiefs and councilors in those areas to educate them about the need to pay the bills to prevent the hospital from closing. Mamohau Hospital changed its policy to accept any amount of payment toward the outstanding balance, including in-kind payments. Before Sister 'Mele's project, only 40% of the patients had paid their bills; after her intervention, more than 85% had paid something to the hospital, cash or in kind.

Lesotho–Boston Health Alliance

As the BU team followed the successes of the PSBHospitals program participants, the need to address the human resource and systemic challenges facing Lesotho's hospitals became more apparent. Dr. Brian Jack, Academic Vice Chair of the BU Department of Family Medicine, who possessed substantial experience in international health, was invited to the first PSBHospitals workshop and quickly became a key member of the Lesotho team. The BU–Lesotho team grew and merged with Boston Medical Center, BU's teaching hospital. The Boston University Medical Campus (BUMC) collaboration established the Lesotho–Boston Health Alliance (LeBoHA) as its NGO based in Lesotho. The LeBoHA team worked with the MOHSW to transform district health services in Lesotho, and in January 2007 the MOHSW was awarded a 5-year grant by the W. K. Kellogg Foundation to implement this transformation, with BUMC as its lead partner.

Goals of the 5-year program are to strengthen clinical services through physician and nurse training and improve the practice environment and related systems through better management. The objective is to lay the groundwork for transforming district health services across Lesotho and provide an environment that increases the return of Basotho physicians to Lesotho and improves the retention of Basotho nurses and physicians. At present, there is not a sufficiently appealing practice environment for young physicians in Lesotho, and few Basotho return home after medical school in other countries. Physicians need to know there will be hospital and health center complexes all around the country where the practice environment gives them a reason to stay. For this to occur, improved management must go hand in hand with clinical training.

The PSBH approach makes sense as a way of introducing rational planning principles to hospital staff and other health workers. Although the workshops are based on an individual problem-solving model, the strategy could also be applied to teams and organizational work units. In fact, the process of analysis and data collection introduced in the PSBH methodology (e.g., analyzing causes and contributing factors to problems, deciding on targets for improvement, and developing an evaluation plan to know when targets have been met) is a key component of traditional quality management efforts. Representatives from all of the proposed partner hospitals involved in the program funded by the W. K. Kellogg Foundation program to transform district hospitals attended the February 2006

DHF workshop. Participants reacted positively to the potential of PSBH for broader use in health systems and management improvement for Lesotho.

Five PSBH workshops hosted in the first 2 years of the hospital program's implementation provided training for 199 participants from Motebang Hospital, Berea Hospital, Maluti Adventist Hospital, Mamohau Hospital, and several clinics. Participants included physicians, nurses, nurse educators, nurse officers, nurse clinicians, public health nurses and other District Health Management Team members, nursing assistants, ward attendants, nutritionists, counselors, administrators, pharmacy technicians, laboratory technicians, accountants, human resources personnel, office assistants, clerks, cleaners, porters, drivers, cooks, gardeners, and maintenance workers. Successful participants from prior workshops served as facilitators and cofacilitators at all five workshops, thereby strengthening the capability in the districts to sustain PSBH without outside assistance.

Two of the workshops were specifically focused on nursing personnel (Problem Solving for Better Health-Nursing™ [PSBHN™]). This type of workshop was carried out with great support by members and leaders of the Nursing Advisory Board, the Lesotho Nursing Council (LNC), and the Lesotho Nursing Association (LNA).

Participants from the five workshops defined significant clinical problems and created solid plans of action toward a solution. Monthly follow-up and tracking of these participants provided an additional source of support to track problem-solving progress and led to a greater likelihood of success. Although some participants inevitably ran into barriers, many quickly solved their first problem and moved on to identify and solve another. A few selected success stories include:

- Mantahli Mahase, nurse counselor at Maluti Adventist Hospital, tackled the issue of decentralizing the chronic treatment of patients on antiretroviral therapy. She developed a system to identify patients who would benefit from receiving their antiretrovirals (ARVs) from local clinics rather than the hospital. She reassigned these patients to local clinics in batches. The patients receiving ARVs at the local clinics are more likely to adhere to their treatment schedules and receive proper care. In addition, the hospital load has been decreased.
- Drivers at Leribe and Berea, Ntutu Lerata and Senekane Ramaokane, each had the same problem: drivers not being trained to handle patients at the scene of an accident. Mr. Nkemele, the hospital administrator in Leribe, contacted Bethlehem Hospital in South Africa to administer paramedic training for the drivers and junior staff in Leribe and Berea. Since the training, managers report improved performance and attitudes among those trained.
- Matsepo Mofokeng, lab technologist at Maluti Hospital, was concerned about emergency blood donors not being told their HIV status after donation. After meeting with the central Lesotho Blood Transfusion Services (LBTS) and her supervisors, Matsepo adapted the transfusion protocol to include testing and counseling for HIV status, developed an emergency protocol and donation form, and is ensuring regular follow-up with LBTS for quality control.
- Tlhoriso Ntlape, an assistant in the supply department at Berea Hospital, focused on reducing cross-infection at the hospital by making clean linens available daily. Tlhoriso worked with suppliers and Berea's administrator to procure the cleaning supplies in order for linens to be cleaned on a regular basis. Tlhoriso now orders the supplies well in advance, and linens are washed on a continual basis.

Sustaining the Growth

PSBHospitals has become an essential component of the improved management activities in the pilot hospitals. In an effort to link the very important hospital-wide clinical problems identified at the workshops, the management team at Motebang Hospital has identified several "Good Questions" to work with and adopt into the hospital's quality-improvement initiatives. The management team at Maluti Hospital uses this approach regularly to solve problems with an overall benefit to management activities. A PSBH committee has formed at Maluti Hospital, and now other hospitals are following suit.

Most members of the management team at each of the hospitals have attended a workshop. As a result, they have been willing to lend assistance and support when they are approached for help on other PSBH projects. In addition, "team leaders" were selected from the participants at recent workshops to take the lead in coordinating follow-up and alerting the LeBoHA support team if assistance is needed when challenges arise. These team leaders are also facilitators at workshops and provide continuing support to their colleagues as they implement their action plans.

In addition to the support networks now in place, considerable effort has been invested to develop a system that will motivate participants to implement their action plans and continue solving problems upon completion of their proposed projects. This has included the use of motivational speakers, PSBH reunion celebrations, and posters highlighting successful projects displayed throughout the hospitals.

There is now growing interest among donors and the MOHSW in further strengthening health systems across the country. PSBH has been a part of these discussions, and a consensus is growing that it has tremendous potential for improving health systems nationwide.

A Nursing Perspective

Alysa N. Veidis

Since the mid-1990s, a human resource crisis has developed within Lesotho. There is a shortage of physicians, nurses, and clinical personnel in general. District hospitals are understaffed, with minimal physician presence and a skeleton crew of nurses. Community health centers are staffed and managed solely by nurses, with disorganized and insufficient physician oversight, if any at all. Nurses account for 90% of all personnel providing health services in Lesotho (MOHSW, 2005). According to data from Médecins Sans Frontières, there are 62 nurses per 100,000 people in the country, far short of the minimum recommended by the World Health Organization of 100 nurses per 100,000 (Médecins Sans Frontières, 2007). While nurses in Lesotho have a proud tradition of excellence, nursing as a profession has weakened due to insufficient staffing, ineffective management, poor regulatory systems, overdependence on unlicensed personnel, and stagnant career paths resulting in low morale and high rates of burnout.

Alysa N. Veidis is Director of Nursing Programs for the Lesotho–Boston Health Alliance.

LeBoHA's Approach

Because of countrywide staffing issues and clearly voiced challenges by the nurses of Lesotho, the LeBoHA nursing team is working to address the needs of nurses. To this end, LeBoHA developed the Inpatient Nursing Competency Program in collaboration with the LNC, the LNA, the Chief Nursing Officer (CNO) from the MOHSW, and two district hospital matrons. The program focuses directly on improving the clinical skills and competencies of nurses, thus empowering nurses, increasing nurse satisfaction, improving patient outcomes, and promoting nurse retention.

Since March 2008, the Inpatient Nursing Competency Program has been underway in two districts of Lesotho. The theoretical framework for the competency curriculum is the nursing process, a problem-solving and critical thinking approach to patient care that focuses on the importance of *thinking and doing*. Each 1-hour session is taught by one of LeBoHA's Basotho nurse educators in a classroom setting, using presentations, case studies, and role playing. The nurses then return to work and receive on-the-ward mentoring from the same nurse educator while actively working. The nurse educator uses a hands-on approach and applies what has been taught in that morning's session to real-time nursing care.

Additionally, in collaboration with the LNC and CNO, nurses at LeBoHA completed an *inpatient hospital policy and procedure manual*. Prior to this compilation, there was no document or reference manual that stood behind the nursing profession in Lesotho. The new comprehensive manual incorporates the most up-to-date clinical procedural information that is relevant and feasible for district hospitals and nurses. It provides a quick view of accepted procedures of care and gives the nurses standards to strive for in their work. This manual has been accepted by the LNC and MOHSW.

In an effort to evaluate and identify hospital-wide system issues, a baseline survey of nursing documentation was conducted on all inpatient hospital wards at three district hospitals. Results demonstrated the need to improve nursing documentation. For example, nurses were not regularly recording input and output volumes, basic vital signs, and medication administration. Subsequently, and in collaboration with nurses and nurse matrons from the hospitals, four new documentation forms were created. The forms include: admission assessment, nursing care plan, vital signs, and intake and output. On-the-ward training by the LeBoHA team has been reinforcing the importance of documentation using the new forms.

Documentation data collected at 6 months and 1 year after documentation mentoring and training for the new forms was conducted and has indicated immense improvement in the recording of vital signs, medication administration, and nursing care plans when compared with the baseline assessment. Each of the three pilot hospitals has adopted these forms as part of the formal patient chart, and nurses are expected to complete these forms as part of their required shift work. The LeBoHA team continues to reinforce the need for nursing documentation and supports the nurses while carrying out ward mentoring.

Problem Solving for Better Health-Nursing

As the director of the LeBoHA Nursing Program, I have had the opportunity to observe, teach, mentor, listen, and collaborate with the nurses of Lesotho not only at an administrative level but also in the field, on the wards of three district hospitals in Lesotho. With many years of hospital nursing experience myself, I had an instant connection with the nurses in the hospitals.

I sensed discouragement and a lack of motivation among the nurses. I felt their hopelessness and frustration. I appreciated that these bright, talented nurses were starved for education, empowerment, and feedback and were struggling in an unsupported profession and broken health system. Despite this, the nurses had the resolve to continue to believe in the true meaning of nursing and had a desire to be proud of their work while striving to make a difference in the health of patients and their families.

The Inpatient Nursing Competency Program addresses some of the issues faced by the nurses in Lesotho, but there was a need to engage these nurses in a way they never had been before. Our nursing team wanted to encourage free, critical thinking and establish a forum that would lend itself to professional brainstorming and problem solving. We wanted the nurses to realize that they are the backbone of healthcare in Lesotho and that without their ideas, motivation, dedication, energy, and service, the people of Lesotho would suffer.

The PSBH approach has been very successful in empowering individuals to identify, plan, and solve workplace problems, as LeBoHA had seen in previous PSBH workshops in Lesotho. In October 2008, with support from the DHF, LeBoHA carried out two PSBHN workshops. PSBHN workshops focus only on nurses and nursing personnel, and this was the first of its kind in Lesotho. Nurses require critical thinking skills on a daily basis, and the problem-solving approach mimics the nursing process.

The workshop was a great success, helping to motivate and support the nursing staff at the selected district hospitals. The LNC chairperson and LNA president gave the opening and closing remarks, respectively, demonstrating support and encouragement from the professional organizations. Facilitators for the workshop included members from DHF (Pamela Hoyt-Hudson and Ruth Chikasa) and Kangwa Mabuluki, minister from Zambia, as well as local Basotho nurses and LeBoHA team members, including myself.

It was incredible to help the nurses along the winding path of problem solving. We took time to discuss nursing and remember why each individual had entered the nursing profession. Throughout the PSBH process, the nurses went through common phases, starting with a sense of initial lack of motivation; moving on to feeling daunted by the challenge; and finally becoming eager, rising to the opportunity, grasping critical thinking, becoming passionate, and sharing their skills in supportive and collaborative ways. Each participant traveled along the problem-solving path at his or her own pace, but most achieved what, prior to the 3-day workshop, they had considered an unattainable goal.

The problems identified during the PSBHN workshop were not solely clinical but were also administrative problems that affect not only nurses and patient care but also the functioning of the hospital as a whole. Recognizing the importance of systematic collaboration, the LeBoHA nursing team has partnered with LeBoHA's Management Strengthening Team at each respective hospital to provide seamless support to the nurse participants and hospital administration in an effort to carry out each participant's action plan.

The LeBoHA nursing program and PSBHN have given nurse participants a sense of self-respect and pride in their profession by fostering patience, encouragement, and belief in one's self, along with strengthening clinical competencies and critical thinking. The nurses have been given the foundation to continue striving to provide competent patient care, and remain active problem solvers. Each of these nurses is a true success story!

References

Babich, L. P., Bicknell, W. J., Culpepper, L., Jack, B. W., Phooko, M. M., Smith, B., et al. (2008). Institutional commitment and HIV/AIDS: Lessons from the first three years of the Lesotho–Boston University collaboration. *Global Public Health, 3*(4), 417–432.

Babich, L. P., Bicknell, W. J., Jack, B. W., & Culpepper, L. (2008). Mutual benefits: Why an academic medical center and Lesotho are partners. *Academic Medicine, 83*(2), 143–147.

Kimaryo, S., Okpaku, J., Githuku-Shongwe, A., & Feeney, J. (2003). *Turning a crisis into an opportunity— Strategies for scaling up the national response to the HIV/AIDS pandemic in Lesotho.* New York: UNDP publication.

Lesotho Ministry of Health and Social Welfare. (2003). *2003 HIV Sentinel Survey Report.* U.S. Central Intelligence Agency. The World Factbook. Retrieved March 2, 2009, from https://www.cia.gov/library/publications/the-world-factbook/print/lt.html

Lesotho Ministry of Health and Social Welfare, Bureau of Statistics, and ORC Macro. (2005). *Lesotho Demographic and Health Survey 2004.* Calverton, Maryland: MOHSW, BOS, and ORC Macro.

Lesotho Planned Parenthood Association. (2003). *Situational assessment for establishing voluntary counseling and testing services.* Maseru: Author.

Médecins Sans Frontières. (2007). *Help wanted: Confronting the health care worker crisis to expand access to HIV/AIDS treatment: MSF experience in Southern Africa.* Johannesburg, South Africa: Author.

6

Malawi

Sebastian J. Milardo and Maureen L. Chirwa

Malawi is a small (118,484 sq km), landlocked, Bantu-speaking country in southeastern Africa that is bordered to the north by Tanzania, the northwest by Zambia, and the southwest and southeast by Mozambique. Lake Malawi, one of the Great Lakes of Africa, extends along much of the eastern border of the country. Home to 14 million people, Malawi is one of the world's most densely populated countries. Eighty percent of Malawians live in rural areas where agriculture is their economic base. The country has a democratic, multiparty government and a rich culture of song and dance. The rising sun on the Malawian flag represents the dawn of freedom and hope for Africa. The Problem Solving for Better Health program is honored to be a part of that hope.

In 2005, the Dreyfus Health Foundation (DHF) was introduced to Fernanda Farinha of the W. K. Kellogg Foundation of Battle Creek, Michigan. After hearing about the work of DHF, Farinha expressed Kellogg's interest in expanding its presence in Africa to improve health in Malawi. DHF saw this as a good opportunity to expand and strengthen its own existing network in sub-Saharan Africa, and Kellogg agreed to fund a new Problem Solving for Better Health® (PSBH®) program in Malawi starting the following year.

Between January and June 2006, DHF's Director of Operations, Sebastian Milardo, and Regional Coordinator for PSBH in Africa, Ruth Chikasa, made several visits to Malawi to establish partnerships with individuals and organizations, create a committee to oversee the work, and determine the best location for the program. Identification of partners and program locations is a critical step in the PSBH program implementation process. The Ministry of Health, the Nurses and Midwives Council of Malawi, the Research for Equity and Community Health Trust, the Lighthouse Trust, Kamuzu College of Nursing (KCN), the Centre for Youth Empowerment and Civic Education (YECE), the Mlanzi Community

Sebastian J. Milardo is Director of Operations at the Dreyfus Health Foundation (DHF). Maureen L. Chirwa is Managing Director of Prime Health Consulting and Services and Director of the Health Management Unit, University of Malawi College of Medicine. She is also Director of the Local Initiative for Better Health, DHF's implementing partner in Malawi, and Problem Solving for Better Health National Coordinator for Malawi.

Initiative for Development, and the United Kingdom's Department for International Development and the Equi-TB Knowledge Programme, were all essential in providing leads.

In July 2006, DHF conducted a meeting in Lilongwe, the capital of Malawi, to introduce representatives from the aforementioned organizations and interested community leaders to the PSBH methodology. In addition, the attendees were trained as facilitators so that they could assist at a future PSBH workshop. At this meeting, the Nurses and Midwives Council of Malawi Registrar and Chief Executive, Dr. Maureen Chirwa, was appointed the coordinator of the PSBH program in Malawi. Local Initiative for Better Health (LIBH) was selected as the name for the new organization that would coordinate the program in collaboration with DHF. Maxwell M'bweza, Evelyn Nyirenda, and Lifah Sanudi were chosen to assist Dr. Chirwa on the steering committee.

The committee held a meeting in September 2006 to establish a team of local facilitators, drawn from the July meeting, which would assist workshop participants in the development of their projects at the upcoming workshop. A facilitator team assumes responsibility for and ownership of the program as a whole and serves a dual purpose. Facilitators are the primary contacts for project leaders, and regular communication and site visits are expected to provide encouragement, information, and assistance when necessary. In addition, the facilitators determine how best to support the projects. The team must be unified in its decisions regarding issues such as project evaluation, funding, and other forms of support.

Led by Dr. Chirwa and the LIBH team, Malawi's first PSBH workshop was held in September 2006 in Mponela. PSBH facilitators from Cameroon, Ghana, Kenya, Zambia, and the United States attended, as well as 30 participants representing a number of local organizations. Since then, LIBH and DHF have held two follow-up workshops to assess the ongoing success of the projects that were generated.

At the initial workshop, participants proposed a number of projects on topics as varied as water and sanitation, food and nutrition, dam construction, literacy training, and microenterprise. The participants prioritized the problems and agreed that clean water and toilets were the major needs in the area. With Nabitia James and Nasikimu Rabson as the leaders, two projects were developed to take place simultaneously: a protected wells project and a sanitary slabs project. A sanitary slab, or "san slab," is a mud, straw, and concrete platform with footmarks and central holes, used to cover pit latrines.

Community members in Chimwaminga and Chilumaminga villages were actively involved in the projects. They carried rocks, sand, and bricks from the surrounding area to the sites, assisted in the construction of the wells and the sanitary slabs, and prepared food for the workers. The residents explained that this was the first time an outside group had helped to develop projects in their community. Many were pleased that the projects would have an immediate impact. They expressed pride in their work and the fact that they were able to find the majority of the necessary resources locally. The residents felt a sense of ownership and responsibility for the projects and a new sense of unity within the village.

The effort of leaders Nabitia and Nasikimu is the primary factor behind the success of the projects. Their continuing desire to make progressive change was recognized and adopted by the rest of the community. Cases of cholera decreased significantly, from 70% during the 2006 rainy season to less than 10% in 2007. During the 2008 rainy season, which saw many neighboring areas hit by cholera, Chimwaminga reported no cases. The success in Chimwaminga resulted in a request from nearby Chimutukudambo village for replication of these water and sanitation projects (Figure 6.1).

At the same workshop, representatives attended from YECE, an organization located just outside of Lilongwe that focuses on human rights, democracy, and advocacy for people living with HIV/AIDS. These participants recognized that although sanitation was not directly related to the objectives of their organization, cholera and diarrheal diseases significantly compounded the health problems of the region in which they operate. The Area 25 Health Centre under the Lilongwe District Health Office noted that approximately 20 out of every 100 people became infected with cholera each year, resulting in many deaths. The population of Mgona, located near Area 25, is approximately 5,500, and most residents suffered from diarrhea due to drinking contaminated water, lack of personal hygiene, improper use of pit latrines, and improper waste disposal.

To address the problems of sanitation and diarrheal diseases in Mgona, several YECE members, with the assistance of the village chiefs, developed a project with local youth focusing on the disposal of waste, including bagged human waste. Rubbish pits were not available and trash was everywhere in the community, which led to poor environmental sanitation. An additional problem was the tendency of residents to dispose of trash on the railway line, obstructing the passage of the train. For the train to pass, it had to stop while the community cleared the tracks. This led to conflict between residents of Mgona and the railway company, resulting in the company asking the government to move all the people out of Mgona.

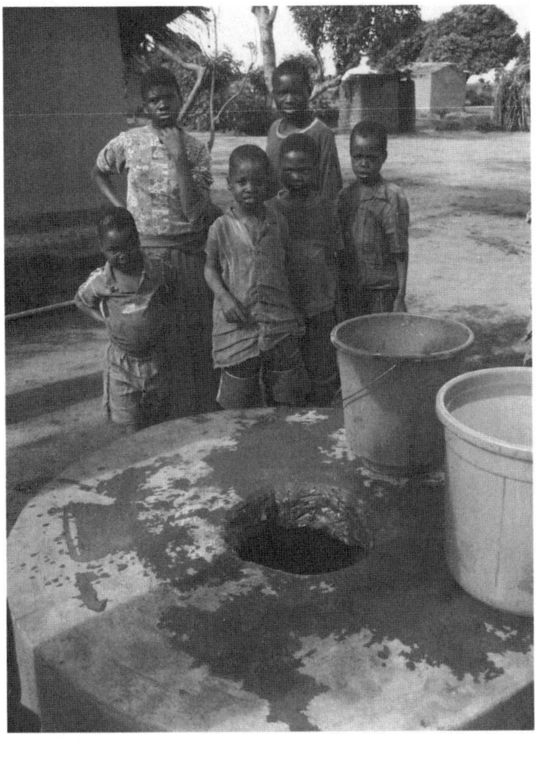

FIGURE 6.1 Chimwaminga villagers await installation of the pump for a protected well built by members of the community and the Local Initiative for Better Health.

To rectify the problem, the YECE team and community members dug large waste pits on the outskirts of the village. They reinforced the pits with brick and chicken wire to protect them from water damage and collapse during the rainy season. A brick fence was constructed to protect children from falling into the pits. Upon completion of the pits, the LIBH team reinforced the importance of proper waste disposal to prevent garbage and human waste from leaching into the ground, affecting water quality.

This simple project had a huge impact on the community. The number of diarrheal diseases, including cholera, decreased significantly, and the people were pleased with the improved living conditions in their village. As in Chimwaminga and Chilumaminga, several residents commented that no one from outside the community had taken an interest in their health before, they were proud to be part of a movement that had made a difference, and the community had gained a new sense of unity. They also indicated that since the project started, not a single case of cholera had been observed. Even during 2008, when Malawi experienced a particularly high incidence of cholera, Mgona experienced better health overall than the surrounding villages.

Further, the project reaped an additional benefit. At the end of the rainy season, local farmers shared the decomposed waste to use as compost. The waste was an inexpensive fertilizer for the farmers, and removing it from the village improved the sanitation problem. For continued support and to maximize the project benefits, the Lilongwe City Assembly's Public Health Department has supplied appropriate equipment to remove waste and convert it to compost.

At the same workshop, KCN identified the village of Kamgumbwe in the Mitundu area as another community in which LIBH could work. The village is situated about 5 miles to the east of Mitundu Community Hospital in the Lilongwe district. It has a total of 170 households and a population of more than 830 people. In 2006, only 51 homes, or 30% of the village, had pit latrines. The local water supply was often contaminated by the common habit of defecating in the bushes. During the rainy season, human waste soaked into the ground and, as a result, most of the residents suffered from diarrheal diseases, including cholera. During the 2 years before the project, the number of cholera cases more than doubled from one year to the next, and the prevalence of diarrheal cases increased due in part to a lack of knowledge of environmental sanitation and hygiene.

One of the workshop participants, Chrissy Mazoni, a health surveillance assistant working in Mitundu, identified cholera and diarrheal diseases as the problems she and her team wanted to address in their project. Ms. Mazoni noted that few of the existing pit latrines were protected from degradation during the rainy season. The team developed a project to dig sturdier pit latrines that were lined with rock, cement, and chicken wire and covered with san slabs. The village chiefs mobilized the residents, insisting that families dig their own pits. The men broke stones and the women carried them to where san slabs were being cast. In addition, the women cooked for the workers and encouraged their husbands to participate in the projects. Every family that dug a pit received a san slab to cover it.

Another issue was that many people obtained water from contaminated streams, due to a lack of wells. The residents were taught to boil the water and add chlorine to it before drinking to make it safe. A "Sanitation Open Day" featured health professionals explaining proper use and maintenance of the protected wells, latrines, and san slabs, as well as the use of chlorine for water sanitation and waste disposal. As project participants, nurses from the KCN gained valuable field and problem-solving experience. The project was successfully carried out in Kamgumbwe and replicated in the nearby Jimu and Chaponda communities.

A second PSBH workshop in Mponela was held in December 2008, for 30 new participants from the Lilongwe and Mzuzu areas. Approximately 25 participants from the 2006 workshop shared success stories from their water sanitation projects, which generated interest in expanding them to more villages. Other projects developed at the new workshop focused on HIV/AIDS awareness, food security, crime reduction, women's and children's rights, maternal and child mortality reduction, tuberculosis education and prevention, and malaria reduction.

The successful implementation of PSBH projects in Malawi can be attributed to a number of factors. First is the PSBH approach, which encourages individuals and communities to identify, analyze, and prioritize health problems and make use of existing resources to solve them. Project management structure starts with community members, who choose an oversight committee to work with the project leader and the LIBH team on all project matters. Village chiefs are invited to be members of the committee, helping with decision making and mobilizing people to work on projects. LIBH organizes training sessions relevant to each project and provides regular supervision. Effective leadership and team spirit among the national steering committee members have also played major roles in project success.

LIBH has experienced challenges ranging from lack of community participation to delays in completing projects. However, they have tackled each challenge with the relevant community and partner institution(s). Delays in delivery of resources often discouraged communities and caused conflict with project coordinators. The situation improved with reorganization of project activities and adherence to a schedule. Project completion was also affected by weather and season. For example, digging of wells is best done during the dry season and not during the rainy season when the water table is high. Sickness increased absenteeism, causing further delays. Health surveillance assistants provided medication and referrals to local doctors, which gave the community a sense of being cared for. When villagers began to benefit from clean water, proper waste management, and improved sanitation, their participation greatly improved.

The LIBH team learned that it is important to encourage community members to take part in identifying and solving their own health problems. Prior to their PSBH training, members of the team had visited communities to tell the residents to dig latrines, yet the problem was not only a lack of latrines; there was an underlying problem that was not being addressed. After PSBH training, the team members realized that those suffering from health problems in their community were not properly utilized in the development of solutions. They realized that community members must be involved in projects that affect them and must use available resources instead of waiting for donors. These tactics lead to self-sufficiency and ownership of projects by the community.

The communities learned several important lessons, and gained unique insights, through their participation in PSBH. Community members learned good hygiene, how to work together for the good of the whole community, and that community development projects bring people together. The most important lesson they learned is that in unity there is power.

7

Niger

Njoki Ng'ang'a

Niger is a landlocked country in West Africa, bordered by Algeria, Libya, Chad, Nigeria, Benin, Burkina Faso, and Mali. Its land comprises desert in the north; a central zone that is home to nomadic pastoral people; and a settled, largely agricultural zone in the south. Niger is home to some 15 million people who include the Hausa and Djerma-Songhai, among other ethnic groups. Niger's culture contains key elements from Islam, the traditions of its ethnic groups, and French influences. The Dreyfus Health Foundation has been privileged to partner with the International Organization for Women and Development to bring Problem Solving for Better Health to Niger as part of a much larger program to strengthen nursing in the country.

In Niger, the average number of births for women who live to the end of their childbearing years is 7.4 (United Nations Development Programme, 2008). The maternal mortality in the country remains one of the highest in the world at 1,600 per 100,000 live births (World Health Organization [WHO], 2005). The health system in Niger is severely under-resourced and overstretched, with the most recent data from WHO (2004) estimating that there are only 296 physicians and 2,818 nurses and midwives in Niger. This results in inadequate coverage of health services. For example, skilled personnel attend only 18% of all births, a leading factor contributing to the development of harmful consequences, such as obstetric fistulae (WHO, 2006).

Obstetric Fistulae

An obstetric fistula is an abnormal connection between the vagina and bladder and/or the vagina and rectum formed when labor is allowed to progress for prolonged periods

Njoki Ng'ang'a is Director of Nursing at the International Organization for Women and Development in New York, Dreyfus Health Foundation's implementing partner in Niger along with l'Hôpital National de Niamey.

(often up to a week) without medical intervention. The soft pelvic tissue is compressed between the descending fetal head and the mother's pelvic bone, cutting off blood supply, causing the tissue to die, and leaving a gaping hole through which urine, feces, or both, leak uncontrollably. As if the physical shame of incontinence is not enough, the psychosocial consequences of fistulae cause serious emotional trauma. The woman suffers from a loss of dignity due to the foul smell and bears the burden of being an outcast and disowned by family and friends. In a society that places considerable importance on marriage and family, the breakdown of these relationships is devastating (Wall, Karshima, Kirschner, & Arrowsmith, 2004). Coombes's (2004) study, conducted at the Addis Ababa Fistula Hospital in Ethiopia, found that 97% of fistula patients reported feeling depressed.

Obstetric fistulae are an international public health problem that exists primarily in developing countries where access to care during pregnancy, labor, and delivery is lacking. Advances in obstetric care have led to the eradication of obstetric fistulae in the developed world. Therefore, it is unbelievable that today, according to United Nations Population Fund (UNFPA, 2010) estimates, more than 2 million cases exist worldwide, with 50,000–100,000 new cases occurring each year. Although the number of cases of fistula in Niger is unknown, the incidence is similar to that in other countries with a high maternal mortality, approximately 2–3 per 1,000 live births (UNFPA, 2010).

Combating the Problem in Niger

"If we do not know how, we cannot help them." Identifying Nigerien nurses' inability to tackle obstetric fistulae, Saadatou Amadou, an operating room nurse, referred to more than 100 fistula patients awaiting evaluation and surgery in an obscure courtyard located at l'Hôpital National de Niamey (HNN) in Niger. Obstetric fistulae afflict more than 1 million young women who are native to a region in sub-Saharan Africa known as the "fistula belt" that stretches from Mali to Eritrea. Poverty, illiteracy, and subordinate status in society prevent women with fistulae from seeking much-needed care for their ailments. Although native healthcare workers like Amadou, with their intimate understanding of local traditions and customs, are best positioned to address this complex problem, the severely deficient healthcare system in Niger is unable to develop and sustain a sufficient pool of well-trained personnel to successfully serve in this role. While few surgeons are trained in specialized pelvic floor repair, even fewer regularly dedicate their expertise to this much-needed service, which forces fistula patients to remain a marginalized and vulnerable segment of the population, condemned to a fate similar to that of lepers. In response to this systemic dysfunction, the international community has sent healthcare workers to endemic regions and donated the equipment and medication necessary to treat fistula-related illnesses and simultaneously train the local workforce. While every effort is commendable, the results are weak largely because periodic fistula camps (short-term medical interventions providing surgery for women with obstetric fistulae) are hardly sufficient to halt or reverse the occurrence. Therefore, attention must be focused on increasing the capacity of existing Nigerien human resources for health (HRH) that can then stimulate significant strides toward eliminating fistulae.

Since 2003, HNN has offered free examinations, surgery, and postoperative care for fistula patients through a collaborative agreement between the government of Niger and the International Organization for Women and Development (IOWD). IOWD is a

New York–based charitable organization committed to a sustainable program for the treatment and care of patients suffering from obstetric fistulae in Niger. Since the program's inception, Amadou and the nurses at HNN have provided comprehensive care to fistula patients throughout their postoperative course, although they lack the relevant training to manage the complex cluster of physical and psychosocial problems associated with fistulae. For example, at a team meeting dealing with issues encountered during postoperative care, a nurse in the postoperative ward attributed the difficulty of freshly postoperative fistula patients maintaining proper hygiene practices to their being "from the village." It was clear that the nurse did not perceive herself as a link to patient well-being. This attitude was not unique to this nurse but was rather the general outlook among Nigerien nurses at HNN. This attitude can be changed if nurses strive to create a caring environment by adopting therapeutic techniques and establishing trusting relationships with their patients to encourage observance of good hygiene habits, while preserving patients' dignity and independence.

If nurses at HNN are to change from passive observers into active participants exercising their power to influence the trajectory of health outcomes for fistula patients, the transformation needs to begin from within. While working with the nurses at HNN, I searched the literature for innovative nurse-led approaches to global health problems and found the Problem Solving for Better Health-Nursing™ (PSBHN™) program. The Problem Solving for Better Health® (PSBH®) methodology offered a strategy to improve quality of care by promoting individual empowerment, endowing a sense of professional responsibility, and expanding nurses' knowledge. In addition, by encouraging reliance on resources that are easily accessible, PSBHN challenges nurses to develop sustainable solutions. PSBHN was the key to fulfilling Nigerien nurses' potential in meeting the healthcare needs of patients suffering from fistulae. Also, merging the principles of PSBH with the overall aims of the fistula treatment program would create a new and powerful opportunity for Nigerien and North American nurses to share ideas on improving the quality of care for fistula patients in a mutually respectful manner. Niger needed PSBHN.

Problem Solving for Better Health-Nursing in Niger

I began by contacting Pamela Hoyt-Hudson, the International Nursing Program Coordinator at the Dreyfus Health Foundation. The well-documented applicability of PSBHN in tackling diverse problems across a wide variety of settings made it especially suited for implementation within the Niger context. Step by step, Hoyt-Hudson was instrumental in her steadfast guidance, steering around hurdles that almost ensured a premature halt to the planned launch. Limited funding, for example, prevented a PSBHN facilitator from traveling to Niamey to conduct the workshop. Instead, Hoyt-Hudson decided to train me as a facilitator, offering indispensable counsel along the way. For this, I remain deeply grateful.

Making the Case for Problem Solving for Better Health-Nursing

To completely understand the need for initiatives such as PSBHN in Niger, background information pertinent to the local circumstances is important to consider.

Humanitarian efforts, such as IOWD's program in Niger, are intended to relieve suffering as well as supplement HRH in areas where critical shortages exist. However, there is evidence that tension can exist between local HRH and visiting health workers (Laleman et al., 2007). In exploring the dynamics of relationships between international volunteers and local health workers, Laleman et al. (2007) found that experienced local medical officers had mostly negative perceptions of expatriate health workers for a variety of reasons, such as their perceived inexperience, unfamiliarity with local epidemiology and healthcare systems, unwillingness to create contextually appropriate interventions, and poor communication. These same expatriates were commended for leaving their comfortable livelihoods in the developed world in exchange for difficult working and living conditions. They were also commended for their contribution to advancement in education and training. But these perceptions can sometimes form barriers to properly executing well-intended health programs, and there is an obligation to resolve them. In Niger, PSBHN offered a mechanism for breaking down these very real barriers.

Another obstacle suppressing the advancement of Nigerien nurses in leading innovative health improvement is the lack of resources to increase the nurses' knowledge. Limited opportunities to pursue higher education have resulted in a largely ineffective nursing workforce. For example, in a study of referral patterns by nurses in rural Niger, Bossyns and Van Lerberghe (2004) found that a poor understanding of the health system contributed to inappropriate management of patients in health centers instead of arranging for transfers to district hospitals. The authors listed nurses' lack of knowledge as a barrier to accessing healthcare in Niger, along with distance and cost.

The Problem Solving for Better Health-Nursing Process

"Be the change you wish to see in the world." We borrowed Mahatma Gandhi's renowned quotation as the theme for our 2007 PSBHN workshop. The seven nurses participating from HNN hailed this meeting as groundbreaking. "We have never been involved in anything like this," they said.

Following a roundtable format selected to promote equality, we introduced the PSBH core principles, utilizing imagery found in popular culture to depict key themes. For example, a photograph of penguins huddling together for warmth during the harsh Antarctic winter symbolized our interdependency. To set the tone for the gathering, we emphasized frank discussion as essential for our problem-solving agenda. Participants took turns identifying impediments that prevented full execution of health promotion activities within their various spheres of practice. Problems included a knowledge deficit regarding the pathophysiology and treatment of fistulae; lack of materials, equipment, and medication; lack of clarity about the social reintegration of fistula patients following treatment; strained Nigerien–American relationships and their impact on work culture; illiterate patients; frequent rotation and replacement of nurses, leading to an inconsistent team; priority assignment of operating rooms and ward beds received by New York–based IOWD for fistula patients; and reliance on U.S. Peace Corps volunteers to conduct patient-related activities that are normally the responsibility of the HNN nurses. Although each of these concerns was deemed legitimate, we agreed to narrow the list down to only those problems with a direct link to nursing practice in the care of fistula patients at HNN. For example, while restoring fistula patients to a normal life is a major goal of treatment, we agreed that the mechanism of social reintegration fell outside the immediate domain of nursing practice at HNN.

Second, we identified an inaccurate view of IOWD volunteers held by the Nigerien nurses. The nurses were astonished to learn that none of the IOWD volunteers, including the executive leadership, receive a salary. In addition, the nurses discovered that all volunteers pay for mission-related expenses using personal funds; forgo vacations with family and friends to travel to Niger to care for fistula patients; and, most important, solicit corporate and personal donations of equipment, supplies, and medications. This information helped the nurses understand the decision to dedicate two out of six operating rooms at HNN for fistula surgery three times a year for 2 weeks at a time. In essence, this arrangement was based not on bias toward one group in favor of another but on the availability of the fistula treatment team. Furthermore, the nurses were reassured that the ultimate goal of IOWD's mission in Niger is to support the creation of a comprehensive Nigerien team capable of treating and preventing fistulae to take over the program.

Third, we eliminated "lack of materials, equipment, and medication" from the list of problems simply because one of the core principles of PSBH requires that solutions optimize the use of readily available resources. In addition, whereas scarcity of these supplies is a valid concern and has great consequences for the quality of nursing care, the supplies are ordinarily provided through IOWD.

Once the list of problems was streamlined, participants shifted gears to address the remaining concerns. The nurses identified poor knowledge about the etiology, pathophysiology, and rationale behind treatment modalities as a major barrier, which limits their contribution to the proper care of fistula patients. In 2005, Kyriacos, Jordan, and van den Heever stressed that advanced knowledge in key areas of the biological sciences in nursing supports a highly effective nurse workforce. Therefore, we (the IOWD team) suggested recruiting Dr. Abdoulaye Idrissa, the chief surgeon in charge of the fistula program at HNN, to conduct lectures relevant to filling this gap in knowledge. Mamoudou Soumana, the chief nurse at HNN, agreed to lead this project. Dr. Idrissa and Soumana collaborated to develop relevant course content and organize a class schedule. With the assistance of Haoua Moussa, a postoperative ward nurse, Soumana developed a protocol for the care of postoperative fistula patients. This protocol served as a tool to standardize and enhance the quality of care. The PSBHN program opened a door for HNN nurses to discover a new way of thinking.

A second problem identified was that the Nigerien nurses found it difficult to assimilate with the IOWD volunteers and shared the concern that their contribution to the fistula treatment effort would go unnoticed. On the other hand, visiting IOWD volunteers identified the language barrier as the main hindrance to building a more cohesive team with local staff. IOWD enlists help from U.S. Peace Corps volunteers, who possess knowledge of local languages and culture, as interpreters in the operating room and in the wards, which is seen to further isolate the Nigerien nurses.

Because of my role as the nurse coordinator for IOWD, I was best positioned to bridge this divide. My main goal was to provide an avenue for Nigerien operating room nurses to not only remain functional within the fistula repair program but also excel. We began by reassigning duties to ensure that Nigerien nurses were included in the roster, and simultaneously emphasized accountability in executing these duties. To further support team building, Soumana Boubacar, the chief operating room nurse, agreed to ensure a consistent supply of materials furnished through the HNN system, eliminating another bottleneck to the smooth day-to-day running of the operating room. Making seemingly minor changes in the distribution of tasks was strategic in creating harmony.

Removing the obstacles that prevented the fistula program from functioning like a well-oiled operation served to provide a foundation for improving the program. But this was only the beginning. We set in motion the means for nurses to step up and take charge of their own lives and those of their patients. In addition, the nurses' self-confidence in tackling future challenges improved through effective communication. When a participant was asked how he saw himself as an agent of change, he responded, *"responsibilité dans la reussite du travail"* (responsibility for a successful job). It is my hope that the groundwork laid during this workshop will be a launching pad for the recurrent use of PSBHN in tackling health problems other than fistulae and developing sophisticated solutions that incorporate scientific measurements.

Finally, in appreciation of their outstanding performance at the PSBHN workshop and lasting contribution to the treatment and care of women suffering from obstetric fistulae, HNN nurses received certificates of recognition. Since then, we have built a system of acknowledgment into every mission as an expression of gratitude to all who have given selflessly of themselves to care for fistula patients.

Conclusion

The remarkable breadth and depth attained by the PSBHN experience at HNN was unparalleled. The ability of PSBHN to mobilize ordinary people into extraordinary action was best manifested through the late El Hadji Sayze. An elderly, well-respected central supply technician at HNN, Sayze confirmed that real power is created when the opportunity to fulfill one's potential within one's professional role becomes accessible. Amazingly, Sayze did not attend the workshop but instinctively responded to the optimistic energy exuded by the participants with a commitment of his own. Taking ownership of the problem and expressing empathy for the anguish that women with fistulae endure serves to demystify any ill-conceived perceptions the healthcare workers may have toward fistula patients, thus contributing to a shift in the branding of fistula patients from cursed to legitimately ill.

If we are to see substantial leaps toward enhancing health, we need to directly invest in increasing the abilities of HRH, especially in resource-deprived settings. Empowering team members to share the burden of ensuring positive health outcomes is vital for realizing those outcomes. Creating a sense of ownership among Nigerien healthcare workers and allied health workers like Sayze leads to a collaborative spirit that is needed to guarantee health for patients suffering from fistulae.

It was impossible to ignore the renewed sense of vitality among the PSBHN participants and the contagious nature of the PSBHN program, which noticeably extended its reach beyond the initial group of participants. Community cooperation, a central concept within Nigerien society, aided the translation of similar ideas for use in the healthcare context. For example, in Niger, duty to the extended family is paramount. If one family member is in need, the others rally around him or her to lend a helping hand. Fostering a similar obligation to one another and to their patients planted a seed of mutual understanding among the nurses, resulting in a symbolic union to overcome health problems.

The most important lesson I learned in the process is the significance of nurturing ambition, hope for better health, and aspiration to be better nurses, which are crucial requirements for the success of PSBHN-inspired initiatives. Commitment to a daily journey of excellence is our promise to the patients we serve. Instead of looking outward for solutions to health problems such as fistulae, we vowed to search inward, to value ourselves and our desire to give all we have to promote the change we want to see around us. Atul Gawande (2007, p. 246) said it best in his book *Better: A Surgeon's Notes on Performance*: "Better is possible. It does not take genius. It takes diligence. It takes moral clarity. It takes ingenuity. And above all, it takes a willingness to try."

References

Bossyns, P., & Van Lerberghe, W. (2004). The weakest link: Competence and prestige as constraints to referral by isolated nurses in rural Niger. *Human Resources for Health, 2*(1), 1.

Coombes, R. (2004). Supporting surgery for obstetric fistula. *British Medical Journal, 329*(7475), 125.

Gawande, A. (2007). *Better: A surgeon's notes on performance.* New York: Macmillan.

Kyriacos, U., Jordan, S., & van den Heever, J. (2005). The biological sciences in nursing: A developing country perspective. *Journal of Advanced Nursing, 52*(1), 91–103.

Laleman, G., Kegels, G., Marchal, B., Van der Roost, D., Bogaert, I., & Van Damme, W. (2007). The contribution of international health volunteers to the health workforce in sub-Saharan Africa. *Human Resources for Health, 5,* 19.

United Nations Development Programme. (2008). *Human development report 2007/8.* Retrieved September 24, 2008, from http://hdrstats.undp.org/countries/ data_sheets/cty_ds_NER.html

United Nations Population Fund. (2010). *Fast facts: Fistula and reproductive health.* Retrieved April 12, 2010, from http://www.endfistula.org/fast_facts.htm

Wall, L. L., Karshima, J. A., Kirschner, C., & Arrowsmith, S. D. (2004). The obstetric vesicovaginal fistula: Characteristics of 899 patients from Jos, Nigeria. *American Journal of Obstetrics and Gynecology, 190,* 1011–1019.

World Health Organization. (2004). *Core health indicators.* Retrieved September 24, 2008, from http://www.who.int/whosis/database/core/core_select_process.cfm?country=ner&indicators=healthpersonnel

World Health Organization. (2005). *Millennium Development Goal 5.* Retrieved September 24, 2008, from http://www.who.int/making_pregnancy_safer/topics/ mdg/en/index.html

World Health Organization. (2006). *World health report 2006—Working together for health.* Retrieved September 25, 2008, from www.who.int/whr/2006/en/index.html

8

Zambia

Ruth Chikasa

Zambia is a landlocked country in the heart of southern Africa with a high-plateau land area of 776,996 sq km and eight neighbors: the Democratic Republic of the Congo, Tanzania, Malawi, Mozambique, Zimbabwe, Botswana, Namibia, and Angola. Its population of 13 million, drawn from 72 Bantu-speaking ethnic groups, resides mainly in the region around the capital, Lusaka, and in the industrially important Copperbelt Region in the north. Zambians are a musically and artistically talented people. They are also great problem solvers, as their participation in the Problem Solving for Better Health process has shown over the past decade.

In October 1994, Adam Greenberger, a former staff member of the Dreyfus Health Foundation (DHF), introduced DHF's Problem Solving for Better Health® (PSBH®) program to Zambia. Adam came to the Zambia Flying Doctor Service headquarters in Ndola to meet with Executive Director Dr. Mannasseh Phiri to discuss a possible collaboration. As Dr. Phiri's assistant, I had the opportunity to join in the meeting and hear about the foundation and its progams. As a result of the meeting, we began preparations to initiate the PSBH program and conduct a workshop. On February 5, 1995, we officially launched PSBH in Zambia and established the Foundation for Better Health (FBH) to coordinate the program with DHF. Dr. Phiri was the first National Coordinator for the Zambia program, and I initially served as the project assistant. In 1998, Dr. Tom Y. Sukwa took over from Dr. Phiri, and in 2000, when Dr. Sukwa left to work with the World Health Organization in Zimbabwe, I became the National Coordinator.

Ruth Chikasa is International President of the Girls' Brigade International Council and Director of the Foundation for Better Health, Dreyfus Health Foundation's implementing partner in Zambia. Chikasa is also Problem Solving for Better Health (PSBH) National Coordinator for Zambia and PSBH Regional Coordinator for Africa.

Programs

Problem Solving for Better Health

Problem Solving for Better Health® (PSBH®) provides individual frontline health workers with skills to identify solutions to health problems they face in their day-to-day lives, using the resources already available to them. Since Zambia's initial PSBH workshop, held in Ndola in 1995, FBH has worked with individuals who want to enhance the health status of their communities. FBH partners with individuals in local communities, churches, and schools, as well as with the national Ministry of Health. While these partnerships work quite well, we have experienced some challenges. For example, the individual who plans a project carries the vision and the burden of success for the project and is responsible for ensuring that work colleagues and the rest of the community believe in the program. If the project leader leaves the community for any reason, the continuity and sustainability of the project are not guaranteed. The project is viewed as belonging to that particular individual, even though the rest of the community could benefit from the outcome.

Despite the challenges, there have been many successful projects implemented by individuals who were motivated and committed to bettering the lives of their community members in Zambia. Mr. Samukwepa Chikuni, from the Mpongwe Mission Hospital in the Copperbelt town of Luanshya, provides a good example (Figure 8.1). Mr. Chikuni was worried about the high number of snakebite cases reported to the hospital. Almost 80% of these cases resulted in unnecessary amputations or even deaths, because the people in the community did not have knowledge of first-aid treatment for snake bites. Also, cultural beliefs relating to snakes hindered some people from seeking effective treatment when bitten. Mr. Chikuni sensitized the community to the dangers involved in delaying a visit to the hospital once one has been bitten by a snake. He also taught community members about the different types of snakes in the area (venomous and nonvenomous) and started first-aid classes on the treatment of snake bites. The project was supported by the community members, because they had experienced deaths of loved ones, as well as numerous amputations, and so were willing to do all they could to address the situation. The success of the project resulted in the implementation of other health-related projects in the community, because community members had learned to unite in order to defeat a common enemy.

Problem Solving for Better Health Initiative

In 1999, FBH introduced DHF's Problem Solving for Better Health Initiative™ (PSBHI™) program to Zambia. A PSBHI links together smaller, individual projects to create a bigger impact on a community or region.

The Kaloko Initiative is an example of a successful community project. The Kaloko community in Ndola did not have safe drinking water, which resulted in a number of diarrheal diseases in children younger than 5 years of age. Each rainy season, there was a breakout of cholera and dysentery. The Kaloko community together with the District Health Management Team and FBH worked with the Kafubu Water and Sewerage Company to build water kiosks, which were then managed by community members. This resulted in the improved health of community members and fewer reports of cholera and dysentery. One of the advantages of the PSBHI program is easier management for FBH

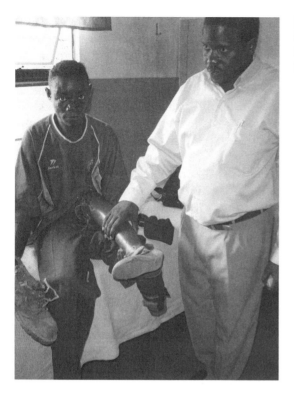

FIGURE 8.1 Samukwepa Chikuni, a Problem Solving for Better Health project leader at the Mpongwe Mission Hospital in Luanshya, attends to a snakebite amputee.

staff, because a community development committee, responsible for all developmental projects, records the program's progress. For the Kaloko project, FBH used the already existing channels of communication in the community and worked with them. The involvement of the entire community ensured transparency and project success. The availability of resources motivated the residents to work together and achieve the desired objective in the Kaloko community—reducing the number of cholera and dysentery cases by providing safe drinking water.

Problem Solving for Better Health-Nursing

In 2004, DHF and FBH introduced the Problem Solving for Better Health-Nursing™ (PSBHN™) program to Zambia and, like PSBHI, it was highly successful. The Ministry of Health, in particular, appreciated PSBHN because the issues raised in the workshops concerned the nurses who handle patient care in the hospitals, clinics, and health centers. Health administrators were happy to work with us to improve the working environment of the nurses so that patient care could be enhanced. The administrators made the welfare of nurses a priority in the hospitals and sought information from us on the challenges described by nurses during the workshop. This information helped the hospital administrators to understand the frustrations the nursing staff faced and how the challenges could be addressed. FBH was invited to give input to the strategic planning of the hospitals, as it was evident that we knew the challenges of the nursing staff first hand, and we could report on their experiences accurately.

One example of a project successfully implemented under PSBHN dealt with the poor attitude some nurses exhibited due to fatigue and dissatisfaction with their working conditions. Hospital administrators had received many complaints from the public on the attitude of nurses toward patients at a local general hospital in Ndola. After attending a PSBHN workshop, one of the matrons of the hospital decided to do something about this problem. Within each ward, she set up a group, including staff nurses, matrons, and human resources personnel, to review nursing practices and guidelines. The meetings served as platforms for the nurses to let their superiors know what was frustrating them. For instance, in addition to long shifts and little time off, nurses had to buy their own uniforms or have them made. Consequently, there was great disparity in the quality of uniforms. There was also a shortage of basic nursing equipment (e.g., blood pressure monitors) and cleaning supplies for the wards. As a result of the meetings, the nursing environment improved. The hospital provided breaks with refreshments during each shift and adequate time off. Also, the hospital began issuing good quality uniforms and providing more equipment and cleaning supplies so that the nurses and the wards did not need to share. This project resulted in better working conditions for the nurses, an improvement in nursing attitudes, and, ultimately, an improvement in the quality of patient care at Ndola Central Hospital.

Conclusion

One of the most outstanding benefits of the PSBH process in Zambia is the changed and renewed mindset of the people involved (as evidenced by testimonies from across the country). Program facilitators, community members, and individuals who come to our workshops are empowered to begin to change their work patterns and their environments in order to realize good health. PSBH energizes and drives them to begin to understand and acknowledge that they themselves can do a great deal to change their own health status, as well as the health status of others with whom they interact.

Another outstanding benefit of the PSBH process is the community mobilization resulting from a PSBHI, as seen in Kaloko. Members of communities unite to tackle a common problem and from there often decide to collectively tackle other local issues. In another community, Roman, in rural Ndola, PSBH helped the residents to establish a cooperative that gave small loans to farmers. In time, the community members lobbied the Ministry of Education to give them a school and teachers, and they also asked the Ministry of Agriculture for technical support with their farming. This community organization and the positive outcomes that resulted began with PSBH.

Over the past 15 years, we have learned that ordinary people can achieve much for their communities if they are empowered and supported to realize the potential that they have. Many people live in abject poverty without recognizing their own worth and that they hold the key to unlocking the wealth within their community. That is why we at FBH in Zambia are very grateful to DHF for partnering with us and the people of Zambia in community development. We salute all who continue to support our programs.

9

China

The People's Republic of China is the world's most populous country, with 1.5 billion people, and one of the largest in land mass. No short introduction can even begin to describe its many-thousand-year history, civilization, or diverse peoples, let alone its achievements in so many arenas since the republic was established in 1949. The success of its hosting the 2008 Summer Olympics captures just where China is in the world today. As this chapter chronicles all too briefly, China is not only the birthplace of the Problem Solving for Better Health program, but also the nurturer of a process that has extended to 20 cities and 10 provinces throughout the country.

Introduction

Barry H. Smith

As previously mentioned, China was the birthplace of the Problem Solving for Better Health® (PSBH®) program; specifically, PSBH was born at West China University of Medical Sciences (now part of Sichuan University) in Chengdu, Sichuan Province, in August 1989. In partnership with the Chinese Medical Board, the Dreyfus Health Foundation (DHF) quickly expanded its programs to several other schools of medicine in China.

To date, PSBH workshops have been implemented in Beijing, Chengdu, Fuzhou, Guangzhou, Hangzhou, Hohhot, Kunming, Lanzhou, Lhasa, Macau, Nanning, Shanghai, Shantou, Shenyang, Shijiazhuang, Urumqi, Wenzhou, Xian, Xining, and Yinchuan. Many PSBH program participants submitted project descriptions for inclusion in this book; space constraints made it impossible to include all of these reports.

From the early initiation of the program in China, nurses and nursing students showed great enthusiasm for PSBH. This led to a special emphasis on PSBH for nurses, a program that came to be known as Problem Solving for Better Health-Nursing™ (PSBHN™). Dean Huaping Liu and senior faculty of Peking Union Medical College School of Nursing (PUMC SON) have led the way toward a national PSBHN program in China. The goal is to mobilize at least 200,000 nurses to take the PSBH message to the people so that the people can take responsibility for their own health and quality of life. To date, nurses in Kunming and Fuzhou have trained more than 1,000 other nurses in PSBHN. In some cases, such as that of Inner Mongolia Medical College in Hohhot, PSBH has been integrated into the medical and nursing curriculum. Hundreds of students have successfully completed projects.

What follows is a description of some of the accomplishments of PSBH in China, in the words of those directly responsible. The approaches of the various reports reflect the unique process of PSBH. *Let one hundred flowers bloom!*

Beijing—Peking Union Medical College School of Nursing

Xiaokun Liang, Jianfen Liu, and Huaping Liu

Since 1996, DHF has sponsored collaborative clinical and basic health research at PUMC SON, and the school continues to serve as the home base for PSBHN in China. PUMC SON offered the first Bachelor of Science in Nursing program in China and plays an important role in teaching nursing students and clinic and community nurses. Under PUMC SON's leadership, 27 PSBHN workshops have been held in China since 1996. Approximately 1,000 nurses and nursing students have participated, developing over 860 projects, 505 of which have been completed.

The PSBHN program facilitates the important role of nurses in emphasizing personal lifestyle change and results in many projects that promote better health. Directed toward all age groups, PSBHN projects have taken place in various settings, such as hospitals, communities, and academic institutions, and have addressed a wide range of healthcare issues.

The projects created included nursing interventions for chronically ill patients and their family members, management and instruction for community people, and health education for nursing students. The following "Good Questions" highlight some of the projects implemented: (1) Will providing assistance devices to 49 patients with active rheumatoid arthritis at a general hospital in Beijing improve their functional ability with respect to, and as measured by, their activities of daily living? (2) Will a health educational program and nursing intervention for 107 hospitalized elderly patients at Fujian Provincial Hospital reduce the rate of falls by 5% in 6 months? (3) Will organizing a blood donation program for 50 university students who have never donated blood increase the blood donation rate to 60% in 1 year?

The PSBHN program improved the hospital and community nurses' and nursing students' ability to identify and solve clients' health problems within various settings. PSBHN was officially incorporated into the PUMC SON curriculum and has enhanced the students' academic experience.

Xiaokun Liang and Jianfen Liu are senior faculty at Peking Union Medical College School of Nursing (PUMC SON). Huaping Liu is Dean of PUMC SON.

Fuzhou—Fujian Provincial Hospital

Hong Lee, Juan Lin, and Xiaoxia Zhang

The PSBHN program began in Fujian Provincial Hospital, Fuzhou, in 2003, with guidance and leadership from PUMC SON. The PSBHN team in Fuzhou has conducted nursing workshops together with PUMC three times since 2003, including a program at Wuyi Mountain Municipal Hospital.

In the initial 2003 PSBHN workshop, 40 head nurses and staff nurses participated; 40 projects were developed and 38 were completed. Juan Lin, one of the head nurses who works in the endocrinology department, proposed a project called "The Systematical Health Education Program to Improve the Effect of Blood Sugar Control Among Type 2 Diabetes Outpatients," which was approved and supported by our leaders and specialists in the division of endocrinology. The project leader developed a club and consultation clinic for type 2 diabetes outpatients. The education club conducted a training program carried out over 7 months each year. The training program has been held five times to date and more than 325 patients have participated. The training uses a variety of education methods, such as lectures by physicians and nurse specialists, group discussions, yoga and Taiji exercise, and cooking contests. Miss Lin summarized the program in two papers, "Outcomes of the Health Education Club for Type 2 Diabetes Outpatients" and "The Analysis of Mental Health Status and Nursing Among the Aged Type 2 Diabetes Mellitus Outpatients," that were published in the *Chinese Journal of Nursing* and the *Journal of Qiqihar Medical College*, respectively. Based on these successes and the experiences of the diabetic patients, a training program was held for 72 clinical diabetes nurse specialists in Fujian Province.

In March 2005, a PSBHN workshop was held at Wuyi Mountain Municipal Hospital. There were 30 participants who developed 29 projects. Xiaoxia Zhang, the head nurse in the operating room, proposed a project called, "Application of Games in the Preoperative Interview to Improve Cooperation Level Among the Children." The project results were published in the *Chinese Journal of Nursing*.

The application of the PSBHN program improved nursing quality. In the first three PSBHN workshops the participants were nurse managers and staff nurses. We then incorporated the PSBH method into the nursing administration curriculum for head nurse preparation. All the head nurses in our hospital were trained with the PSBH methodology, and patient care was improved. To reward their achievements, we selected 54 projects from the more than 300 projects in our hospital to receive prizes. Some of these projects focused on management of safe medication among inpatients, a self-made box for medical sharps waste, intestinal nutrition by infusion pump, formulation of optimal operation room arrangement, emergency preparation in the event of a power failure in the intensive care unit, and prevention of falls in elderly patients. Nursing supervisor Ruilan Li published her work, "The Analysis of Dangerous Factors and Preventing Methods in Tumble Accidents Among Aged Patients" in the *Fujian Medical Journal.* "The Self-Made

Hong Lee is Vice President of Fujian Provincial Hospital. Juan Lin is Deputy Director and Xiaoxia Zhang is Nurse in Charge at Fujian Provincial Hospital and Wuyi Mountain Municipal Hospital, respectively.

Box for Medical Sharps Waste" by Fen Li and her colleagues won the golden prize. The development of such continuous quality improvement projects is highly valued by leaders in our hospital.

One of the most important education objectives for undergraduate nursing students is the development and cultivation of nursing research abilities. The PSBHN program provides a method for teaching clinical research skills. We have utilized the PSBHN program in the clinical nursing research education for undergraduate nursing students since 2005. We use examples from the PSBHN projects developed in our hospital. Through discussion, each student selects a topic for study, develops plans for solving the problem, identifies potential samples and evaluation indices and methods, and projects expected results. Student evaluations of the program are positive.

To evaluate the effectiveness of the program in depth, Chen Chen, a student who graduated in 2008, conducted a project called "Self-Assessment About Research Ability Among Undergraduate Students." She demonstrated statistically significant differences between the students who have been trained by the PSBHN program and those who have not in recognizing problems and writing theses. The articles, "The Exploration of the Methods for Cultivating the Ability of Clinical Nursing Research Among the Undergraduate Students" and "Using the Method of Problem Solving to Guide Students to Develop Nursing Research," written by Shuang Jin, were published in the *Journal of Nursing Science* and the *Chinese Journal of Nursing Education*, respectively.

Since June 2005, 210 students have been trained in PSBHN. They developed 180 projects, and all of the students completed their theses. In order to raise awareness and develop the problem-solving ability among nurses, we incorporated the PSBHN training program into the new nurse pre-employment training in 2007. Since that time nurses have been enthusiastic about developing projects and publishing their results. Between 2004 and 2005, 55 nursing articles were published, and between 2006 and 2007, 143 articles were published, 21 of them in publications such as the *Chinese Journal of Nursing*, the *Chinese Journal of Nursing Education*, *Chinese Nursing Management*, and the *Journal of Nursing Science*. The PSBHN program cultivates both the ability of problem solving and nursing research among nurses and students.

Hohhot—Inner Mongolia Medical College

Yongqiang Cai, Wenxing Han, Ying Han, Shuang Kang,
Xiaohe Li, Zhijun Li, Wanling Liu, Jing Meng, Guoqiang Wang, Jianwei Wang,
Zhenfeng Wang, Na Wei, Wenhua Xin, Lidong Zhang,
Man Zhang, Yan Zhao, Yuxia Zhong, and Na Zhuo

Madame Yuling Zhou has been instrumental in the expansion of PSBH to the northwest region of China. Zhou continues to foster DHF's ongoing partnership with Jiaotong

---

The authors are administrators, nurses, physicians, professors, and students who have participated in Problem Solving for Better Health workshops at Inner Mongolia Medical College.

University in Xian and is responsible for the development of two new partnerships with Inner Mongolia Medical College in Hohhot and Xinjiang Medical University in Urumqi. Sebastian Milardo, DHF Director of Operations, has worked closely with Zhou to extend the reach of PSBH to this region. What follows is a brief description of the program at Inner Mongolia Medical College in Hohhot. The program began in 2003 and has already involved more than 6,000 college and middle school students, more than 10,000 peasants and herdsmen, more than 100 administrative units, and more than 80 social organizations.

Led by the Student Affairs Division and the Committee for Cooperative Projects of Inner Mongolia Medical College, PSBH teams were set up by the Academic Affairs Division, the Technology Department, and the Foreign Affairs Office of the college. The initial chairman was the former President of Inner Mongolia Medical College, Dr. Lifu Bi. An organized system was founded, led by the Students, Scientific and Technological Renovation Association, with the project teams as the basic members. This provided the organizational framework for a sustainable PSBH program.

The PSBH office collects project topics from all the students in the college every December. Students choose the health or social matters that they care about as their subjects, including medical and pharmaceutical matters, health and fitness, and community medicine. Most topics are closely related to the students' academic majors, although some students choose the health problems that commonly exist in Inner Mongolia today. The specialists and professors then assess the feasibility of the submitted projects. Those projects with high feasibility are discussed with the DHF facilitators at the PSBH workshop to determine which projects should proceed to the implementation phase. Project teams are required to hand in quarterly progress reports and conduct quarterly seminars to problem-solve challenges encountered during the implementation phase. Upon project completion, follow-up seminars are held to report progress and obtain feedback from DHF site visitors.

Several participants of the PSBH workshops have submitted their work to national and regional competitions and received substantial recognition. The PSBH project group led by Lidong Zhang and Yuxia Zhong was awarded the national honorable title of The Hundred Excellent Associations in 2006. Two PSBH projects were highlighted in special issues of *Acta Academiae Medicinae Nei Mongol*, an Inner Mongolian medical journal. The project that focused on lead content in children's hair won third prize in the College Students Academic Science and Technology Achievement contest. The awards and recognition help to illustrate the effectiveness and the necessity of the PSBH projects.

Through the PSBH process, students learn to think independently and creatively. The college places special priority on certain nonintellectual factors, like the spirit of PSBH, participation, commitment, responsibility, and confidence in completing tasks successfully. PSBH projects provide students with practical choices for recognizing public health issues. This hands-on process is a good way to appropriately determine public health needs. In addition, many professors also have the opportunity to apply theories to practice by taking an active role in the projects. Teachers are readily on hand to oversee the development and implementation of the projects. We at Inner Mongolia Medical College are motivated by the entrepreneurial spirit that has been stimulated in us by the PSBH program and are determined to keep the mission to improve health in Inner Mongolia moving forward.

Kunming—First Affiliated Hospital of Kunming Medical College

Guixian Liang and Jin Shen

The First Affiliated Hospital of Kunming Medical College (KMC) was founded in 1941 near the Da Guan River in the western part of Kunming city. It is a comprehensive hospital that combines medical service, teaching, research, and healthcare for government officials. There are more than 2,000 staff members in 50 departments including surgery, internal medicine, and medical technique. The hospital has 1,900 beds with a usage rate of 103%–110%, and the average annual number of inpatient cases is 45,000. The number of outpatient cases is more than 1.5 million. The hospital has 19 clinical teaching sections, and teachers from the sections are responsible for the clinical courses and internships at KMC.

With support and direction from DHF, the hospital launched the PSBH program in 2000, and the nursing department has since incorporated PSBH into its operations. The program was implemented by training all head and staff nurses. One hundred sixty-five projects have been completed. In the first phase, the hospital team completed projects on medicine, nursing, and psychology. Projects expanded to the Second Affiliated Hospital, the Preventive and Treatment Center for Drug-Dependents of Yunnan Province, and Yunnan Normal University. The projects affected patients, students, and substance abusers and their parents. In the second phase, the hospital team completed projects that expanded to regional, county, and municipal hospitals. The number of health education programs increased and reached larger areas.

Through the PSBH process, the hospital has enhanced nursing techniques to promote health. Additionally, the hospital improved the health education plan and handbook and provided free health education to patients in the outpatient department. The reputation of the hospital has improved, and every clinical nursing unit provides health education to inpatients to assist in their recovery.

As a result of the PSBH program, hospital staff visited patient wards, villages, and schools, and provided needed services by executing their project action plans. They showed their love and passion. They learned a method of how to identify issues, raise questions, develop hypotheses, and make plans to solve problems. This has proven to be effective. For example, doctors from the physiotherapy department began health education for cervical spondylosis (disease of the vertebrae) patients. This education helped the patients improve their quality of life and decrease their symptoms. Obstetricians provided education to women and their family members about postnatal self-care and newborn care. Cardiologists visited patient wards, communities, and villages to provide residents with more knowledge of the risk for hypertension. Patients benefited from all these projects. The relationship between doctors and patients improved because patients trusted and respected their doctors. These doctors set a good example for other doctors and other medical workers.

Included in the hospital's plans for the next 5 years are expansion of health education for communities, factories, and schools, and additional nursing projects. Two issues of concern are substance abuse treatment and prevention and HIV/AIDS awareness. As part of the 5-year plan, the hospital staff will study the cultures of the ethnic minorities

---

Guixian Liang is a nursing director, and Jin Shen is a physician and professor, at the First Affiliated Hospital of Kunming Medical College.

living in the area to provide better patient care and education and to understand how their lifestyles affect their health.

Macau—Kiang Wu Nursing College

Andrew Leung Luk

Macau is a very small city situated near Hong Kong. It has a population of 538,100, estimated at the end of 2007, with more than 95% of residents of Chinese origin (Statistics and Census Services, 2008). We have participated in the PSBH program for more than 5 years. This section includes our city's healthcare goals, a history of how we became involved with DHF and how our programs evolved over the past 5 years, and examples of some of our programs.

The Macau Special Administrative Region (MSAR) is committed to promoting public health. One of the targeted healthcare goals is to develop Macau as a healthy city as defined by the World Health Organization (WHO). A healthy city is continually creating and improving physical and social environments and expanding community resources to enable people to mutually support each other in performing all functions of life and in developing to their maximum potential (WHO, 2004). In 2004, the chief executive of MSAR pledged to build Macau into a pleasant and harmonious healthy city (Department of Health, 2008a). The objectives of the Healthy City project in Macau are to raise the level of participation of citizens, mobilize citizens to take part in various activities that benefit health, and eliminate or diminish those risk factors affecting the physical and social environment. The Healthy City project aims to improve health status and welfare, beautify the physical environment, and advocate healthy lifestyles, thereby achieving healthy people living in a healthy environment (Department of Health, 2008b).

Based on the healthcare statistics, the standard of public health in Macau is quite high. However, the development of a healthy city is still in its infancy stage. There is a long way to go for the implementation of different programs initiated by the Healthy City subcommittees. For instance, the law to enforce smoking control in public areas is still being drafted.

In 2003, clinical nurses in the Kiang Wu Hospital and some student nurses from the Kiang Wu Nursing College (KWNC) were invited by PUMC SON to participate in the first PSBH program in Macau. There were 43 participants with 11 projects completed, 3 from clinical nurses and 8 from student nurses. Due to the positive responses from the first program, the second program was held in 2005 with a quota of participants allocated to nongovernmental organizations (NGOs) in the community. Representatives from seven NGOs joined the second program.

In 2007, the PSBHN program was officially integrated into the third year of the curriculum at KWNC. In 2008, 41 third-year student nurses participated in the PSBHN program. With the experiences gained from the implementation of the PSBH methodology, we affirm that it is a highly effective problem-solving approach to managing health problems. The PSBHN projects completed in Macau included projects in hospitals, clients' homes, and schools in the community. All projects were administered on a small scale aimed at solving manageable health problems. Some examples follow.

Andrew Leung Luk is professor of Nursing at Kiang Wu Nursing College.

One of the projects initiated by the student nurses was "Teaching Correct Hand-Washing Method to Children." From 2002 to 2003, the occurrence of hand–foot–mouth disease increased in Macau, primarily in children younger than 10 years. Given that using the correct hand-washing method is an effective strategy for preventing infectious disease, a PSBHN project was designed for 39 kindergarten children to minimize their risk of being infected through contaminated hand–foot–mouth disease. Students received information on the mode of transmission of the disease and demonstration of correct hand-washing methods. The expected goal was that within 2 weeks the children could perform correct hand washing; 40% of participants had hand washing in both morning and afternoon sessions in the kindergarten. The results showed that all the children could perform correct hand washing within 2 weeks.

Participants from KWNC also initiated a health project, "The Study of Visual Acuity of Primary Students in Macau," that received financial support from the Education and Youth Affairs Bureau. Studies show that increasing numbers of children have myopia. The project goal was to explore the visual ability and myopia of primary students in Macau and recommend appropriate health measures for protection. Through random sampling, 14 out of 66 primary schools were selected. A total of 84 classes were selected with 2,381 primary students, representing 6.8% of all the primary students in Macau. Methods employed included visual examinations and questionnaires. The results showed that the visual ability of 45.9% of participants (1,093) was below the normal standard, and 32.8% of participants (781) had myopia. The eyesight of the children in the upper grades was worse. Some factors relating to eye health, such as reading when lying down, walking, or traveling on a bus, and long hours of computer use, were identified and informed the design of health promotion activities. The study raised the awareness of teachers, school administrators, and government officials regarding the health of children's eyes.

Based on the findings of that project, KWNC carried out a follow-up project, "Promotion on Eye Health in Schools Series." From 2006 to 2007, 87 classes on "Eye Health Exercises" were delivered to 42 primary schools for 8,148 students. Four "Eye Health Trainer Courses" were delivered to 132 teachers to increase their eye health knowledge so that they could help supervise and guide their students in proper eye health exercise. A booklet on care of eyes and eye health exercises was published and sent to schools for distribution to teachers, students, and parents. A promotion day on care of the eyes was also held for 10 primary schools, with the participation of parents and teachers. This represented collaboration between home and school, an effective way to improve health promotion.

Through the years of implementing PSBHN projects conducted by clinical nurses, student nurses, and our faculty, we have found that the methodology is a simple, practical approach to solving manageable health problems. Though the problems may be small, they are not unimportant. Some projects can have great impact on the existing health condition of the targeted population, which will gradually change its health concept and behavior. The rationale behind PSBH is easy to learn and put into practice. The support of colleagues and administrators is crucial to making PSBHN a success.

We believe that small programs are a good way to train our students in this approach and prepare them for health promotion in their nursing careers. Based on our experiences, a health and research center was established as a response to the spirit of promoting health with collaboration and partnerships in the community. We hope in the future we can continue to work with schools and NGOs, hand in hand, to promote health in the community of Macau.

Nanning—First Affiliated Hospital of Guangxi Medical University

Jianmei Cai, Yunchao Chen, Xia Dai, Xiaohong He, Muhong Huang, Yihua Huang, Yuzhu Huang, Kui Jia, Jianmei Li, Weiwei Li, Rong Liang, Zhanghua Lin, Hengli Ling, Guimei Liu, Ruxiang Luo, Tiesheng Que, Mingjun Wang, Ruili Wei, Yongfeng Wei, Hanchun Wen, Zengming Xiao, Ningxian Yu, Jin Zeng, Xiaofen Zeng, Huaping Zhang, Jincai Zhong, Aimin Zhou, Xiaomin Zhou, and Jinge Zhu

The PSBH program in Nanning began in the mid-1990s. The first PSBH workshop for nurses and doctors at the First Affiliated Hospital of Guangxi Medical University led to a series of many more workshops and projects in the region led by the PSBH team in Nanning. We have included just a few project highlights to sample the fine work that has been done by so many of our local team leaders.

The first project that will be described was led by Yihua Huang and colleagues, and focused on cervical disease. Cervical disease, like cervical erosion, is very common in Chinese women and is one of the main factors that can cause cervical cancer and do harm to women's mental and physical health. Currently, there are treatments of cervical disease with technology, for example, laser, cryosurgery, and microwave. Another effective measure is applying medicine (known as "dust") to the cervix. Given the anatomical location of the cervix, we found a simple and effective measure for application of the dust using a rubber aspirator, an improvement on the traditional application method, which is complex and wasteful. We compared the two measures, and found that the new method is better than the traditional method in accuracy, time spent on applying medicine (dust) to cervix, and quantity of the drug used. Subsequently, this new measure has been widely applied in practice. Since 2005, when the project began, it has evolved from scientific research into routine clinical work.

The second project described in this section relates to end-of-life care. Life and death education may help terminally ill cancer patients to become less anxious, frightened, lonely, depressed, and suicidal. Not only can death education help the patient, but it can also help family members adapt to the patient's condition and the death process. Such education also helps the family members to understand that the person's social value continues and his or her significance survives.

This project was led by the following PSBH team members: Weiwei Li, Zhanghua Lin, Tiesheng Que, Yongfen Wei, Huaping Zhang, Jincai Zhong, and Xiaomin Zhou. To implement the project additional human resources were recruited to participate, including several medical professionals, one driver, and 200 volunteers. Patient visits were held in the home environment and were respectful of culture and religious beliefs, which can help to support the patient and family members through the death process. Education was provided to patients and families with the purpose of helping them through the grief process and facing end of life.

Participants included 158 patients with advanced cancer for the observation group who accepted the treatment at the First Affiliated Hospital of Guangxi Medical University during 2006–2007, and 71 patients for the control group who accepted general medical services in

The authors are administrators, nurses, physicians, and professors who have participated in Problem Solving for Better Health workshops at the First Affiliated Hospital of Guangxi Medical University.

the internal medicine department of the hospital during the same period. The observation group treatment method was based on logotherapy, the belief that striving to find a meaning in one's life is the primary motivating force in man and in our country's culture.

The Life Attitude Profile (LAP), as established in 1990 by Taiwan scholar and Professor Yingqi He, was selected for assessing the meaning of life. The scale is used to evaluate the following six factors: the will to meaning, the frustration level, the purpose of life, life control, suffering accepted, and death accepted. Results show that LAP scores of the observation group were significantly increased compared with those of the control group. Logotherapy improved the sense of the meaning of life as it ameliorates negative feelings. For patients with advanced cancer, it is an important psychological treatment of palliative care.

Additional projects were initiated to apply and extend the results. Our staff created a hospice service pattern with Chinese characteristics. Student and community volunteers are trained to work with terminally ill patients and their families through a "Hospice Medical" course. After study and training, volunteers utilize components of logotherapy to understand what the patient is experiencing and instruct patients and family members about diet and life, personal hygiene, and the observation of pain-relieving drug efficacy. This helps the patient and the family members face death together, and find significance and value in life.

Jinge Zhu, PSBH participant, shared her project experience as well as a personal statement about the program:

> I have taken part in three studies about PSBH since it came to our hospital. And I finished them all successfully. In 2002, I started my first study. My study was with women who underwent surgery for infertility. I gave them education and instruction about how to become pregnant. After this, the rate of becoming pregnant increased. Also, in 2003, we started human-based nursing and studied the effects of this new model of care on patient satisfaction. As a result, patient satisfaction increased from 90% to 96%. Health is so important for everyone. I hope I can make a contribution in human's health hand in hand with PSBH.

Shanghai—Shanghai Medical Workers College

Ye Shen, Gongliang Tao, Tai-zhen Tao, Weirong Wang, Youhua Yao, Weiping Yu,
Weihua Zeng, Hua Zhang, Weibo Zhang, and Shitai Zhu

Shanghai Medical Workers College (SMWC) was established in 1979 under the jurisdiction of the Shanghai Municipal Health Bureau. DHF has worked closely with Jianzhen Yu and Xie Jun at SMWC to organize PSBH workshops for health professionals who work in the community. Since 1997, Jianzhen Yu and Xie Jun have played a critical role in involving health professionals at the grassroot level in the PSBH process. To date, a total of six workshops have been held for approximately 200 participants. In total, 160 community-based better health projects have been implemented and benefited over 30,000 residents in 14 districts of Shanghai. Several PSBH projects were developed to solve community

---

The authors are administrators, nurses, physicians, and professors who have participated in Problem Solving for Better Health workshops at Shanghai Medical Workers College.

health problems brought about by poor living conditions (Figure 9.1). Health promotion is a common thread throughout the Shanghai PSBH program. For example, a total of 12 health clubs were established to teach the residents the importance of presentation and self-care (Figure 9.1). Additionally, the leaders at SMWC have made an effort to spread workshop participants' successes in promoting health in the area. As a result, 155 articles were written, and more than 80% of them were published in the national or provincial journal. Over the past 12 years, the program implemented at SMWC has made a positive impact on strengthening health professionals' problem-solving ability, improving quality of community health services, and promoting health of the people. Several PSBH participants, for example, organized a project to provide more education and mental health support for middle school students in Changqiao community, southeast of Shanghai. Ye Shen and Weirong Wang studied hearing loss among students at SMWC. Yet another PSBH team focused on the use of traditional Chinese medicine (TCM) for patients with hypertension. We have highlighted in detail one project, implemented by Weiping Yu and colleagues, that addressed the problem of access to rehabilitative care in the community.

Community-based rehabilitation is advocated by WHO and is a major concern for both developed and developing countries. It is in its infancy in China. The Chinese government has mandated the provision of rehabilitation services for the disabled by 2015, which is a challenge because China has no professionals devoted to community-based rehabilitation who have the necessary credentials.

A survey conducted in our community indicated that of the six functions of community-based health service—prevention, treatment, healthcare, rehabilitation, family planning, and health education—rehabilitation lagged behind the others because there was no systematic process for the transfer of treatment between the regional medical center and the community-based health service center. The lack of qualified personnel in

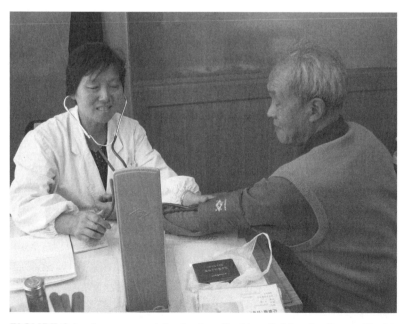

FIGURE 9.1 A nurse participating in a Problem Solving for Better Health project on hypertension prevention and treatment for the elderly in Shanghai.

Shanghai has become a serious problem because there are 500,000–1,000,000 people in need of rehabilitation services.

A PSBH workshop was held for the Executive Committee of SMWC. One participant developed a project focused on this issue of community-based rehabilitation. He noted that patients with cerebrovascular accident (CVA) do not have consistent and effective rehabilitation training. After conducting research on the needs of people with disabilities caused by CVA, the project team built a strong network for community-based rehabilitation and developed effective techniques with a team of professionals to upgrade the level of the community health services.

In the past, when CVA patients were discharged from the hospital, community-based rehabilitation organizations could not intervene in time because they had not received the necessary information to provide treatment and rehabilitation. To solve this problem, a reporting network for the neighborhood involved training 280 people in the community to identify those patients requiring services. As a result, intervention time can be shortened from 9–12 weeks to 4–6 weeks. Community doctors can immediately conduct home interviews and evaluations, and provide rehabilitation as soon as they receive the reports. For most discharged patients, rehabilitation can be completed in a timely manner and ensure the continuance of patient improvement. The PSBH project team developed an instruction manual for rehabilitation professionals specifically focusing on the training for CVA patients. The manual is easy to understand and suitable for community home health visitors. The manual also serves as a reference book for the patients, their family members, and home caregivers. Patients can practice exercises with the help of the home caregivers, family members, or housemaids. As a result, knowledge of community-based rehabilitation has improved.

In order to ensure the quality of community-based rehabilitation, every year the project team offers education and additional training for general practitioners, massage therapists, acupuncturists, and physical therapists. A therapy team has been developed to provide rehabilitation with general practitioners as the backbone. PSBH project team personnel participate in academic conferences at home and abroad, and have had papers published in medical journals annually. The research has been incorporated as an important component of the primary healthcare programs of Shanghai Health Bureau, and as a featured community healthcare project.

Wenzhou—Wenzhou Medical College and Mount Sinai Medical Center

Kathleen Leask Capitulo, Ian R. Holzman, Jing Lin, and Diane Stanton

Wenzhou, China, is an industrial city of over 14 million people in Zhejiang province, which has a population of over 46 million people. Healthcare in Wenzhou is provided at more than 10 hospitals and numerous neighborhood clinics. Wenzhou Medical College is the academic hub of the healthcare system.

The authors are members of a healthcare team in New York who initiated a partnership with Wenzhou Medical College.

In 2004, Jing Lin, a neonatologist at Mount Sinai Medical Center's Kravis Children's Hospital in New York, asked Diane Stanton, a nurse colleague; Ian Holzman, a physician colleague; and Kathleen Capitulo, a hospital nurse executive, to go to Wenzhou, China. Dr. Lin was born and had attended medical school in China, and he returns several times a year, working with Wenzhou physician and nurse leaders, to collaborate on research and clinical projects and participate in medical education.

Many people in China have no access to care simply because they cannot afford it. Hospitals charge patients a fee per service, but the price is tightly regulated by the government. No money equals no healthcare. For those who can afford care, hospitalizations are long. With fee for service as the payment system, there is no focus on reduction of length of stay. In Yuying Children's Hospital, an affiliate of Wenzhou Medical College, most babies have no health insurance. This 350-bed tertiary children's hospital has greater than 500,000 outpatient visits a year and greater than 10,000 hospital discharges per year, including 1,900 from the neonatal intensive care unit (NICU). Some of the challenges facing perinatal, neonatal, and pediatric healthcare in Wenzhou include the lack of regionalization of care, the lack of public funding, and the disparate education of physicians and specialists.

American neonatal units are filled with infants who were born between 24 and 28 weeks of gestation. In the United States, improved obstetrical care and the decision to monitor and deliver such tiny infants before they severely asphyxiate has led to many of these infants surviving. Such tiny babies are not often seen in Chinese NICUs, but the Chinese neonatology community wants to move ahead and change that reality. To move to the next step will take changes in philosophy and training. Medical personnel are prepared to do this and exhibit courage and commitment to quality care.

During our visit to the NICU at the Second Affiliated Hospital of Wenzhou Medical College, we met with nurses to discuss policies and practices regarding patient care. The Chinese nurses' instincts for care were consistent with American standards of care, but the nursing staff did not feel empowered to convince their medical team about the care needed. This visit laid the groundwork for a PSBHN program for nurses in Wenzhou. The program was designed to encourage nurses to tap into their leadership potential and ability to influence practice based on evidence.

In Wenzhou, we met Liping Jiang, Dean of the School of Nursing at Wenzhou Medical College. We also met nearly 100 nursing leaders who were eager to discuss professional issues and collaborate on practice, education, and research. Wenzhou's hospital and university leaders were eager to support nursing and healthcare collaboration between Wenzhou and New York, and so, over the next year, through DHF, we built a partnership between nursing and healthcare leaders in Wenzhou and New York. The Transcultural Nursing Leadership Institute (TNLI) was designed with support from the Robert Wood Johnson Executive Nurse Fellowship. The purpose of the TNLI is to promote scholarly and professional collaboration between nurse leaders in the United States and international nursing leaders.

In early 2006, the team returned to Wenzhou with a delegation of nursing and healthcare leaders and held a TNLI conference and PSBHN workshop. More than 200 healthcare professionals attended the conference, and 60 registered nurses attended the workshop. At the conclusion of the workshop 57 nurses had developed clear, practical, evidence-based, and measurable project proposals, and all participants completed evaluation forms. The evaluation report was extremely positive; all participants rated the workshop, teaching methods, and content as excellent.

To ensure sustainability of the program, a local steering committee was established in Wenzhou, consisting of the Dean of Nursing and the Chief Nursing Officers of the affiliated hospitals. An advisory board was also established to advise the steering committee and to support collaborative research, publications, and practice initiatives. In the year following the initial PSBHN workshop in Wenzhou, the steering committee met three times to discuss the work of the TNLI. Contact between the steering committee and all the workshop participants was frequent via email, providing ongoing consultation to participants about their projects. As such, participants were connected to expert nursing leaders who were available to mentor them in their work.

Many of the projects involved creation of patient education programs, particularly for vulnerable, underserved populations, including factory workers, parents of NICU babies, and the elderly with osteoporosis. Wenxian Zheng, LePei Jiang, Lu Juan Yang, and Jinji Guo Junyi, from the Orthopaedics Hospital of Wenzhou Medical College, initiated an osteoporosis project. They organized one outreach event attended by more than 500 people and their project is ongoing. Another project, "Promoting Colorectal Health in Rural Populations," by Aihua Chen, included a survey with an intervention study, which resulted in improved colorectal health in underserved areas. Ms. Chen presented this project at an international conference, the World Union of Wound Healing Societies, in Toronto, Canada, in June 2008.

Many projects addressed issues of health disparity, particularly with poor and uninsured people. All projects were framed within a cultural context. In populations of Chinese descent, hypertension, nutrition, osteoporosis, cancer prevention, and the health of children are of major concern. Most of the nurses' projects used health education as an intervention to positively impact health disparities. Health education programs were designed with the recognition that many of the clients had low literacy skills. In addition, a major focus was crafting the programs to be culturally congruent, acceptable, and welcomed in the Chinese cultural groups.

On May 7, 2007, the TNLI hosted the chair of the steering committee and four major leaders of university hospitals at North Shore University Hospital in New York. All participated in a major health policy program and Nurses' Week activities at North Shore. Attending were more than 100 members of the North Shore University Hospital nursing staff and major health system administrative and clinical leaders. Discussions included creating programs to address health disparities; creating culturally congruent healthcare environments to promote health and healing of mind, body, and spirit; and promoting self-care for health professionals.

In October 2007, key members of the TNLI Advisory Board returned to Wenzhou. We met with the PSBHN project leaders so they could formally report on their project progress to date. We ran a "Facilitator Workshop" the following day, outlining the methodology for those conducting future PSBHN workshops in the province, to provide ongoing program expansion and sustainability. The facilitators have since run PSBHN programs throughout the province; Wenxian Zheng has personally conducted 12 workshops.

Forty nurses in Wenzhou completed projects, many of which reported significant results. For example, the colorectal outreach project resulted in improved colorectal health, with decreased rectal fissures, decreased hemorrhoids, and the detection of two early-stage rectal tumors. In addition to the project outcomes, the participants reported in focus groups that they felt more empowered, could effect positive change, and could have input into important healthcare policies. Of the initial participants, five published their work in nursing journals, and three presented their projects at an international conference in Canada.

The PSBHN nurses in Wenzhou were eager to collaborate with American colleagues, participate in joint research, and present at conferences. Although faced with their own nursing shortage, more severe than that in the United States, and a drain of educated registered nurses seeking more lucrative employment abroad, China's nursing education systems are expanding to produce more graduates. Successful transcultural partnerships require respect for each other's cultures, acknowledgment of differences, celebration of cultural traditions, and sharing of knowledge and self. The partnership between colleagues in Wenzhou and New York has been exemplary.

The PSBHN method has strengthened the bridge we have built between Wenzhou, China, and New York, United States. Prior to PSBHN, healthcare leaders invited American professionals to come to Wenzhou to speak about advances in healthcare. Now PSBH's method has empowered healthcare leaders in China to identify and solve their own problems. Our partnership continues with opportunities to collaborate on research, practice, education, and safety. It has been a privilege to learn from our colleagues in Wenzhou, China.

Conclusion

China is an incredibly dynamic country—a country with a wonderfully rich past and also a magnificent future, with a world leadership role that continues to grow. PSBH was born and grew up in China at a propitious time. From the small sampling of project reports provided in this chapter, it is clear that PSBH has struck a resonant chord with Chinese physicians, nurses, administrative personnel, and medical and nursing students. For many of the participants, PSBH represents a tool to help address the problems they face in their work on a daily basis. It also trains them to think clearly and present their ideas and results in a precise manner. PSBH helps participants develop the habits of critical thinking and the self-assurance that comes with knowing that one can accomplish goals.

More important, PSBH and the projects it generates represent a transformational process that causes Chinese health professionals to see themselves as having the capability of making change for the better. The role of health professionals is not simply in the treatment of disease but in being agents of change within their communities. Physicians and nurses must accept an additional charge—to enable the people to take responsibility for their own health and change it for the better.

The DHF program in China could not have progressed without the leadership of Madame On Ning, DHF's National Coordinator for China. We are deeply grateful to Madame On Ning, and to her family, as they have all contributed to PSBH in one way or another. We are fortunate to work with Hsin-Ling Tsai, who is currently leading the PSBH program forward with assistance from Madame On Ning and input from our institutional partners and local leaders throughout China.

References

Department of Health. (2008a). *Healthy city.* Government of Macau Special Administration Region: Department of Health. Retrieved January 10, 2008, from http://www.ssm.gov.mo/design/NEWS/ health_city/index.c.htm

Department of Health. (2008b). *Healthy city.* Government of Macau Special Administration Region: Department of Health. Retrieved January 10, 2008, from http://www.ssm.gov.mo/design/NEWS/ health_city/index.e.htm

Statistics and Census Services. (2008). *Estimates of Macao resident population.* Government of Macao Special Administrative Region. Retrieved September 30, 2008, from http://www.dsec.gov.mo

World Health Organization. (2004). *A glossary of terms for community health care and services for older persons* (Vol. 5). WHO Centre for Health Development, Ageing and Health Technical Report, Retrieved January 10, 2008, from http://whg/ibdoc/ who/int/wke/2004/WHO_WKC-Tech.Ser._04.2.pdf

10

India

India is the world's seventh largest country in land area (3,166,414 sq km), is second only to China in population (1.2 billion people), and has the world's largest democracy. With a rich and complex history dating back thousands of years, the country has an incredible diversity of ethnic groups, cultures, religions, and at least 100 languages and many more dialects. It is the birthplace of Hinduism, Buddhism, and Sikhism. The Problem Solving for Better Health program has thrived in almost half of the country's medical education institutions. Shaped, reshaped, and led by the Indian people themselves, PSBH is helping to change the face of health in India.

This chapter is dedicated to Dr. C. R. Soman, former President of Health Action by People and Problem Solving for Better Health National Coordinator in India.

Introduction

Barry H. Smith

In 1993, Dr. G. N. Menon, a specialist in clinical pharmacology and a pioneer of the international clinical development of drugs, introduced the Dreyfus Health Foundation (DHF) to Dr. C. R. Soman, Chairman of Health Action by People (HAP) in Trivandrum, Kerala, India. Since then, Dr. Soman and his colleagues, Drs. Raman Kutty, Ram Das Pisharody, K. Vijayakumar, K. P. Aravindan, and C. C. Kartha, among others, have helped to shape DHF's Problem Solving for Better Health® (PSBH®) program in India. The HAP team developed a particular PSBH model involving the education of medical and nursing students that has incredibly broad implications in India and around the world. These academic leaders and members of HAP soon became our teachers, colleagues, and friends, and gave more to PSBH (Hoyt, 2007; Smith, 1993) than we at DHF could have imagined.

The first PSBH workshop in India was held in collaboration with HAP at the Trivandrum Medical College in 1993. It is impressive that, in a place that had achieved so much already, the HAP leaders and participants were open to this simple process. The atmosphere in the first workshop was electric and exciting. Many of the participants already knew they could create change and were eager to do even more to build their society. Since that first workshop, under the leadership of Dr. Soman and his team, there have been more than 160 workshops in India, with approximately 15,000 participants and close to that many better-health and quality-of-life projects.

The diversity and scope of the implemented projects have been vast. The participants and project beneficiaries have included men and women from all walks of life and professions; children of all ages; students at all levels, including graduate medical and nursing students; academicians; and the elderly. Problem areas addressed have included communicable and infectious diseases, economic issues, healthcare and policy issues, health promotion and healthy lifestyles, mental health, noncommunicable and chronic diseases, nutrition, social issues and services, and women's health.

Since 1999, the HAP team has conducted PSBH workshops specifically for medical students and, since 2004, nursing students. What began as a modest one-school program has extended to 75 medical and 4 nursing colleges in India. The total number of students who have participated in the process is now more than 15,000, while more than 100 faculties, have been involved in the process of introducing the students to this innovative method of learning community medicine. Since the inception of the program, students have completed approximately 4,200 projects.

Problem Solving for Better Health for Medical and Nursing Students

V. Raman Kutty and K. Vijayakumar

By focusing on medical and nursing students, Dr. Soman and his HAP colleagues have provided an important component to PSBH. They recognized that sensitizing medical and nursing students to the program's problem-solving philosophy and methodology, and encouraging teamwork in developing, implementing, and evaluating practical, multifactorial solutions to problems, will ensure their future roles as public health leaders.

Community Medicine

The Medical Council of India (MCI) requires a community medicine course for all medical college students. Often, however, a college's community medicine department is organized solely to meet the MCI requirement and not to accomplish the fieldwork it should. In many colleges, the administration shows little support for the course and its faculty once the MCI inspection has taken place. The importance of social and environmental origins and dimensions of illness and the role of nonmedical interventions in reducing the burden of disease are frequently sidelined. As a result, medical students are often not

V. Raman Kutty is a professor at the Achutha Menon Centre for Health Science Studies, Sree Chitra Tirunal Institute for Medical Sciences and Technology, Trivandrum, Kerala. K. Vijayakumar is a professor in the Department of Community Medicine, Medical College, Trivandrum. V. Raman Kutty is Chairman of Health Action by People (HAP), the Dreyfus Health Foundation's implementing partner in Trivandrum. Kutty is also Problem Solving for Better Health National Coordinator for India. K. Vijayakumar is Secretary of HAP.

conversant with skills in preventive medicine and health promotion. When these new health professionals are later called upon to advise policy makers and implementers in initiating health action, their training has not equipped them to fulfill these obligations with confidence and competence. The PSBH process assists medical and nursing students in acquiring these missing skills and gives them the confidence to develop innovative approaches to solve health problems of local relevance. Sowing the seeds of PSBH philosophy in the impressionable minds of young medicos can reap benefits long after they have ventured out into the realms of medical practice.

The MCI's 1997 revised education curriculum emphasized that medical education should be learner oriented and community based rather than teacher oriented and hospital based. To accomplish this and provide medical students enough time for ample learning experiences through different learning methods, "theory" hours were reduced and practical learning sessions were doubled.

The revision posed a challenge for community medicine departments to effectively utilize the increased learning hours to provide students with unique learning experiences. The PSBH process in community medicine provided new learning experiences through an intensely participatory process. Participants were encouraged to think of health problems that needed urgent attention and to create innovative approaches to solving them.

The Problem Solving for Better Health Process

The PSBH process is a progression of steps from identifying a problem to implementing a solution. The first step in our program for medical students involves a 2-day workshop organized for 100–200 students by a department of community medicine. Students are divided into groups of 10–12 with a faculty facilitator. After introductions, each group member identifies and lists problems; individual or group priority problems are then selected. The students refine their problem, determine a solution, frame the PSBH "Good Question," and develop a protocol.

The mode of implementation of the projects is left to the discretion of individual community medicine departments. Some departments incorporate implementation during practical sessions and others require students to carry out their projects after classroom hours. Departments also differ as to which semester project implementation takes place, whether it is compulsory, and whether it is graded. Some projects are undertaken individually, but most are carried out by groups of students. Examples of project topics are gestational diabetes, the prevalence of antimicrobial resistance, and stress among medical students. The students are encouraged to generate information on health through cross-sectional surveys or analysis of hospital records. Students may present their completed projects at department sessions or at various state and national conferences.

Early in the PSBH process, students' responses are usually mixed. Some of them enthusiastically respond to the work, while others simply see it as a requirement to complete. A small number think that doing projects without marks during the student period is not useful. During the process, some find exposure to field circumstances exciting and some experience hardships, such as adverse environmental conditions in the field or pressure in terms of time. After project implementation and presentation, many are often relieved and amazed that they accomplished their goals and could present before an audience. The students develop confidence in carrying out projects and sharing their experiences.

They learn how to work in teams and gain experience in thinking about problems from different points of view.

National Conference of Problem Solvers for Better Health

Two national conferences for student problem solvers have been held to date, and students from all participating colleges attended. The students presented their findings to audiences of distinguished faculty, visiting international PSBH program coordinators, and DHF representatives. After each presentation, faculty drawn from different medical schools remarked on the work that had been accomplished. The students who attended these conferences said they were unique experiences; the students were excited to see peers from all over India involved in the PSBH process and sharing similar experiences. The conference instilled confidence in these students and inspired them to continue seeking new approaches to solving health problems. They cherished the event for both the academic feast and the friendships forged.

One project presented was "Interventional Study on Dental Hygiene Practices Among School Children in the Age Group of 10–13 Years," developed and implemented by Arun Kumar, Balaraman, and Arun—students from the Kilpauk Medical College, Chennai. Their "Good Question" was, "Will a dental health education programme, using dentists at the First Level, for 110 students of Class VI and VII, aged 11–13 years, in a school in Chennai, result in modification of their existing oral hygiene practices, at least by 40% in two months interval time?" The objectives of the project were to assess the oral hygiene practices of the students, identify those with dental problems, provide necessary treatment, and teach students good oral hygiene practices. First, a survey was conducted to assess the dental hygiene practices of the children and to identify those who had problems. Students diagnosed with dental problems were given one-on-one counseling and encouraged to perform proper dental hygiene to avoid problems in the future. Health education classes were held every other week to instill the importance of proper dental hygiene. At the end of the project, the percentage of students brushing their teeth twice daily increased from 30% to 65%, and the students who cleaned their tongues increased from 61% to 85% (Figure 10.1).

"A Study of Change in Knowledge and Attitude About Common Childhood Illnesses One Month After a Health Talk Among Women Residing in a Slum Area of Surat City of Gujarat," conducted by Dhaivat, Bhadra, Nilesh, Namrata, Yajuvendra, Nilesh, Jayraj, Sumit, and Prashant, was another project presented. The project leaders' "Good Question" was "Will a health talk of 90 minutes about childhood illnesses like fever, diarrhea, and the common cold result in an increase of knowledge and hence change in attitude among 56 women residing in a slum of Surat city of Gujarat when tested again after a month using a common questionnaire?" The objective of the project was to assess the knowledge about common childhood illnesses and the inclination among women of urban slums to run to the doctor for mild symptoms. The 56 women involved in the project were asked to complete a questionnaire on their knowledge of fever, diarrhea, and the common cold. The women attended a health talk that provided information on these childhood diseases, and after a month they completed another questionnaire to assess their level of knowledge and their attitudes toward managing symptoms at home. The results of this project indicate that regular health talks for women can significantly

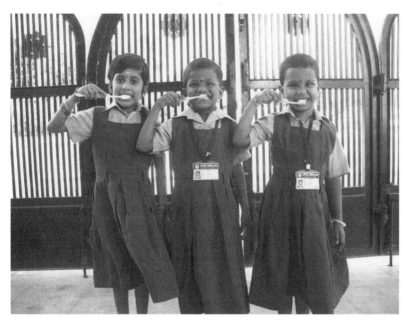

FIGURE 10.1 Schoolgirls in Coimbatore, Tamil Nadu, demonstrate proper dental care.

increase their knowledge of childhood illnesses, raise their confidence in providing home healthcare, and contribute to creating a healthier society.

New Attitudes

With the program firmly established, students now demand the PSBH experience. The PSBH process has also proven rewarding for the faculty. Initially, because there was flexibility regarding execution of projects, some faculty were apprehensive about how to encourage 100 students to develop and carry out 20–30 different projects in ways that would be exciting to them. Therefore, the process was a unique learning experience for the faculty as well. Faculty and students needed commitment and patience with each other; faculty spent many hours with students outside work time, discussing their projects and advising them on project implementation and preparation of their presentations. PSBH lessened the divide between faculty and students and forged a bond between them.

PSBH also sharpened the epidemiological and research skills of the faculty. Dr. Sairu Philip, Associate Professor in the Department of Community Medicine at the Government Medical College in Kozhikode, Kerala, described the "thrill and excitement" faculty experience while carrying out projects in the field. She also valued the "reverse learning" process whereby faculty participating in the program actually learned from their students. For the faculty, the most satisfying moment usually arrives after the projects are completed. The students realize that the experience was rewarding, and they call to thank their teachers and tell them of the success of their PSBH projects.

Dr. Tapasvi Puwar, Assistant Professor in the Preventive and Social Medicine Department at the Smt. NHL Municipal Medical College in Ahmedabad, Gujarat, described his experience with PSBH as follows:

> The [PSBH] process taught me how to lead, how to handle various situations, and how to solve various problems. … I think that the strength of PSBH is the process; it makes every workshop successful. Here the process is important and not the individuals. I gained personally, professionally, and academically through PSBH.

Everyone achieves something through PSBH, and no one is a loser. It is a win–win situation for all stakeholders. It gives preventive and social medicine (PSM) departments necessary recognition among students. Students admit that these subjects were a "bitter pill" before PSBH. But the process gave them an understanding of the importance of public health and research. Because the process demands thorough interaction between facilitators/teachers and students, it also makes these relationships more cordial and improves the academic environment. Faculty members gain academically because of the intense interaction with the students. It helps them to sharpen their practical and research skills. Resource-scarce PSM departments also benefit from PSBH via increased infrastructure.

Medical and nursing students in India find PSBH very interesting because of its participatory and student-centric nature. They gain skills necessary for research, such as teamwork, developing and implementing protocols, using various instruments for research, reviewing literature, analyzing and interpreting results, applying statistical tests, writing reports, and more. Students also learn the arts of communication, making scientific presentations, and contributing to scientific and rational arguments. Many students present their work at various professional gatherings and conferences, and some also publish their projects in local journals.

It is well said that the PSBH process is the beginning and not the end of learning. PSBH motivates all to make a difference. In India, it has shown us a path through which we can solve the health problems of mankind innovatively and locally. It is our goal to extend our reach to more medical and nursing schools in India, so that more students, and ultimately, more people, can benefit from the process.

References

Hoyt, P. (2007). An international approach to Problem Solving for Better Health-Nursing™ (PSBHN). *International Nursing Review, 54,* 100–106.

Smith, B. H. (1993). Optimizing the use of available resources: Problem Solving for Better Health. *World Health Forum, 15*(1), 9–15.

11

Indonesia

Alex Papilaya, Aisyah Maulina, and Taufik Pramudja

Indonesia stretches 5,100 km along the equator, from the Indian Ocean to the Pacific Ocean, with a north–south reach of 1,800 km. The country is composed of 17,508 islands, of which 6,000–7,000 are uninhabited. As the world's fourth most populous country, Indonesia is home to 240 million people of varied ethnicities, including Javanese, Sundanese, and Malay. With the median age of its population at 28 years, it is a young, vigorous country with enormous potential. Given the program's ability to take on the shape and direction of local health and community leaders, and to be sustained locally, Problem Solving for Better Health is well suited to this nation of far-flung and varied health and quality-of-life outposts.

Indonesia is the fourth-largest country in the world in terms of population, but the public expenditure on health is low. The number of doctors, nurses, and health workers is inadequate compared with other countries in the region. In the face of these challenges, when it comes to healthcare the Indonesian people expect the government to enact clear guidelines on the responsibilities of various institutions in both the public and private sectors. There are strong political movements toward reforms in the functioning of the public sector. Changes in these areas may have a major effect on the health sector.

One significant initiative developed to this end is called "Healthy Indonesia 2010." The goal of the program is to initiate and provide a health component to national development; Johns Hopkins University/Population Communication Services, Indonesia's Ministry of Health, and various nongovernmental organizations (NGOs) monitor the effort. The program works to maintain and enhance individual, family, and public self-reliance in improving the environment; maintain and enhance quality of life and equitable and affordable health services; and promote public self-reliance in achieving good health.

Alex Papilaya is Director of the Indonesian Foundation for Better Health (IFBH), the Dreyfus Health Foundation's implementing partner in Indonesia, and Problem Solving for Better Health National Coordinator for Indonesia. Aisyah Maulina and Taufik Pramudja are senior staff members of IFBH.

Food and nutrition policies aim to empower poor families and other vulnerable groups to develop self-sufficiency through community-based activities. As this chapter illustrates, the Problem Solving for Better Health® (PSBH®) program has proven to be an apt precursor to the strategic plan, in line with its goals and the goals for Healthy Indonesia 2010.

History and Evolution of Problem Solving for Better Health

PSBH was introduced to Indonesia in 1996. Dr. William Sawyer, the Executive Director of the China Medical Board (CMB), then in New York, introduced Dr. Barry H. Smith, Director of the Dreyfus Health Foundation (DHF), to Dr. Alex Papilaya, Director of the Center for Family Welfare at the University of Indonesia. CMB had a long relationship with the Center and the Faculty of Public Health at the University. During the same trip, Dr. Smith visited the Faculty of Public Health at Hasanuddin University in Makassar, South Sulawesi, and the Faculty of Medicine at Airlangga University, East Java. Subsequently, these three institutions, among others, became involved with PSBH. The Center for Family Welfare was identified as the coordinating institution for the PSBH program in Indonesia, and Dr. Alex Papilaya was designated National Coordinator.

PSBH workshops were promoted by sending invitations to a variety of institutions in the health field. The projects generated at the workshops covered subjects such as improving services, staff knowledge and skills, education and training curricula, and community participation in health. International facilitators from Poland, India, England, Vietnam, Jordan, Ghana, and the United States attended the workshops.

Problem Solving for Better Health-Nursing

Problem Solving for Better Health-Nursing™ (PSBHN™) started in Indonesia as a collaboration between the Center for Family Welfare and the Faculty of Nursing at the University of Indonesia. At the time, the university was the first and only institution in Indonesia providing bachelor's and master's-level courses in nursing. As an advocate for PSBHN, the Dean of Nursing, Dr. Elly Nurachmah, was personally involved in the planning and implementation of the first Indonesian PSBHN workshop, held in Jakarta. Workshop participants included nurses from hospitals, health centers, and nurse training institutions, including Faculty of Nursing teaching staff.

PSBHN projects focused on improving the quality of nursing services and record keeping, shortening the length of hospitalization for burn patients, registering newborns accurately, developing an educational program on self-care for chemotherapy patients and breast care for postcaesarean patients, registering and following up on patients with preeclampsia, and improving the nutritional status of malnourished children younger than 5 years.

One nurse from the Fatmawati General Hospital in Jakarta developed and implemented her plan of action and went on to complete five additional projects in collaboration with her fellow nurses. She initiated PSBHN in the hospital and influenced and motivated the hospital director to adopt the PSBH approach to solving healthcare problems in the hospital. Doctors and other hospital staff also became involved. In 2003, the hospital was awarded the first Problem Solving for Better Health Hospital Award by DHF. Currently, Fatmawati General Hospital has more than 108 ongoing PSBH projects.

The second PSBHN workshop was held in Surabaya in collaboration with the East Java chapter of the Indonesian National Nurses' Association. Participants were mainly from hospitals, district health offices, and nurse education institutions. Projects included teaching self-care methods to gangrene patients, improving patient satisfaction with nursing care, improving intravenous (IV) care techniques, developing a system for separating medical and nonmedical waste, and increasing hand washing among nurses and doctors in surgery rooms.

Problem Solving for Better Health Initiative

The Center for Family Welfare also implemented three district-wide Problem Solving for Better Health Initiative™ (PSBHI™) workshops. The first one took place in Jakarta; the second in East Jakarta; and the third in Batu Sangkar, West Sumatra. The East Jakarta PSBHI workshop was focused on the central theme: "Is East Jakarta healthy?" Personnel from the East Jakarta mayor's office attended the workshop, as well as participants from a variety of sectors such as health, housing, transportation, park management, market management, labor, and NGOs. The participants then developed action plans to solve the problems they perceived as "not supporting health" in their sector. Projects included educating mothers on the importance of using sanitary latrines, improving cleanliness standards of food vendors through training and certification, decreasing the incidence of diarrhea and typhoid, improving wastewater drainage in communities, and improving the environment by planting trees and community gardens.

The Batu Sangkar workshop used the same focused approach and generated projects to improve administration of the Posyandus (community-based, integrated, health service posts), increase tomato planting and maintenance to augment tomato farmers' income, improve discipline and productivity of government staff, decrease cases of rabies, and improve national examination scores of junior high students.

Problem Solving for Better Hospitals

As a result of the growing number of hospital staff attending PSBH, PSBHN, and PSBHI workshops, Dr. Papilaya coined a new program title—Problem Solving for Better Hospitals (PSBHospitals)—for initiatives focused on improving the quality of patient care. A PSBHospitals workshop is held as an in-house activity. The hospital setting guarantees success and sustainability of as many hospital-related projects as there are workshop participants, because the hospital management follows up on, monitors, and evaluates each project. Nineteen hospitals have held workshops, with staff from approximately 140 hospitals participating and more than 1,700 projects implemented. The PSBHospitals program will be further discussed in this chapter.

Problem Solving for Better Disease Prevention

In 2003, Dr. Papilaya initiated yet another special PSBH program, called Problem Solving for Better Disease Prevention (PSBDP), to focus specifically on decreasing the incidence of tuberculosis (TB) in Jakarta. As the capital province of Indonesia, Jakarta has resources and a developed health sector that serves as a benchmark for the other provinces. Nevertheless, TB in Jakarta is on the rise. There are managerial as well as technical problems in dealing with TB, and neither community nor private practice doctors do much to combat the problem.

The PSBDP program was implemented in 52 health centers and five municipal health offices of Jakarta. Participants were health center doctors, nurses, analysts, and municipal health office coordinators. Some of the TB projects include increasing the number of health center staff who treat TB patients, training the elderly to recognize TB symptoms, improving sputum examination in satellite health centers, improving new doctors' knowledge about TB management, increasing case detection rates by using leaflets and a "TB hotline," and improving TB patients' knowledge and awareness about the importance of completing their medication. More than 100 TB projects were carried out. Because of the success of the TB program, it was introduced in three additional provinces in collaboration with the Ministry of Health and funded by the World Health Organization.

Problem Solving for Better Education

A number of participants from the PSBHN workshops worked in nurse education institutions, paramedical training institutions, and faculties of medicine and public health. These participants targeted problems focused on issues of education that they encountered in their daily work. Based on this experience, the Indonesian Foundation for Better Health (IFBH—established by Dr. Papilaya in 2004 to operate and expand the PSBH program in the country) organized a third special PSBH-based program, Problem Solving for Better Education (PSBE), for staff of educational institutions. Projects generated at PSBE workshops focused on increasing writing skill activities for teaching staff, enhancing teaching activities through group lectures, expanding academic counseling, decreasing overscheduling of lecturers, and strengthening neurosurgery education through collaboration with district hospitals.

The Indonesian Foundation for Better Health

The IFBH, an independent nonprofit and registered NGO, was established in September 2004 to perpetuate PSBH in Indonesia. Its aim is to empower the Indonesian people to reach better health. The IFBH founders were all staff at the Center for Family Welfare, and all PSBH activity was transferred to the foundation. Trained facilitators and associates from various backgrounds support PSBH activities.

At present, IFBH's primary focus is PSBHospitals. The program objectives are to improve service quality, patient safety, and management efficiency. These three objectives must be accomplished to have a significant effect on the overall improvement of hospital services and administration. To participate in the program, a hospital is required to establish coordination to monitor, supervise, and follow up on projects. This function has become a permanent entity in the organizational structure of participant hospitals. After 6 months, IFBH facilitators and senior hospital management staff conduct a final evaluation. The six best projects are awarded a trophy and five additional projects receive Certificates of Excellence.

Staff from almost 140 Indonesian hospitals have been, and still are, involved in PSBH. The hospitals, both public and private, serve 11 provinces. Nineteen hospitals have conducted in-house workshops because the hospital leadership and staff are committed to improving their hospitals. PSBHospitals is an important component of their hospital quality improvement programs, and this fact guarantees sustainability of the projects. It is estimated that the number of PSBHospital projects in Indonesia is more than 1,700, with the greatest number in Dr. Sardjito General Hospital in Yogyakarta (112), Fatmawati General Hospital in Jakarta (108), and Pantiwilasa Citarum Hospital in Semarang (82). These numbers will only increase because many projects are being replicated in other units within all the hospitals and new projects are being developed.

Project sustainability is a major part of the PSBHospitals process and is addressed by the problem solver as well as by the hospital administration. The problem solver develops a clear plan for sustaining the project, and the hospital is responsible for ensuring that the plan is implemented. All new tools, forms, and procedures developed as a result of the project should be approved by the hospital director and incorporated into routine hospital practice. In addition, every project report is developed into a "Success Story." These stories play a significantly important role in improving hospital accreditation and International Organization for Standardization ratings. Because of successful project sustainability, problems solved 3–4 years ago have not reoccurred. Hospital projects have focused on improving medical and nonmedical waste management, decreasing postcaesarean section infections, enhancing nutritional care of diabetes patients, increasing use of gloves among nurses, improving ultrasound procedures for abdomen and gynecology patients, improving presurgical procedures, and decreasing the incidence of phlebitis in pediatric patients.

Several hospitals involved in the PSBHospitals program have developed an extraordinary number of quality projects. With the agreement of DHF, a set of criteria was developed to award outstanding hospitals with the PSBHospitals award. To qualify for the award, a hospital must have implemented and sustained 60 projects and replicated at least five in other areas of the hospital. In addition, the hospital must have incorporated PSBH into its system by establishing a PSBHospitals unit and appointing a coordinator. The award was given to Fatmawati General Hospital in Jakarta in 2003 and to Dr. Sardjito General Hospital in Yogyakarta in 2007.

Success Stories

Decubitus Ulcer Cases in the Perinatal Intensive Care Unit

In January 2004, 2 out of the 19 patients in the perinatal intensive care unit (PICU) at Dr. Sardjito General Hospital in Yogyakarta were diagnosed with decubitus ulcers (bedsores). At the time, the PICU did not have a procedure for bedsore management; however, the incidence of the condition is one of the indicators for measuring the quality of nursing care, and bedsores should not occur. Clinical symptoms of decubitus ulcers can range from blistering and edema to deep tissue ulceration and necrosis of the skin.

The PSBH process requires each workshop participant to ask a "Good Question," which for this project was, "Will … a new standard operational procedure for decubitus ulcer management, [including] improvement of personal hygiene of patients, for a period of two weeks, implementing the new procedure with at-risk patients at the PICU, Dr. Sardjito Hospital, Yogyakarta, decrease the occurrence of decubitus ulcers from 10.52% to 0% in three months?" The new procedure to prevent bedsores required nurses to provide skin care three times a day—at 8:00 a.m., 4:00 p.m., and midnight—as opposed to the previous morning-only care. In addition, the nurses were required to mobilize their patients regularly and monitor them for signs and symptoms of sores. All PICU nurses participated in the project, which was supported by the hospital. Results were amazing: In 3 months, decubitus ulcers in infants in the PICU were eliminated. This was a first for the PICU. When the IFBH staff visited the hospital in June 2008, no new decubitus ulcer cases were observed, meaning that the project had been, and continues to be, sustained.

Stocking Supplies in the Emergency Trolley

Tugurejo District Hospital in Semarang, Central Java, is a 245-bed hospital with 508 staff members. Amaryllis Ward II has 19 rooms with one patient per room. The ward has an emergency trolley stocked with injectables, IV drips, and medical devices. Based on monthly observations, the trolley was only 60% stocked. This caused problems in providing services to patients in emergency situations and threatened patient safety. The lack of supplies was caused by staff using the injectables, drips, and devices from the trolley and failing to request replacements from the pharmacy. In addition, the replacement supplies were not placed directly in the trolley.

The "Good Question" for the resulting project was "Will developing a procedure for the use of injectables, IV drips, and medical devices from the emergency trolley, which includes ... sending [replacement] requests to the pharmacy, coding supplies ..., reporting their use, and training the nurses in the Amaryllis Ward II of the Tugurejo District Hospital in the procedure, increase stock of supplies from 60% to 100% in four months?"

The project team coordinated with the Pharmacy Department to develop a standard procedure for immediately restocking supplies in the emergency trolley and instituted a checklist for recording the number of supplies available in the cart. The nurses received training in the new procedure and were monitored by management after each work shift. After 3 months, there was an increase to a full stock of supplies in the trolley. Services could be provided appropriately, and patient safety increased. This project became part of the standard operating procedure for Amaryllis Ward and has been replicated in the other hospital wards.

Postcaesarean Section Wound Infection in the Third-Class Obstetric Ward

Dr. Soeradji Titonegoro District Hospital in Klaten, Central Java, has three in-patient wards. One ward has three sections, one of which is a third-class obstetric unit with 22 beds and 22 cribs. The bed occupancy rate as of 2007 was 76.64%. Between August and November 2007, 10 wound infection cases from 85 postcaesarean section patients occurred in the obstetric ward (a rate of 11.76%). This was due to the lack of a standard operational procedure for the care of postcaesarean wounds. The same wound care kit was being used for several patients, and not every nurse was using protective equipment, such as a mask and/or gloves during postcaesarean section wound care. As a result, prolonged treatment and hospitalization occurred, along with patient dissatisfaction and a negative hospital image.

The "Good Question" for this project asked, "Will developing a post–caesarean section wound care procedure, [including] a procedure for use of a wound care kit; bedside teaching for wound care; coordination with the ward supervisor in monitoring, evaluation, and provision of guidance; and information dissemination about these procedures for two weeks, to 14 nurses and midwives … decrease infections from 11.76% to 5% in three months?"

The project team assessed the number of postsurgery patients with infections on the third day after surgery and during their first visit to the Obstetric/Gynecology clinic. Postcaesarean wound infections decreased from 11.76% (August to November 2007) to 1.09% (May to September 2008). The procedures for wound care and the proper use of the wound care kit were adopted into the standard operating procedures of the hospital, including the mandatory use of masks and gloves and regular monitoring by a ward supervisor and primary nurse. The new procedures have since been replicated in the surgery ward.

Conclusion

The success stories described above are just a few examples from the Indonesia program to date. Dr. Alex Papilaya has long recognized the need to build the capacity of Indonesian citizens to become changemakers in their society and, ultimately, the need for both individuals and whole communities to take responsibility for their own health and well-being. In collaboration with DHF, Dr. Papilaya carried PSBH and its capacity-building methodology to communities, hospitals, and medical universities throughout Indonesia's many islands. Today, with the establishment of the IFBH, Dr. Papilaya and his team are ensuring that the PSBH programs in Indonesia will continue to grow and expand, while also meeting the goals set forth by Healthy Indonesia 2010.

12

Kyrgyzstan

Sebastian J. Milardo

Kyrgyzstan, in Central Asia, is bordered to the north by Kazakhstan, to the east by China, to the south by Tajikistan, and to the west by Uzbekistan. Mountains cover about 80% of the country, and the majority of Kyrgyzstan's 5.5 million people, 69% of whom are the Kyrgyz, live in the mountains and valleys consistent with their nomadic history. In the cities and towns, Russians, Uzbeks, Tatars, Uighurs, Tajiks, Kazakhs, and others join the Kyrgyz. The Kyrgyz people have had major interactions with the Mongols, the Chinese, the Uighur khanates, and the Russians of both Tsarist and Soviet days. With the breakup of the Soviet Union, the Kyrgyz became independent in 1991. The Problem Solving for Better Health program has been inspired by the enthusiasm of Kyrgyzstan's people.

In June 2003, the Dreyfus Health Foundation (DHF) attended a conference organized by ECOLOGIA (Ecologists Linked for Organizing Grassroots Initiatives and Action) for Central Asian delegates to observe and learn from innovative antismoking and alcohol/substance abuse programs carried out in the United States. The delegates represented a wide range of public health occupations, from nongovernmental (NGO) workers to family doctors to a vice rector of the Kazakhstan School of Public Health.

At this conference, the DHF representatives identified a Kyrgyz delegate, Aibek Mukambetov, as a resourceful, hard-working, young professional who showed a strong desire to see how DHF's Problem Solving for Better Health® (PSBH®) program could impact his work and community. At the time, Aibek was 26 years old, a PhD student, and a full-time social worker at a youth center called Sotsium in Bishkek, the capital of Kyrgyzstan. Sotsium was the first NGO in Central Asia to introduce region-wide, innovative programs to reduce harmful consequences associated with high-risk activities. Sotsium has strengthened the capacity of the workforce within the existing healthcare system to prevent chemical dependencies. It has also worked to develop and ensure the availability of the following programs: rehabilitation services, needle exchange points,

---

Sebastian J. Milardo is Director of Operations at the Dreyfus Health Foundation.

the first self-help groups in Central Asia based on 12-step programs for anonymous drug and alcohol users, 24-hour phone hotlines, and preventive education centers. Aibek's enthusiasm and professional work led me, along with Dr. Jan Sobotka, DHF's Regional Coordinator for Eastern Europe, Central Asia, and the Middle East, to pursue the possibility of initiating a PSBH program in Kyrgyzstan.

Over the course of the next several months, Dr. Sobotka and I corresponded with Aibek regarding how to set up a new PSBH program in Bishkek. Aibek also attended a PSBH workshop in Ukraine in late 2003 in order to get a better sense of how to organize such a workshop and how to recognize potential partners in Bishkek. By March 2004, he had contacted many organizations, institutions, and government agencies regarding the PSBH program. The Director of Sotsium, Ms. Batma Estebesova, agreed to partner with DHF to start a PSBH program in Kyrgyzstan, with Aibek serving as the National Coordinator.

For the next 6 months, Aibek continued to meet with organizations in and around Bishkek in order to maintain enthusiasm and recruit participants for the first workshop, to be held in October 2004. Aibek had, by then, developed a team of young Kyrgyz men and women to organize the program and facilitate the workshop. Several members of the team were chosen because they had good English skills to help with interpretation and communication. A group of international PSBH facilitators attended the workshop to assist the local team: Jan Sobotka and Kasia Broczek from Poland, Giedre Donauskaite from Lithuania, and Maryana Sluzhynska from Ukraine. The international team of facilitators was important for this first workshop because none of the local team members, other than Aibek, had participated in a PSBH workshop. Each international facilitator partnered with a local team member in order to share his or her PSBH facilitation skills and workshop experiences.

Aibek and the local PSBH team chose the participants for the first workshop. They consisted of doctors, NGO workers, lawyers, psychologists, nurses, researchers, and other members of the public actively working to improve their communities. Over the course of two and a half days, both the international and local facilitators assisted the participants through the problem-solving process. Each participant identified a community health or social problem and developed a project that he or she believed could help solve the issue. Because of its close proximity to Afghanistan and its opium fields, Kyrgyzstan faces the many social problems that drugs create. Thus, many of the projects developed at the first workshop focused on these problems. Prisons in Kyrgyzstan are filled beyond capacity and tend to have high incidence rates of HIV/AIDS and tuberculosis (TB), mostly due to drug use. One project focused on educating prisoners about intravenous drug use, HIV/AIDS, and TB. Another participant noted that Kyrgyzstan has a high number of homeless children and that these youth often turn to crime and drugs, sometimes leading them to prison. This project leader developed an initiative with several psychologists at a local rehabilitation center for homeless children; the program included counseling, therapeutic activities, and educational sessions on various health issues. Early in the development of the PSBH program in Kyrgyzstan, it became clear that these three issues (drug use, HIV/AIDS, and TB) and their interrelatedness were monumental concerns in Kyrgyzstan.

In July 2005, a second PSBH workshop was held in Bishkek with a new group of participants. Again, the majority of the resulting projects addressed HIV/AIDS, TB, drug use, and youth. One participant, Alina Ibraeva, found through her work at a local NGO that drug use was common at nightclubs in Bishkek. She observed, "Some of the people come there in order to try and forget about their life and its problems; some come to listen to famous rock groups singing. However, they do not think about the future harm of unprotected sex, drug use, and alcohol." Over the next several weeks following the workshop, Ms. Ibraeva found partners, including the Red Crescent Society of Kyrgyzstan, and developed an educational program to be used in the nightclubs. The program included games, competitions, and prizes, as well as the provision of informational booklets about HIV/AIDS and drugs; free condoms; and contact information for psychologists, doctors, and substance abuse therapists. Two specific nightclubs, Zeppelin and Tekilin, agreed to host the educational programs prior to their evening entertainment. After distributing the literature, Ms. Ibraeva and her team proceeded with games and competitions. Part of the competitions included questionnaires for participants to complete concerning their lives, the harms of drug use and unprotected sex, and the possibility of contracting HIV from these risky behaviors. After each competition, participants received pens, pencils, condoms, and t-shirts with emblems representing a drug-free life.

Over 5 months, Ms. Ibraeva and her team conducted eight educational programs in each of the clubs, educating more than 300 people on the dangers of drugs, unsafe sex, and HIV/AIDS. Ms. Ibraeva also used the educational program in the Kazibek, At-Bashi, and Alish village schools in Narin province, one of the poorest provinces in Kyrgyzstan. The project reached approximately 350 students at the schools. Ms. Ibraeva explains:

> Tests showed that we improved education on [the dangers of drugs and unsafe sex] by 30%. We gave [the students] tests at the beginning and end of each program in order to measure their improved knowledge, but I think that it is not enough. I would like to continue to work in the poorer regions of Kyrgyzstan, like Narin, Talas, and Issyk-Kul. During this project we received various kinds of help from different organizations including DHF, the Global Fund, the Red Crescent Society of Kyrgyzstan, Partnership Net, as well as even private financial support from individuals involved. I want to say a big thanks to all these organizations and people who helped make this all possible, and I hope we can continue to work together.

Ms. Ibraeva's health initiative is an illustration of the effectiveness of a well-designed and executed PSBH project. Her plan of action was thoroughly outlined, allowing her to develop partnerships with strong institutions. Individuals from these institutions were eager to support the program and promote the lessons. The efficacy of her program was proven not only by the increase in knowledge measured in the participants through pre- and posttesting but also by the desire expressed by individuals in the community to learn this important health information.

Asel Temirova, a manager for the Red Crescent Society of Kyrgyzstan, also developed an effective project at the second PSBH workshop. Kyrgyz Ministry of Internal Affairs (MIA) statistics show that a very large number of children aged 3–16 live on the streets of Bishkek. In large part, this is due to drug and alcohol addictions of parents who have either orphaned these children or driven them from their homes. Often these children have suffered physical, emotional, and sexual abuse, either at home or on the streets. These children often come from the poorer regions of the country. They come to the capital hoping to find a job and to escape their unhappy homes. At the workshop, Mrs. Temirova spoke about the issue, saying "I have always wondered how they could survive on the streets and how they could stay alive even in the cold winters without clothes and food. I have since realized that they survive by trying to forget. They try to forget about their difficult lives and their problems, and to do this, they begin to use and abuse alcohol, to sniff glue and gasoline, and to become part of the commercial sex trade."

Prior to the workshop, Mrs. Temirova had visited a center for the rehabilitation and behavior modification of street children in Bishkek, the Juvenile Collection and Distribution Center. As employees of the MIA, the workers there are responsible for finding and gathering street children. For 30 days, children stay at the center while the MIA staff, the majority of whom are police officers, try to find the children's homes and their parents, if they have either. Unfortunately, after 30 days the children can leave of their own volition, if they have not done so already, legally or otherwise. During her visit there, Mrs. Temirova discovered a negative psychological atmosphere among not only the children but also the MIA workers. The police officers had difficulty interacting with almost all of the children. They treated the children with disdain and, as a result, the children became silent and unresponsive.

After participating in the PSBH workshop, Mrs. Temirova began the process of instituting a program at the center to tackle the communication issues and negative atmosphere, while educating the children on risky behaviors. To carry out her plan, she found three volunteers who were experienced with communicating and working with street children and could effectively explain to them the harms of drugs, unprotected sex, and HIV/AIDS, as well as the benefits of good hygiene. Together, they created a program plan for the children and workers to teach them how to better interact with each other. The team planned bimonthly visits during which they would use various psychological techniques, games, tests, and art therapy, as well as just plain fun, to help the group improve communication skills.

From the very first meeting at the center in October 2005, Mrs. Temirova and her team encountered problems in communicating with the children. The children were not at all open with them and had difficulty speaking about their personal lives. They refused to reveal their names and some refused to speak at all. Furthermore, about 80% of the children were not able to read or write. Despite these issues, the team worked toward overcoming their communication difficulties by playing games with the children as well as continually reassuring them of their safety. During art therapy, children had the opportunity not only to display their talents but also to express their feelings and concerns. In addition, lessons in reading and writing and harm reduction proved successful. Through the use of pre- and post-intervention surveys, the team determined that the children's knowledge about the harm of unprotected sex and HIV/AIDS grew by 50%.

Although the team saw great improvement in the children, the adults were more of a challenge. The primary goal of the project was to reduce the negative psychological atmosphere between the workers and the children and help them build positive and beneficial relationships with each other. At first the MIA workers were not at all interested in the project. However, the team found a solution to this problem through tests and games that the workers and children could do together. In playing with the children, a whole world opened up for the workers and helped them overcome some of the barriers in their relationships.

As a result of the project, the workers have become friendlier with the children, and the children and the workers eagerly await visits from Mrs. Temirova and her team. The team plans to continue its work at the center on a regular basis, using the same program. Mrs. Temirova was attracted to the PSBH program because:

It helps to solve the problems around the world. This program educates you on how to write a project by using questions and discussions, but the most wonderful thing in the program is that it improves the emotional, physical, and spiritual health of everyone involved. Also, it gave me an opportunity to realize the differences we all can make as individuals; even the MIA workers expressed their surprise and appreciation for seeing that they could do more and better work with the children. It was very empowering. Through this program, we were able to use our ideas and make a valuable contribution to our society.

Following the second workshop, the Kyrgyz PSBH team realized that specific health issues had come up repeatedly in the workshops. The team found that funding was most readily available from both local and international organizations when PSBH addressed specific, topical issues. Because the vast majority of the projects developed in the first workshops dealt with issues that directly or indirectly affected youth, the team decided to focus on healthy lifestyles among youth and adolescents through education on substance abuse, HIV/AIDS, and TB.

At the beginning of 2008, the Kyrgyz PSBH team received a grant from the World Bank to develop a youth center in Bishkek. The team hoped to establish a gathering place that could provide shelter, education, and activities for youth in an impoverished area of the city with a large number of homeless street children. The youth center is now up and running, providing hundreds of youth every month with free psychological support, educational programs, and sports and leisure activities. Volunteers from all facets of the community, including youth advocates, student peers, nurses, doctors, and parents, commit time and resources to the center. Free Chinese and English courses are available along with the PSBH educational health trainings on prevention of substance abuse, HIV/AIDS, and TB. Leadership courses, dance classes, wrestling, and computer courses are also offered at the center.

The success of the PSBH program in Kyrgyzstan is due, for the most part, to the strong, focused efforts of Aibek and his team. The team identified the major issues confronting their communities and eventually focused their attention on one particular, vulnerable target group that was adversely affected by a range of these problems. Their initial success led to the World Bank grant that then enabled them to tackle many problems from the centralized location of one youth center. Participants from the first workshops collaborated on these later efforts as well, as they saw the opportunity to scale up the work they were doing by tapping into the resources at the youth center. Finally, the center has also drawn attention from the city government, including the education and health departments, and is now a model for youth centers throughout Kyrgyzstan.

13

Vietnam

Tran Duc Thai, Le Thi Luc Ha, and Jill B. Derstine

Vietnam is the easternmost country on the Indochina Peninsula in Southeast Asia. Bordered by China to the north, Laos to the northwest, Cambodia to the southwest, and the South China Sea to the east, it is home to over 89 million people. Vietnam's forests, highlands, mountains, and coastal lands contain 16% of the world's species, making it a rich source of biodiversity. The long, complex history of the Viet people has included both Asian and European/Western influences. Their struggle to build a nation after the end of the Vietnam War in 1975 has been characterized by great economic and diplomatic success, with a major drop in the percentage of the population living in poverty. Nursing has been the emphasis of the Problem Solving for Better Health program in Vietnam.

The Vietnamese government designed a national healthcare strategy for the years 2001 through 2010, the goals of which include improving the health of all people, preventing disease, combining modern medicine with traditional medicine, and socializing healthcare. Health Volunteers Overseas (HVO), an international organization, sponsored the initial health project in Vietnam that served as a foundation for a subsequent partnership with the Dreyfus Health Foundation (DHF). This initial project began in 1991 and centered on introducing rehabilitation nursing and medicine to health professionals (O'Toole, Melli, Moore, & Derstine, 1996). The international nurses involved in the rehabilitation project observed that Vietnamese nurses had little or no rehabilitation in their basic nursing education. The rehabilitation project consultants then expanded their focus to a nursing curriculum project that eventually developed into an affiliation between

Tran Duc Thai is the former Dean of the Faculty of Nursing at Hue University College of Medicine and Pharmacy (HUCMP). Le Thi Luc Ha is a Lecturer of Nursing at HUCMP. The Faculty of Nursing at HUCMP is Dreyfus Health Foundation's implementing partner in Vietnam, and Tran Duc Thai is Problem Solving for Better Health National Coordinator for Vietnam. Jill B. Derstine is a Clinical Associate Professor at Drexel University and Professor Emeritus, Temple University.

Temple University in the United States and the nursing program at Hue University College of Medicine and Pharmacy (HUCMP) in Vietnam.

The association between these partners and DHF began in 2003. Building on their shared commitment to global health, the Temple University–HUCMP project staff, in partnership with DHF, considered implementing the Problem Solving for Better Health-Nursing™ (PSBHN™) program within the curriculum of the nursing program at HUCMP. The Dean of the Faculty of Nursing at Hue, Dr. Tran Duc Thai, was already familiar with the global programs of DHF and enthusiastically embraced the idea of a collaborative venture with Temple University, HVO, and DHF. During an assessment site visit to explore a potential collaborative effort, Dr. Thai suggested integrating the PSBHN program into the third-year nursing curriculum that included a community-based course.

As part of the visit, Dr. Thai introduced Dr. Jill Derstine from Temple University and Pamela Hoyt-Hudson, the International Nursing Program Coordinator at DHF, to several of the outlying minority villages in Nam Dong district, Thua Thien Hue province, that students and faculty would visit to identify local health needs and problems as part of their coursework. Following the community health assessment, DHF facilitators would conduct the PSBHN workshop with the goal of developing project action plans to address the health problems identified in Nam Dong. Nam Dong has a main clinic to serve several villages, and each village has a small, one-room "clinic" that is not always staffed. Health professionals from the main clinic visit the smaller villages on a monthly basis to provide immunizations and address other health-related issues.

Hue Problem Solving for Better Health-Nursing Workshop I

The first PSBHN workshop was held in Hue in March 2004. Forty third-year nursing students, six Hue University nursing faculty, two Temple University nursing faculty, Pamela Hoyt-Hudson, and two trained DHF facilitators from Indonesia attended. The Problem Solving for Better Health® (PSBH®) model was introduced at the workshop, and plans were made for follow-up site visits. The program's impact on nursing education and the communities in Nam Dong district would be determined on the basis of outcome criteria and evaluation tools developed for each project.

Each student came to the workshop with a community problem in mind. Students and facilitators met in groups to focus on issues that were solvable by the students themselves. Eventually, each group took one issue to work on in detail. Projects generated included improving garbage management; improving nutrition of children younger than 5 years of age; and implementing an education program on the importance of immunizations, their potential side effects, and how to manage care of the child postvaccination. Details from the immunization project are provided as an example.

The immunization project grew out of an observation by students that mothers were not familiar with side effects of immunizations and were treating the side effects as a separate illness, often bringing their children back to the health center for treatment. Therefore, the students focused the project on educating women with children younger than 1 year of age about the importance of immunization and possible side effects. The students contacted local health workers at the Nam Dong Health Center to obtain their support and permission to conduct the project. From August 2004 to February 2005, the students interviewed 100 women to assess their knowledge of the immunization program, the side effects of immunization, and normal reactions to immunizations. Interventions then took place for 3 days each month for 6 consecutive months, using brochures, posters, and recorded messages that were broadcast over a loudspeaker in the village. To evaluate the outcomes of the project, students returned to the village for 3 months, March through May 2005, and interviewed the same 100 women. Using a series of charts, the students presented their outcome data. Improvement was shown in the percentage of women taking their children to get vaccinations (4%), knowing about the benefits and side effects of vaccination (16%), and knowing the vaccination schedule (28%). Costs of this project included student transportation to the village, cassettes and a cassette player, posters, and brochures. The project has been sustained by local health workers at the center.

Hue Problem Solving for Better Health-Nursing Workshops II and III

For the next 2 years, two DHF facilitators (faculty members from Temple University), together with several nursing faculty from Hue trained in the PSBH process, conducted an annual problem-solving workshop with current third-year students. Prior to each workshop, DHF facilitators visited the villages to evaluate the results of the previous year's projects. Throughout the 3-year period of PSBHN, Hue nursing faculty undertook more and more of the responsibility for running the workshops. It was gratifying to see the transformation among not only the involved nursing students and faculty but also the participating community members from the various ethnic minorities. The community members were proud of their participation in the projects and enjoyed working with the students to improve the quality of life of people in their district.

Several of the second-year projects focused on children in preschool, elementary school, and secondary school. Projects included dental hygiene for preschoolers, hand washing for 4-year-olds, sex education for high school students, and first aid treatment, just to name a few. Dr. Derstine and Hoyt-Hudson conducted an evaluation visit in 2007, traveling to several village schools to see the projects still in action. The nursing students taught children at all levels, including 4- and 5-year-olds who were learning hand washing and teeth brushing.

Each of the PSBHN workshops in Vietnam received positive evaluations by participants. As summarized by Hue University nursing faculty, "The PSBHN program is an excellent framework on which to build transcultural collaboration." The nursing students gained cultural knowledge of minority groups and worked with these communities to impact health and quality of life in Nam Dong district. By the third workshop, Dr. Derstine and Hoyt-Hudson observed that the Hue University nursing faculty were capable facilitators and no longer needed assistance from the international DHF team. One of the nursing students from the first PSBHN workshop is now a faculty member and facilitates new workshops. The dean and faculty were encouraged to move toward self-sustainability. The problem-solving workshops continue to be an important part of the curriculum for nursing students at Hue, using the resources of the university and the surrounding area (Figure 13.1).

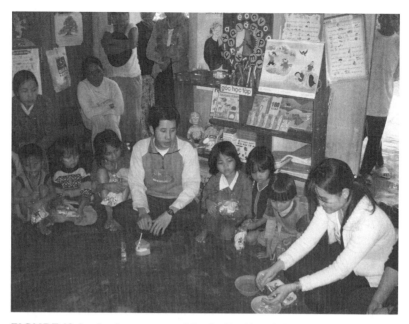

FIGURE 13.1   Student nurse and faculty Problem Solving for Better Health project leaders demonstrate basic hygiene practices to schoolchildren in the rural highland district of Nam Dong.

Program at Da Nang Orthopaedic and Rehabilitation Hospital

In 2005, having seen how PSBH's problem-solving methodology had enhanced nursing students' academic experience and impacted community health, the coordinators of HVO requested that a PSBH workshop be held at the Da Nang Orthopaedic and Rehabilitation Hospital for a variety of health professionals. HVO had been working with therapists, nurses, and physicians to implement needed changes at the hospital, but the plans had lost momentum. The HVO coordinators were hopeful that a PSBH workshop would encourage concrete action plans to improve quality of care at the hospital. During the ensuing 3-day problem-solving workshop, three DHF coordinators worked with hospital staff, and more than 25 projects emerged. Dr. Derstine and Hoyt-Hudson visited this hospital as part of their evaluation site visit in 2007.

One project from the hospital focused on developing a program for eight staff members on using computers to manage patient information. Evaluation compared the use of the database system and the paper system; the staff demonstrated proficiency with the new system and stated that it enabled them to work more efficiently. Other projects included establishment of a training program for physical therapists to improve use of home exercise, a program to maximize activities of daily living skills for stroke patients, an education program on intermittent self-catheterization patients with spinal cord injuries, and a health education program to provide counseling on the use of prosthetics for amputee patients.

In summary, the PSBH methodology has been successfully applied and sustained not only in the academic and community setting, as evidenced by PSBHN at Hue University, but also in the hospital setting at Da Nang Orthopaedic and Rehabilitation Hospital. The next step is to explore potential new sites for program replication and expansion in Vietnam and secure the necessary resources for implementation of additional initiatives.

Reference

O'Toole, M., Melli, S., Moore, M., & Derstine, J. (1996). Global gladiators: A model for international nursing education. *Nurse Educator, 21*(1), 38–41.

14

Bulgaria

Evgenia Dimitrova and Yanka Tzvetanova

Bulgaria borders Greece, Macedonia, Romania, Serbia, Turkey, and the Black Sea. Situated in southeastern Europe at the crossroads of Europe, the Middle East, and Asia, Bulgaria is one of the oldest states on the European continent. Ancient Greece, Rome, and Byzantium were important influences, and centuries of Ottoman dominance and, more recently, Soviet influence and policy also left strong marks on the Bulgaria of today. With its mix of East and West, Bulgaria, home to 7.6 million people, is a "worldly" country. Shaped by the Bulgarians themselves, the Problem Solving for Better Health program has spread throughout the country, and in the process, has been transformed and enriched.

Each day people are challenged to solve problems varying in nature and complexity, and success depends on the problem solvers and the environment in which problems are solved. The Problem Solving for Better Health® (PSBH®) program in Bulgaria is run by the Association for Better Health (ABH), a nonprofit organization in Pleven, with close collaboration and support from the Dreyfus Health Foundation (DHF). PSBH in Bulgaria began in 1994, in the midst of the country's transition toward democracy and a market economy. These changes in the country were characterized by high unemployment; high emigration rates; stress; increased domestic violence, crime, and drug abuse; and many people living at the subsistence level. This was a period of decline in the health status of the population as well as a demographic crisis. There were low birth rates and high morbidity and death rates, including unacceptably high infant and maternal mortality.

The first PSBH workshop was held in Pleven. Projects focused on prevention of drug and alcohol abuse among adolescents between the ages of 14 and 19 years, education of asthma patients, prevention of spinal deformities in primary school children, first

Evgenia Dimitrova is Senior Lecturer in Nursing and Yanka Tzvetanova is Senior Lecturer of English in the Department of Foreign Languages, Medical University–Pleven. Tzvetanova is also Director of the Association for Better Health, Dreyfus Health Foundation's implementing partner in Bulgaria, and Problem Solving for Better Health and Communications for Better Health National Coordinator for Bulgaria.

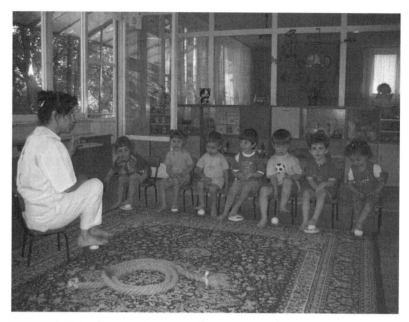

FIGURE 14.1   Rositza Cherneva, a nurse project leader, directs an activity to prevent flatfoot deformities at a crèche in Kazaniak.

aid training, prevention and secondary prophylaxis of acute myocardial infarction, antismoking programs, promotion of breast feeding, and early diagnosis of breast cancer. Many of these projects were extended to regional programs or replicated in other parts of the country. Between 1994 and 2007, many more PSBH workshops were organized throughout Bulgaria. The participants included doctors, nurses, educators, social workers, psychologists, nonprofit organization activists, university students, and administrators, who developed and implemented more than 400 projects. Participants presented their progress and results at follow-up workshops, site visits, and meetings.

The PSBH team in Bulgaria includes facilitators from the Medical University–Pleven, the Medical University–Varna, and the Faculty of Medicine in Stara Zagora, and local coordinators from university, district, and specialized hospitals throughout Bulgaria. Over the years, ABH has established collaboration with the university hospitals, the Ministry of Health, local governments, professional associations, regional health promotion centers, Bulgarian-Swiss Hospital Hygiene project leaders, and the Children's Help Net Foundation, Inc. in New York

Facilitators play an important role in the process. Since the first workshop in 1994, a team of 14 local facilitators has implemented the program. To achieve program effectiveness, team members were carefully selected from various regions of Bulgaria. Potential workshop facilitators first attended a workshop and implemented a project. Then they were further trained in the problem-solving methodology. During the training the participants were exposed to various tools, such as conflict management, and they engaged in role play to practice their facilitation skills. Upon completion of the training, participants led workshops under the guidance of an experienced facilitator. Assuming they received positive feedback on their performance, they were invited to participate in future workshop activities.

The Problem Solving for Better Health Initiative™ (PSBHI™) program began in Bulgaria in 1999. Approximately 300 projects were developed. The PSBH team and local organizers in each location organized and carried out follow-up workshops. In 2002, DHF launched Problem Solving for Better Health-Nursing™ (PSBHN™) to encourage nurses to take a leadership role in improving global health. In Bulgaria, the program has provided nurses with the opportunity to act as catalysts for better health using the PSBH approach. The PSBHN program initially involved nurses from all over the country who were pursuing their bachelor's degrees at the Department of Healthcare, Medical University–Pleven.

From 1998 to 2007, PSBHN workshops and follow-up workshops were held throughout the country and over 500 projects were implemented and completed; 51% were patient oriented and 25% focused on further training for health staff, especially nurses. Projects covered topics such as prevention of infections (particularly nosocomial), improvement of communication skills among nurses, application of new nursing techniques, training in computer skills, and resource management.

Some of the PSBHN workshops were specifically focused on children's health and the prevention and management of nosocomial infections. Four workshops were held in collaboration with an organization that coordinated all activities within the Bulgarian-Swiss Hospital Hygiene Program. The PSBHN program provided an opportunity to involve nursing staff in efforts to solve many problems in the hospital. The Bulgarian-Swiss Hospital Hygiene Program funded over 100 nursing projects, including covering some of the workshop expenses.

A large number of these projects focused on children and their parents, and were implemented in kindergartens and crèches (day nurseries; Figure 14.1). PSBHN participants worked with parents to conduct education on oral hygiene and prevention of caries, increase physical activity and reduce childhood aggression, improve early diagnosis and rehabilitation of spinal and foot deformities, manage respiratory illnesses, and encourage healthy eating habits. Nurses also developed projects on health education, sexually transmitted infections, reproductive health, and contraception. Additional projects focused on reducing stress in children admitted to the hospital, especially those with severe and chronic diseases requiring frequent admission and long hospital stays. Project leaders received assistance from parents, teachers, psychologists, and school administrators.

In our experience in Bulgaria, projects that focus on children's issues tend to foster a great deal of interaction among participants during the workshop and throughout the project implementation phase. The Bulgarian team also had success in obtaining support for these projects from local governments and health promotion departments in Varna, Pleven, and Stara Zagora, as well as from the Children's Help Net Foundation, Inc.

Since 1997, information about the PSBH/PSBHI/PSBHN programs in Bulgaria has been reported in the *Bulgarian Health Information Digest*, published in collaboration with DHF's Communications for Better Health® program, the Medical University–Pleven, and the ABH. Through this medium, PSBH participants have access to information about health issues addressed at workshops and project outcomes. Over the years, the published materials have given participants recognition for their contributions to improving health, provided information on health issues, and introduced potential participants to the PSBH program.

Evaluation of the PSBH approach to solving health-related problems is a major focus of the Bulgarian team members. They study the opinions of workshop participants, including what changes or advantages occurred in their work environment as a result of their participation in the program. The team distributed questionnaires to participants that included questions about workshop activities, issues discussed, expectations, communication processes, and suggestions for organizers. The team then analyzed more than 100 questionnaires and collected documentation for all projects.

Seventy-six percent of the participants who completed the questionnaires felt that small-group sessions were the most useful part of the workshop. This outcome could be attributed to the characteristics of the small group itself: a kind of "community" that remains the same throughout the workshop, in which participants can communicate freely. It is in the small group that problem-solving strategies are discussed, and the group members often gain knowledge and encouragement from one another. Participants also stated that the PSBH handbook utilized during workshops was a useful tool guide for the problem-solving process.

Participants indicated that presentations of problems and "Good Questions" in the large-group session consumed too much time during the workshop. This response may be attributable to the more "secure" atmosphere of the small-group session in contrast to the large-group/plenary session. According to 84% of the participants, the most difficult task during the workshop was defining the problem. In addition, they found it difficult to pinpoint the most important problem, feeling that all problems are important. Results from the questionnaires revealed expectations regarding communication and collaboration with the organizers. More than half of the participants wanted to work together during the implementation phase and recognized the importance of follow-up.

A cumulative review of all project topics indicated that project leaders are addressing the country's major health issues. Many projects focused on patients with severe and chronic diseases such as cancer, cerebrovascular disease, cardiovascular disease, diabetes, tuberculosis, asthma, and chronic renal disease. These projects incorporated a wide range of intervention activities aimed at preventing complications and relapses, managing disease, and improving quality of life. Local health authorities, health promotion specialists, and nongovernmental organizations assisted the workshop participants. Medical and nursing college students participated in the health education programs. These collaborations could not have been achieved without training received during PSBH workshops.

A majority of the participants reported that their communication skills had improved as a result of the workshops. Their skills improved in the following ways: using communication for the purposes of patient and family education, building consensus to work as a team, and developing techniques for fundraising.

The PSBH process can help frontline health workers gain professional experience and motivate them to solve health-related problems. PSBH provides people with a unique opportunity to take responsibility and become agents of change. Through the PSBH process, individuals are transformed from mere observers to real problem solvers.

15

Lithuania

Giedre Donauskaite-Tang

Lithuania shares borders with Latvia, Belarus, Poland, and Russia, as well as the Baltic Sea. It is the southernmost of the three Baltic states, which include Latvia and Estonia. Lithuania's 3.5 million citizens are committed to the advancement of their home country. A strong history and a wonderfully rich folklore, music, and arts culture have provided a solid foundation for a national identity. Since 1992, Lithuanians have worked hard and successfully to transform their country from a former member of the Soviet Bloc to a constitutional republic. Problem Solving for Better Health has made sense to them, and they have used it as a tool to help with their transformational process.

The Problem Solving for Better Health® (PSBH®) program in Lithuania was launched in 1999, after Dreyfus Health Foundation (DHF) representatives visited several hospitals and health centers and met with a variety of medical professionals and laypeople. As a result of these meetings, the DHF representatives recognized that many Lithuanians had serious concerns about healthcare in their country and were ready to become involved in solving some of the problems. They were ready to act; they just needed guidance. DHF offered a tool to help people solve existing problems and prevent future ones. In Lithuania, DHF partnered with ECOLOGIA (Ecologists Linked for Organizing Grassroots Initiatives and Action) to promote PSBH.

The first PSBH workshop was held in December 1999. Organizing this workshop was not an easy task. Lithuanians are reserved and cautious people, and it was not easy to convince heads of health institutions to allow their employees to participate. Administrators were skeptical, asking "What else can our people learn that they don't know yet? If they learn, will they really act to make a change?" To make the situation more accessible to potential participants, the first and subsequent workshops were held on weekends.

In Lithuania, we have a proverb: "The first pancake always is burnt." But this was not the case for the first PSBH workshop. Fifty-five participants, eager to learn, clearly

Giedre Donauskaite-Tang is the National Coordinator of the Problem Solving for Better Health program in Lithuania and from 1993 until 2007 was the Director of Baltic Programs for ECOLOGIA (Ecologists Linked for Organizing Grassroots Initiatives and Action), the Dreyfus Health Foundation's partner in Lithuania.

understood the main points of the PSBH process and left the workshop with realistic visions of how to solve their identified problems. Lithuania is small enough to spread the word about a practical and very useful program such as PSBH. The result was the unexpected difficulty of organizing more workshops and choosing new participants. Group work cannot be productive if the groups are too large. In this case, community spirit helped. Participants from the initial workshop were willing to share their experiences with colleagues, so the methodology and spirit of PSBH were spread to a much larger audience than PSBH workshops alone could reach.

Priority for hosting the new workshops was given to the smaller towns and rural areas, where people have fewer opportunities to participate in training programs than the health professionals in the capital city, who often are overwhelmed with invitations to attend different conferences. The majority of PSBH program participants at these workshops were nursing care specialists and social workers. Other participants included psychologists, psychiatrists, teachers, and representatives of health and environmental nongovernmental organizations (NGOs).

The problems that PSBH participants faced in the workshop were no different from the problems people face in the rest of the world: diabetes, hypertension, cancer, thyroid diseases, sexually transmitted diseases (STDs), social isolation of people with physical disabilities, and increasing numbers of young people who smoke and use drugs. Most of the projects generated at the workshops dealt with mental health, improvement of youth and children's health, and improvement of the social environment.

In addition, a number of PSBH participants identified diabetes prevention and treatment as health issues in Lithuania. Effective diabetes management is crucial in order to prevent complications. Recognizing the symptoms of diabetes early is important, because untreated diabetes can lead to kidney failure; blindness; heart disease; and foot problems, such as nerve damage and poor blood flow that may lead to amputation. Several PSBH projects in Lithuania were devoted to this topic. In the Pakruojis District, residents lacked information about diabetes. Adele Dobiliene, Chairwoman of the Vita Diabetes Club, recognized the need for diabetes awareness and implemented a project aimed at reducing the number of complications experienced by diabetics. She organized 12 classes on diabetes management for 403 club members and covered many relevant topics. Doctors and pharmaceutical company representatives participated as guest speakers. The project received media coverage and reached a much broader audience than the target group of 403 people. Feedback from the club members who attended the classes revealed that 95% of them felt that educational campaigns and lectures are necessary to continue raising diabetes awareness.

PSBH workshop participants from Atgaja, the Siauliai Society of Kidney Patients, initiated "Let's Learn to Live With the Illness," a project designed to teach dialysis patients healthy lifestyles and eating habits. These good habits increase the effectiveness of the dialysis procedure and reduce patients' pain both before and after a kidney transplant. Similarly, participants from the Lithuanian Kidney Patients Association, GYVASTIS, implemented "Providing Dialysis Patients With Information on Proper Nutrition." The purpose of this PSBH project was to produce printed materials on proper nutrition for dialysis patients in order to avoid nutrition-related health complications, such as uremia (a toxic condition resulting from kidney disease in which there is a retention in the bloodstream of waste products that are normally excreted in urine) and high levels of potassium that can cause death.

After one PSBH workshop, Ugne Shakuniene of GYVASTIS, initiated a project, "You Can Save Our Lives," to create a web page publicizing an organ donor program in Lithuania and to encourage people to become organ donors. Many young people visit the site, ask questions, and consider showing their benevolence to those whose lives can be saved by organ donation. However, this project achieved far more than its original goal of setting up a website and raising awareness. Mrs. Shakuniene wrote a letter to the President of Lithuania, Valdas Adamkus, asking him to support the organ donor idea by announcing the importance of the matter. At a social event attended by a number of governmental representatives, the President made a speech about the importance of compassion and charity, and how one can save the life of another person by making the decision to sign a donor card. Going even further, both the President and the Minister of the Interior announced that they had personally signed donor cards and encouraged other government officials, military officers, soldiers, and the general public to do the same. This shows how a PSBH workshop inspired a participant to take action with a small idea that led to far-reaching benefits for many. Mrs. Sakuniene said, "I wanted to implement this project for a long time, [I] just did not know how to start. And I was shy. After the PSBH workshop I was sure: I know how to do it, and will do it immediately."

Since 1999, psychologists, psychiatrists, and nurses have also developed a wide range of PSBH projects to address the fact that Lithuania has one of the highest suicide rates in the world (World Health Organization, 2009). The projects included assisting depression patients to overcome their illness, educating family members on taking care of the mentally disadvantaged, disseminating information about mentally ill people to counteract stigma, and preventing alcoholism and drug use among young people by involving them in community activities. Project leaders explained how various groups enjoyed participating and enthusiastically joined in all the activities.

One project, "Psycho-Educational Support Groups for People With Schizophrenia," was implemented at the Republican Vilnius Psychiatric Hospital. According to existing practices, schizophrenia patients receive medical treatment but not the psychosociological support needed for their total health. They do not receive enough information about their disease, and are not taught how to live with the condition and how to control it. They become more and more isolated, and lose their social skills and self-confidence. As a result, these patients are being rehospitalized frequently. Workshop participants from the psychiatric hospital developed a 2-month program of biweekly meetings to educate the patients on the psychosocial aspects of their disease by providing theoretical and practical information. In the end, the program achieved success in decreasing readmittance rates.

Many people, especially the elderly, experience social isolation in rural areas and urban settings alike, and several PSBH projects dealt with this topic. A nurse in Vilnius wanted to teach people to control their blood pressure. This project developed into a social club for the elderly where they not only check their blood pressure but also gather together for daily talks and various activities. A similar project was developed at Kaunas University Clinical Hospital. There are more projects of this type that at first look like social projects but, because of the physical as well as emotional benefits of companionship, actually assist in preventing not only problems of social isolation but also physical diseases and psychological disorders.

Measuring the success of a project is a part of the PSBH process. When the goal of a project is to reduce the incidence of specific illnesses, it is not difficult to evaluate the success of the project. One simply compares measurements before and after project implementation. But when dealing with social isolation or mental illness, it is not as easy to assess the success or failure in terms of a percentage change. These projects deal with lonely or mentally ill people, and it is difficult to measure either decreased levels of loneliness or improved mental health. However, such projects are not less successful than projects for which there are quantifiable results; we have received positive comments from many of the individuals involved about their appreciation for PSBH and feelings of wellness as a result of the projects.

During the implementation of a project the project team seeks volunteers and supporters. Important for the sustainability of projects are the partnerships that are formed, some lasting for the duration of the project, others continuing into the future to support the replication of existing projects or the development of new projects.

Perhaps the most important moment in the PSBH process occurs when participants realize that they can effect change and improve health for themselves, for their families and communities, and for the country. These individuals know what their goals are, and continue taking small steps to reach those goals. A program participant, Rima Petruseviciene from Jonava, expressed this sentiment when she said:

> Participating in the program I learned how to implement big works with minimum amount of money. I understood that I am the main person when starting any kind of work, because success of all works started will depend on my capacity to organize and to convince other people. Activity should not stop when the project was implemented. I have new projects in mind already.

The biggest joy was meeting a project leader after he completed his project and hearing him say, "This project is finished. But I will not stop. I have so many ideas now—so many problems need to be solved. This is just the beginning."

Reference

World Health Organization. (2009). *Mental health: Suicide rates per 100,000 by country, year and sex (Table)*. Retrieved April 28, 2010, from http://www.who.int/mental_health/prevention/suicide_rates/en/index.html

16

Poland

Jan Sobotka, Katarzyna Broczek,
Malgorzata Leznicka, and Jacek Zyrkowski

Poland borders Belarus, the Czech Republic, Germany, Lithuania, Russia, Slovakia, and Ukraine. The country's central location in Eastern Europe has been both a curse and a blessing for its nationhood. The end of World War II brought the Soviets to Poland, but in the 1990s, courageous Poles changed their country into a market-based democracy. Today, Poland is a strong nation moving forward to a bright future for its 40 million people. Led by the Polish team, more than 550 Problem Solving for Better Health projects have been implemented, and the Kujawsko-Pomorskie Province has adopted PSBH as one of its key methods for improving the health of its two million citizens. Poland has also, befitting its strategic location, been the stimulus for the development of PSBH programs throughout Eastern Europe.

In the last decade of the 20th century, Poland, as the western border of the Eastern European Bloc, faced health problems similar to those in other countries with healthcare systems lagging dozens of years behind those in Western Europe in terms of financing and management. The main health problems were high cardiovascular morbidity and mortality, late diagnosis and treatment of cancer, obesity, addictions, and accidents. There were also health issues related to specific population groups, for example, physical and psychological problems of schoolchildren and rehabilitation needs of the growing population of elderly people. Working conditions and underpayment of medical staff at

Jan Sobotka is an assistant professor in the Department of Preventive Medicine and Hygiene, Institute of Social Medicine, Medical University of Warsaw, as well as Problem Solving for Better Health (PSBH) National Coordinator for Poland and PSBH Regional Coordinator for Eastern Europe, the Middle East, and Central Asia. Katarzyna Broczek is an assistant professor in the Department of Geriatrics, Medical University of Warsaw. Malgorzata Leznicka is an assistant lecturer in the Department of Healthcare Organization and Management, Ludwik Rydygier Collegium Medicum in Bydgoszcz, Nicolaus Copernicus University, Torun. Jacek Zyrkowski is a physician in internal medicine at TORMED, Torun.

all levels of care had a significant negative impact on effectiveness and quality of care. Healthcare goals included redirecting care from therapeutic to prophylactic activities, as well as tackling inequalities in health, especially between rural and urban areas. It was in this context that Problem Solving for Better Health® (PSBH®) came to Poland.

History and Evolution of Problem Solving for Better Health

The PSBH program in Poland began in 1992, when The Health Foundation (THF), now the Dreyfus Health Foundation (DHF), visited Poland to seek potential partners in Eastern Europe. Poland was in economic and political transition and facing challenges in all areas of public life, including healthcare. Political transformation initiated by the workers' union, Independent Self-Governing Trade Union ("Solidarity"), in 1980, and systemic transition to democracy in 1989, shed light on many hidden health problems. These developments also provided new opportunities for individual activity and learning from the experience of others in the field of healthcare. The PSBH philosophy, uniting realistic and creative approaches to solving health problems, was a perfect tool to facilitate individual participation and responsibility. Thus, the Secretary General of the Polish Society of Hygiene, Dr. Jan Sobotka, responded enthusiastically to the proposal of future cooperation with THF (DHF) and its PSBH program.

The Polish Society of Hygiene

The Polish Society of Hygiene (*Polskie Towarzystwo Higieniczne*) was officially registered in 1898 and is one of the oldest associations in Poland dedicated to preventive medicine. Jozef Polak, founder of the society, and publisher of the periodical *Zdrowie Publiczne* (*Public Health*), co-organized two expositions dedicated to hygiene. Dr. Polak's motto was, "Health education is a powerful means for the protection of the health of the nation and the hygienic culture of the population" (Demel, 1970, p. 105). The society played a significant role in developing the healthcare system in Poland in the early 20th century. Today, it dedicates its activities to health education and preventive medicine in schools, workplaces, and the public health sector by organizing conferences, publishing periodicals (currently *Problemy Higieny i Epidemiologii* [*Problems of Hygiene and Epidemiology*]), and cooperating with other organizations on national and international levels. During the last two decades, cooperation with DHF has been one of the most important activities of the society, and many of its members have been engaged in the realization of PSBH workshops and projects.

Problem Solving for Better Health in Practice

The first PSBH workshop was organized in 1993 in Bialobrzegi, located approximately 30 km from Warsaw. The 55 participants included doctors, nurses, public health representatives, sanitary and epidemiological station workers, and teachers from 12 areas of Poland. Projects developed during the workshop included a broad spectrum of topics, including school health, oncology screening, addiction prevention, and preserving the environment. The proceedings of the workshop with outlines of the projects were published in a periodical, *Problemy Higieny* (*Problems of Hygiene*), and distributed to participants and members of the Polish Society of Hygiene (Sobotka, 1994).

The fascinating quality of the PSBH program is that it is never static. Each workshop is a new experience for participants and facilitators and opens new possibilities for learning and cooperation. From 1993 to 2007, 20 PSBH workshops were organized in Poland, with approximately 1,000 participants creating over 800 projects. In addition, more than 40 follow-up workshops were organized to evaluate the results of the projects. The progress of the projects was also presented in publications of the Polish Society of Hygiene and DHF, including *Problem Solving for Better Health—Polish Health Information Digest*.

The National Coordinator for PSBH in Poland is Dr. Jan Sobotka. Dr. Katarzyna Broczek assists in the organization of the program as a co-coordinator, and Ms. Malgorzata Leznicka and Dr. Jacek Zyrkowski have coordinated programs in the Kujawsko-Pomorskie Province and Silesia regions, respectively. A team of more than 10 local facilitators includes members of the Polish Society of Hygiene, the Medical University of Warsaw, and the Polish Nurses Association; all of these local facilitators began their adventure with PSBH as workshop participants.

Impact of Problem Solving for Better Health

Projects developed during the first years of PSBH in Poland were small initiatives, implemented in local communities, schools, and health centers and driven by enthusiasm, creativity, and the dedication of project leaders who used local resources in the best possible way. In many cases, the overall significance of the projects exceeded the specific results since the projects covered intangible issues such as comfort, happiness, and relief from suffering. Saving even a single life is priceless, as is putting a smile on one child's face. An example is a project developed in 1997 by Dr. Lilianna Lechowicz, who organized a playground for mentally and physically handicapped children attending a special-care preschool in Lomza, a city in northeast Poland. The mother of a handicapped child herself, Dr. Lechowicz gained support from a local nongovernmental organization (NGO), the Association for Help for Children with Brain Dysfunction, as well as from the local administration. The new playground, named after her son Adas, serves 14 children with physical disabilities who, in this safe environment, could interact with nondisabled peers. What did this mean for the disabled children's well-being and future development? It meant a whole new world to discover, where numbers and letters simply did not matter.

PSBH provides a simple, effective, and flexible tool for solving problems of various origins and levels. The flexibility of the methodology was proven during a PSBH workshop dedicated to the consequences of a 1997 flood in Central Europe and Poland. The workshop was held several months after the flood in the town of Swieradow Zdroj in southern Poland, the area that had experienced the worst damage. The main topics addressed by participants included posttraumatic stress disorder, the cooperation of rescue services during disasters, and the quality of water in rural areas. PSBH projects that were successfully implemented for those affected by the flood included psychological support, collection and distribution of food and clothing, organization of a vaccination program, and early prophylaxis of addictions.

The importance of allies in the implementation of health-related programs is especially emphasized in PSBH methodology. The philosophy of the program motivates participants to dismiss the idea that health problems should be solved only by health professionals. There are many examples of other professionals and nonprofessionals developing successful projects. Kazimierz Marciniak, a customs officer working on the Polish–German border, developed an educational program on the early prevention of drug use. He organized a series of presentations for schools and conducted a survey on initial drug use among youth. Nonmedical and medical staff of the Sanitary and Epidemiological Station in Zgorzelec set up a program, led by Dr. Jacek Zyrkowski, for addiction prevention by bringing together public institutions, NGOs, and community members in a network of cooperation. This was the beginning of a more comprehensive approach to problem solving that was further enhanced in the Kujawsko-Pomorska Initiative (KPI).

Innovative Solutions

A Problem Solving for Better Health Initiative™ (PSBHI™) workshop, covering a specific region of the country and uniting many partners to reach mutual health goals, was the next step for Poland. The first PSBHI workshop was held in Warsaw in 1999. At that time, Malgorzata Leznicka developed a plan to disseminate the concept of PSBHI to the Kujawsko-Pomorskie Province. In 2000, the regional parliament accepted a long-term program designating the province as a "Health Promoting Province," and in 2001, a document entitled "Strategy of Health Policy for the Kujawsko-Pomorskie Province" was approved by the parliament. The main goals of the Health Promoting Province program are to promote health knowledge and awareness, develop individual responsibility for health, adjust healthcare action to local health needs, and redirect healthcare from therapeutic to prophylactic activity. Changes in healthcare policy created a suitable environment for introducing PSBHI as a method to achieve these goals. Since 2000, nine KPI workshops have been held and 424 participants have developed 366 projects (Figure 16.1). The KPI has led to increased activity of local government agencies in the area of public health and significant changes in the health indices of the province (Leznicka & Stolarz, 2006; Sobotka, 2001).

The Marshal's Office of the Kujawsko-Pomorskie Province has adopted the PSBHI methodology to serve as a tool for implementation of health policy in the province. The Marshal's Office initiates cooperation with local self-governments in counties, municipalities, and local communities and coordinates regional programs in these locations (Leznicka, 2007). There is also cooperation with NGOs, patient-oriented organizations, universities, and other institutions. Local mass media play significant roles in popularizing participation in the regional programs.

Community Level

Projects developed at KPI workshops include many implemented at the community level in cooperation with local organizations. Diverse groups benefit from the projects in settings such as schools and nursing homes. Successful initiatives include projects on early detection and prevention of postural disorders in preschool children (Kindergarten No. 2 in Torun, project leader, Ms. Aleksandra Szlendak) and primary school students (in the

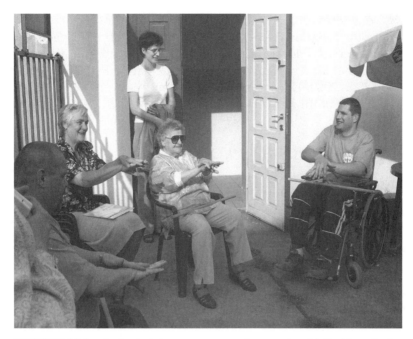

FIGURE 16.1 A physical therapy program for people with Parkinson's disease, a Problem Solving for Better Health project led by the nongovernmental organization Flandria in Inowroclaw in the Kujawsko-Pomorskie Province.

rural community of Zla Wies Wielka, project leader, Dr. Jacek Tejza). The latter program evolved into a larger initiative that enabled screening for postural disorders among all schoolchildren in the region.

Hospital Level

Hospitals have been settings for KPI projects that are larger than those implemented in the community setting. An example is a screening program for sleep apnea among professional drivers. The project leader, Dr. Malgorzata Czajkowska-Malinowska from the Kujawsko-Pomorskie Center of Pulmonology in Bydgoszcz, conducted a survey and a sleep laboratory study to diagnose this dangerous condition, which causes daytime sleepiness and increases the risk of traffic accidents. The results of the study led to adequate treatment of diagnosed cases of sleep apnea, and the recognition of sleep apnea as a "hot topic" at the international conference of the European Respiratory Society held in Glasgow, Scotland, UK, in 2004.

Regional Level

A network of regional programs for communities in the Kujawsko-Pomorskie Province was developed based on the local programs from the first editions of the KPI and analysis of the epidemiological situation of the province. In 2006, the regional parliament approved seven long-term programs and included them in the official health policy of the province. Initially, the programs were financed from the central budget of the Kujawsko-Pomorskie Province and 17 local municipality and rural community self-government budgets. The number of local self-governments participating in the program increased to 115 in 2008 and 173 in 2009. The seven programs continue to be active and are financed by the Marshal's Office of the Kujawsko-Pomorskie Province.

Problem Solving for Better Health-Nursing

Representing the largest group of professionals in the healthcare system in Poland, and in many other countries, nurses are an integral part of the PSBH process and account for a significant number of the workshop participants. Nurses have a special opportunity to educate and promote good health practices while working closely with their patients. Through PSBH, nurses also develop ways to help themselves and each other with specific challenges of the nursing profession, such as work overload, time scheduling, and interpersonal communication. Nurses have made great contributions to the PSBH process, and they have benefited from the process in return.

In 2000, 2005, and 2006, leaders of the Polish Nurses Association, Krystyna Wolska-Lipiec and Dorota Kilanska, worked together with Malgorzata Leznicka to organize three KPI/Problem Solving for Better Health-Nursing™ (PSBHN™) workshops. DHF's International Nursing Program Consultants, Dame Sheila Quinn and Shelagh Murphy, both from the United Kingdom, shared with participants their own extensive knowledge, a practical approach to solving health-related problems, and examples of solutions from other countries.

Project Examples

Developed by nurses from all levels of the nursing profession, PSBHN projects range from preclinical and postgraduate training to patient-oriented programs and social intervention. The following examples come from the 2006 PSBHN workshop in Lodz.

Mariola Bartusek, from the Department of Nursing at the Medical University of Silesia in Katowice, developed an educational program titled "Exposure of Hospital Ward Nurses to Ionizing Radiation and Magnetic Fields." This project included training for all nurses working in the Medical University Hospital, a conference and workshops for 400 nurses, and the formation of a group of experts to develop methods of protection for nurses and midwives in the workplace. Since 2007, the program has become an integral part of the educational activities of the Medical University of Silesia (Bartusek, 2007).

Jadwiga Gnich, a member of the Polish Nurses Association, developed "Metamorphosis," an educational program for adolescents in Warsaw, aged 13–15 years, including modules about diet, hygiene, first aid, safety, and substance abuse. The project is implemented in cooperation with the Medical University of Warsaw, a police department, and local organizations (Gnich, Olejniczak, & Duda-Zalewska, 2007).

Challenges

Many PSBH participants experience challenges in the implementation phase of their projects; however, nurses often face difficulties that make reaching their goals impossible. In particular, two aspects of the nursing profession account for this failure to fully implement a project: working under supervision and being dependent upon the decisions of others. In developing their projects, nurses must recognize the importance of professional cooperation. In addition, physicians, and society in general, must recognize the importance of the role of nurses in the healthcare system. All participants of the program, even those who have not completed their projects, have stated that participating in PSBH workshops, adopting the PSBH philosophy, and undertaking PSBH methodology have equipped them with new skills that are important in their professional and personal lives and enabled them to replicate or develop new projects successfully.

International Exchange of Solutions in Healthcare

International Team of Facilitators

The international exchange of facilitators for PSBH workshops is a significant feature of the program and a motivating factor for workshop participants who have the opportunity to learn from experiences in other countries. In addition, participating in a PSBH workshop in another country is a valuable experience for facilitators, giving them a clearer view of problems and a better understanding of factors influencing health in different settings and circumstances. Workshop facilitators serve as moderators who motivate activity and the creativity of PSBH participants.

The experience of conducting PSBH workshops and programs for almost 20 years has created a strong bond among the international facilitators. These members of DHF's PSBH "family" are grateful for the opportunity to learn together, and they feel a responsibility to share their acquired knowledge. In the contemporary world of rapid technological progress and novel methods in science and medicine, the human face of health seems to have become less important. The PSBH program reminds us that it is *people* who are at the center of any health-related issue.

International Exchange of Experience

Results from the PSBH program in Poland have been presented during national and international conferences, including the European Interprofessional Education Network's first international conference, "Learning Together to Work Together," held in Krakow in September 2007. The PSBH presentation, given by Dr. Katarzyna Broczek and Dr. Jan Sobotka, evoked interest and a lively discussion among the several hundred educators, scientists, and conference organizers. Also in September 2007, the Department of Health Policy of the Marshal's Office of the Kujawsko-Pomorskie Province in Torun organized an international conference on "Building Partnership in Prophylaxis and Health

Promotion," in cooperation with DHF and the Polish Society of Hygiene. Participants included PSBH national coordinators and representatives from public health institutions in Holland, Lithuania, Bulgaria, Romania, and Armenia. Examples of PSBH/PSBHI projects in Poland led to the development of new ideas for international cooperation in the field of preventive medicine.

Sustainability of Problem Solving for Better Health

The Kujawsko-Pomorska Initiative

The KPI is the best example of how PSBH programs in Poland have expanded and become sustainable over time. Adoption of existing PSBH programs and methodology by the local health organizations responsible for planning and distributing funds for healthcare programs has ensured their continuity. Workshop participants who have acknowledged the usefulness of PSBH methodology have coordinated regional programs developed on the basis of their PSBH projects. In addition, the KPI has gathered more than 400 participants from various backgrounds who have successfully implemented their projects and acquired skills that have made them more efficient in solving health-related problems. In summary, the KPI has improved cooperation between different levels of public health service and is considered a tool for cooperation between central and local self-governments of the Kujawsko-Pomorskie Province.

Future Expectations

PSBH methodology would be a valuable tool for solving health problems in other provinces of Poland. However, the provinces must first experience and thoroughly understand the principles of PSBH before these programs can be successfully adopted and implemented. Learning how to approach problems with the PSBH methodology is a step-by-step process, and it takes time and the dedication of participants. Developing PSBH as a sustainable program in other provinces would require starting from the very beginning in each location and would include organizing basic PSBH workshops, and experiencing and learning from both successes and failures. In 2004, Poland became a member state of the European Union (EU), and as a result has gained access to many public health programs supported by the EU. Regardless of the thousands of initiatives implemented by the government, Ministry of Health, and NGOs, the Polish PSBH team believes that there continues to be a need for the PSBH program in Poland.

References

Bartusek, M. (2007). Exposure to ionizing radiation and magnetic field of nurses working in hospital wards. Assumptions, aims and implementation of the project in the Medical University of Silesia. *Problems of Hygiene and Epidemiology, 88,* 242–243.

Demel, M. (1970). *W sluzbie Hygei i Syreny. Zycie i dzielo dr Jozefa Polaka* [In the service of Hygeia and Sirens. The life and work of Dr. Jozef Polak]. Warsaw, Poland: PZWL.

Gnich, J., Olejniczak, D., & Duda-Zalewska, A. (2007). Health education in schools—We can do it! *Problems of Hygiene and Epidemiology, 88,* 240–241.

Leznicka, M. (2007). The role of the regional self-government in solving health problems of the population—An example of Kujawsko-Pomorskie province. *Problems of Hygiene and Epidemiology, 88,* 499–506.

Leznicka, M., & Stolarz, J. (2006). Evaluation of quality and effectiveness of projects developed in the frame of the program "Problem Solving for Better Health—Kujawsko-Pomorska Initiative." *Problems of Hygiene and Epidemiology, 87,* 146–149.

Sobotka, J. (1994). Rozwiazywanie problemow dla poprawy zdrowia [Problem solving for better health]. *Problemy Higieny, 43,* 1–275.

Sobotka, J. (2001). 10 lat wspolpracy pomiedzy DHF i PTH [10 years of cooperation between DHF and PTH]. *Problemy Higieny, 72,* 1–240.

17

Romania

Ana Florea and Paul Florea

> Romania is located in southeastern Europe and shares borders with Moldova, Ukraine, Hungary, Serbia, Bulgaria, and the Black Sea. Its landscape of mountains, forests, hills, and plains, in roughly equal parts, is home to 21.5 million people of Dacian and Roman ancestry and Eastern Orthodox faith. As a crossroads of Eastern Europe, the country has a rich and varied history and culture. With the fall of Communism in 1989, Romania became a constitutional market democracy and entered the transitional period experienced by all the formerly Communist Eastern European countries. Problem Solving for Better Health has been a part of this transition.

The Problem Solving for Better Health® (PSBH®) program in Romania is coordinated by the Andrea Foundation, a nongovernmental organization (NGO) that supports social, educational, and health-related programs benefiting children. In 1998, the Andrea Foundation established a collaboration with the Dreyfus Health Foundation (DHF) at the suggestion of Dr. Daniel M. Levine of The Rogosin Institute in New York. Dr. Levine is also president of the Children's Help Net Foundation, Inc., which works closely with the Andrea Foundation on many projects promoting child welfare in Romania. PSBH has enabled the Andrea Foundation to initiate more projects in different regions of the country and involve many more people.

When PSBH was launched in Romania, the country was in transition to a market economy. There was a high rate of unemployment, many people lived at a subsistence level, and there was a great deal of emigration. High levels of violence and drug abuse existed among youth. Children were abandoned at birth because of poverty and the inability to provide adequate education. Programs for proper hygiene and the prevention of communicable diseases were nonexistent.

Ana Florea is President and Paul Florea is Vice President of the Andrea Foundation. Paul Florea is also Problem Solving for Better Health and Communications for Better Health National Coordinator for Romania.

The first PSBH workshop took place in Bucharest in 1999, with 43 projects developed. Project topics included community integration of orphans and children with disabilities and HIV/AIDS, counseling for parents of children with HIV/AIDS, prevention of HIV/AIDS among teenagers, reduction of morbidity caused by respiratory diseases among children, and education for ambulatory patients with burns. These programs were later replicated in other parts of the country, and some even expanded into regional programs.

In 2001, the first of two additional PSBH programs was initiated in Romania. That year, a Problem Solving for Better Health-Nursing™ (PSBHN™) workshop was held in Bucharest. Nurses from nine hospitals in Bucharest, Craiova, and Cristuru Secuiesc developed 56 projects focused on prevention of illnesses and infections in hospitals, improvement of nurse communication, and professional training for nurses. A second PSBHN workshop was held in Craiova in 2005, in collaboration with the Craiova County Clinical Emergency Hospital, the University of Medicine and Pharmacy of Craiova, and the Dolj branch of the Romanian Nursing Association. Nurses and student nurses developed 40 projects related to various health issues.

In 2002, a Problem Solving for Better Health Initiative™ (PSBHI™) workshop was held in Targoviste, resulting in 61 projects. One project was a health education program for 25 children in School No. 8, a local primary school. Veronica Istrate, a public health nurse, knew that dentists were treating a growing number of patients who were experiencing tooth decay as a result of poor oral hygiene. She developed a program to educate parents and teachers about the correct way to brush teeth and the need for regular dental check-ups, so that they, in turn, could educate the children about the importance of tooth brushing. The teacher and a dentist, under the supervision of Veronica, conducted twice-weekly in-class training sessions. They taught the schoolchildren correct tooth brushing techniques, and the teacher assisted the children in brushing their teeth after their lunch break. A dentist agreed to monitor the children for bacterial plaque over a 3-month period. Parents completed questionnaires before and after the training, and responses indicated that the children were brushing their teeth regularly and, as a result, were preventing plaque buildup. The Colgate–Palmolive Company provided bacterial plaque indicators, toothbrushes, and toothpaste for this project. Veronica obtained additional support from Colgate–Palmolive to duplicate this project with an additional 1,500 children in four more schools in Targoviste.

Andrea Maria Popescu, a high school student in Targoviste, developed another project at the 2002 workshop to reduce the number of teenage pregnancies and abortions among girls attending her school. Working with 27 of the high school students, Andrea first asked them to complete a questionnaire about their knowledge of contraception, sexually transmitted diseases (STDs), pregnancy, and abortion. After reviewing the responses, Andrea held a meeting with the students, at which she provided educational materials about different methods of contraception and STDs. She held an open dialogue with the students to discuss concerns and ask questions. At the end of this session, Andrea asked the students to complete a project evaluation form and learned that the students gained significant knowledge and, as a result, changed their behavior. The success of this project led to its expansion to all the classes at the high school.

Between 1998 and the present, more than 15 PSBH workshops have been held in nine cities throughout Romania. A team of local workshop facilitators has developed from participants who implemented successful projects of their own and can, therefore, share their experiences and knowledge. This team includes psychologists, nurses, doctors, and social workers from hospitals, public health departments, educational institutions, and the Romanian Nursing Association. Workshop participants have included psychologists, nurses, doctors, social workers, educators, and students. In total, they have developed and implemented approximately 700 projects. The team of local facilitators conducts site visits to assess project activities, and the results of these projects are presented at follow-up meetings. In addition to those already mentioned, partners who contribute to the organization of workshops and the monitoring of projects include the public health authorities of Cambovita, Prahova, and Vrancea; the Marie Curie Children's Hospital and the Central Military Hospital, both in Bucharest; the Slobozia County Emergency Hospital; and the School Inspectorate of Vrancea, among other educational and medical institutions and organizations.

Information about the Romanian PSBH program and projects generated at workshops is contained in the *Romanian Health Information Digest*, published by the Andrea Foundation in collaboration with DHF's Communications for Better Health® program. Medical personnel from the Institute of Health Services Management (now the National School of Public Health and Health Services Management), the Colentina Clinical Hospital, the Romanian Nursing Association, the Children's Help Net Foundation, Inc., and the Andrea Foundation have all prepared articles for the *Digest*. The publication is distributed at no charge to the National Library of Romania, hospitals, medical centers, public health departments, and workshop participants.

PSBH is a process that encourages participants to reconsider health and social issues in their homes, workplaces, and communities from their own points of view. The flexibility of the program allows them to identify a variety of problem-solving tools that they can manage themselves to produce positive results and reach their desired objectives. The successes of already implemented projects have inspired a lengthy list of prospective participants for upcoming workshops. More background about the steps that led up to the birth of PSBH in Romania and the relationships that have developed as a result will be described in Chapter 19.

18

Ukraine

Oleksandra Sluzhynska

Ukraine is the easternmost of the Eastern European nations and is bordered by Russia, Belarus, Poland, Slovakia, Hungary, Romania, Moldova, and the Black Sea. Its largely level plain is home to 46.2 million people, three quarters of whom are ethnic Ukrainians, with smaller numbers from each of the bordering countries. A resource- and agriculturally rich land that had long seen domination by some of its neighbors, Ukraine became fully independent as a nation in 1991 and helped to form the Commonwealth of Independent States. With its rich culture of literature, music, art, and the performing arts, among its other strengths, Ukraine is moving forward to a bright future. Problem Solving for Better Health is privileged to be part of that forward movement.

In the late 1990s, I heard, by word of mouth, about the Dreyfus Health Foundation's (DHF's) Problem Solving for Better Health® (PSBH®) program. I contacted DHF and expressed my interest in learning more about its activities in Eastern Europe. DHF's program coordinator for the region kindly invited me to attend a workshop in Slovakia, where the foundation had been working with the Roma people since 1997. There, I met the PSBH Regional Coordinator for Eastern Europe and National Coordinator for Poland, Dr. Jan Sobotka, and the National Coordinator for Slovakia, Dr. Maria Butkovicova. I was impressed with the workshop program and the facilitators who attended from around the world to present the health issues in their countries and share their experiences with PSBH. I hoped that one day Ukraine would become part of the DHF network of problem solvers.

Upon my return to Lviv, I continued to correspond with Dr. Sobotka and DHF's Program Coordinator for Eastern Europe, Lenin Gross. In 2000, both came to Lviv to meet my colleagues, Maryana Sluzhynska and Mariya Telishevska, and to visit possible workshop sites and Ukrainian nongovernmental organizations (NGOs). Later that year,

Oleksandra Sluzhynska is President of the SALUS Charitable Foundation, the Dreyfus Health Foundation's implementing partner in Ukraine. She is also Problem Solving for Better Health and Communications for Better Health National Coordinator for Ukraine.

the PSBH program in Ukraine was established through a partnership between DHF and the SALUS Charitable Foundation in Lviv.

Education For Better Health Initiative

Health education was introduced into the school curriculum in Ukraine; however, teachers lacked illustrative materials and interactive education methods to use in their classrooms. To unite Ukrainian educators in the quest to improve the health curriculum in their schools, the SALUS Charitable Foundation, in partnership with DHF, launched the innovative Education for Better Health Initiative (EBHI). This first Ukrainian Problem Solving for Better Health Initiative™ (PSBHI™) that focused on education was held for 2 days in April 2006. Participants included 27 teachers and psychologists, 4 health education specialists, 2 representatives from NGOs focusing on child and adolescent health, and 2 physicians. Representatives from the Lviv Department of Education also attended.

Topics addressed during the workshop included HIV/AIDS and other physical health issues, mental health, spiritual health, healthy lifestyles, and social aspects of health. Participants separated into groups, with each group focusing on one of the identified topics. Ultimately, the participants generated a total of 12 project proposals, which included support for the creation of educational materials, such as visual and audio aids, computer games, and CDs.

One group of seven participants created a project to develop an educational CD for children on safety precautions and procedures. The CD alerts children to possible dangers during normal activities, such as swimming, crossing a street, or cooking, as well as emergency situations, such as an explosion, a flood, or finding oneself in a pressing crowd. Each participant contributed his or her own ideas on how to make children aware of dangerous situations without alarming them and explain safety procedures that they can understand clearly. Copies of the completed CD have been distributed free of charge to schools where they are shown each school year to students at all age levels.

Another project involved hands-on teaching of animal science while providing good nutrition to children in a community of poor families. Mr. Andriy Kiyko, a representative of the Association of Children's Ecological Centers, was instrumental in developing this project and providing the location for raising Japanese quail at the Lviv City Children's Ecological Naturalistic Center. The target children are taught how to raise the quail and how to harvest their eggs. Special care must be taken in collecting and handling quail eggs because their shells are thin and break more easily than chicken eggs. In spite of their small size, the nutritional value of quail eggs is three to four times higher than that of chicken eggs. They do not have "bad" cholesterol (LDL) and are very rich in "good" (HDL) cholesterol. Because these eggs contain nutritional ingredients useful for strengthening the immune system, the children are encouraged to eat two of the eggs that they harvest each day. In the first 3 months of the project, the children raised 65 young birds. It took another month for the quail to produce eggs. At that time, three sets of eggs were incubated in order to raise more birds, setting the stage for a sustainable project. The children are enthusiastic about the project, as they enjoy learning about and working with the birds, in addition to eating the eggs that their birds produce (Figure 18.1).

EBHI's achievements are due to the successful associations between the SALUS Foundation and the Lviv Regional and City Departments of Education, along with project support from DHF, the Elton John AIDS Foundation, the Poland–America–Ukraine Cooperation Initiative, and the European Commission. The workshop was different from the standard PSBH model, which follows the principle of "one participant, one project," in that the initiative emphasized group collaboration in order to achieve maximum results.

Commemorating World AIDS Day

In line with its focus on sexually transmitted disease and HIV/AIDS prevention, the SALUS Charitable Foundation participates in commemorating the annual World AIDS Day in Lviv. PSBH projects resulted in two events that were organized in collaboration with DHF. In November 2003, SALUS held a designer fashion show at the Hnat Khotkevych City Palace of Culture in Lviv. The purpose of this project was to raise awareness, using the fashion industry to convey anti-AIDS messages. Eighteen designers and 28 models participated in the show. The event was well attended and received full coverage by the local media. In addition to DHF, sponsors were the Poland–America–Ukraine Cooperation Initiative, the Eurasia Foundation, and the Elton John AIDS Foundation.

In December 2005 the Khotkevych Palace hosted an art event dedicated to raising HIV/AIDS awareness. Two PSBH projects resulted in an "Anti-AIDS Photography and Pantomime" competition and exhibition. Approximately 250 Ukrainian artists, 12 photographers, and 9 theater staff members from all over the country participated. Artwork, photographs, and pantomime performances addressed AIDS prevention, misconceptions

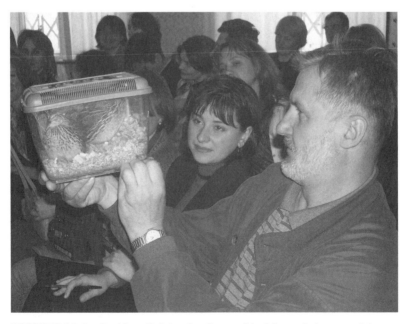

FIGURE 18.1 Problem Solving for Better Health workshop participants admire Japanese quail raised by children in Lviv during a project to promote good nutrition.

about those living with HIV/AIDS, and high-risk groups. SALUS distributed informative brochures and pamphlets on HIV/AIDS prevention and antiretroviral therapy as well as a program calendar to promote year-round awareness.

This is my PSBH story and the story of 30 Ukrainian PSBH facilitators and partners in cities throughout the country. It is the story of close to 1,000 Ukrainian PSBH workshop participants and their achievements. It is a success story, and I do appreciate the support that has been given to Ukraine to carry on the PSBH program.

Note: In collaboration with DHF's Communications for Better Health® program, SALUS and the Ukrainian Medical Association in Lviv have published the Ukrainian Health Information Bulletin, *in which information about the country's PSBH program and projects has been presented.*

19

A Personal Perspective

Daniel M. Levine

With this book, Dr. Barry H. Smith invites the reader to join a global revolution for better health. I am one of those people who answered the call by volunteering to be an international facilitator for the Dreyfus Health Foundation (DHF) Problem Solving for Better Health® (PSBH®) programs in Eastern Europe. My goal in writing this chapter is to impart to the reader what it is like to serve in this capacity and the passion and exhilaration that one experiences in the process. First, I will present my experiences as an international facilitator, with a special emphasis on identifying a potential partner in Romania to host PSBH and the steps toward establishing a successful program there. Second, I will show how a very small grassroots nongovernmental organization (NGO), originally established for the specific purpose of providing basic necessities to children in need in Eastern Europe, was able to work synergistically with DHF to the benefit of both.

In 1995, my wife and I made a life-changing decision to adopt two children from Eastern Europe. In 1996, we adopted our first child, and in 1998 we adopted the second, both from the Republic of Moldova. We met Paul Florea and Ana Pitu Florea (who would later become coordinators of the PSBH program in Romania) in the process of making two trips to Moldova for each child, as required by Moldovan law. Paul served as the adoption attorney and represented Spence-Chapin, a well-known, established, and respected adoption agency in New York. We stayed in Chisinau, the capital city of Moldova, for about 10 days on the first trip for each adoption. We visited the orphanage daily; we, and the families we traveled with, were horrified by the conditions we saw. There was no central heat or hot water, and without money donated by adoptive parents passing through, the children ate only cooked potatoes with beets and bread. Medical supplies and healthcare were scarce, and the children had diseases caused by vitamin deficiency.

In the midst of all of this, Paul asked every parent to become involved with him in creating a long-term plan to help the children in the orphanage. During my third trip to Moldova, a group of children ran up to me shouting "Daddy! Daddy!" as they surrounded me outside the orphanage, and it broke my heart. Paul, who had witnessed this

Daniel M. Levine is Chief Information Officer, Director of the Clinical Research Laboratory, and Co-Director of the Lipid Research Laboratory at The Rogosin Institute in New York. He is also Director of the Children's Help Net Foundation and a Problem Solving for Better Health International Facilitator.

event, said quite plainly, "It has to be you. No one else will do it." Together, Paul and I established the Andrea Foundation in Romania, the Charitable Foundation Andrea in Moldova, and the Children's Help Net Foundation, Inc. (CHNF) in the United States. Paul himself was an adoptive parent, having adopted his daughter Andrea in Romania.

We now had three foundations in three countries. The Andrea foundations in Romania and Moldova would promote adoption, place children, and provide humanitarian aid when possible. CHNF would raise money in the United States to support all activities, although it would not be directly involved in adoptions. (Later, the Romanian government changed its laws regulating NGOs, no longer permitting them to be involved with adoption, so PSBH eventually became the main activity of the Andrea Foundation in Romania.)

But Paul and I wanted to have a greater impact on children and families. By this point, I had worked at The Rogosin Institute (DHF's parent organization) for 12 years and knew about DHF and its PSBH programs, so I approached Dr. Smith about the possibility of a PSBH program in Romania. After meeting Paul, Dr. Smith invited me to help establish the program. This turned out to be one of the most exciting and rewarding experiences of my professional career at The Rogosin Institute.

We held the first PSBH workshop in Romania in Bucharest in February 1999, with 50 participants. This was trial by fire for me. I had only what I had read about the program, the advice of other facilitators I had just met, and the seat of my pants. Perhaps the most relevant advice came from Dr. Smith, who told me to remember that it is all about the participants and the success of the program, and not about us as facilitators.

Two events with my workshop group are illustrative of what DHF often encounters when beginning PSBH in a new country or region. There were three female physicians who worked together and were very outspoken and generally negative about the philosophy of PSBH. After listening to a colleague and me walk them through examples of "Good Questions" from other countries, the most aggressive of these women stood up and said to me, "You are just a stupid American who has no understanding of the problems we face here!" Dr. Smith's words of wisdom flashed through my brain at that moment and without hesitation I replied, "You are right. Perhaps you can help me understand the problems you face and together we can formulate solutions." She was so shocked that she stumbled backward and took her seat. I had her attention.

At another point, an accountant from the same hospital as the three physicians proposed a project working with physicians to cut operating costs without sacrificing the quality of patient care. The same woman turned to him and said in an angry and arrogant tone, "What can you possibly hope to accomplish—you are not even a physician!" I replied to her, "Isn't that, in fact, the whole point? He understands issues that you don't, and you understand issues that he doesn't. That is why this is a perfect project."

The next day, the three female physicians came in with a completely different attitude. The night before, we had sent them home with the task of writing a "Good Question" and encouraged them to read ahead in the PSBH handbook. Now they were cooperative, ready to work, and came in with their "Good Questions." After this initial workshop, Paul and I never looked back and never questioned what we were doing again.

A small group from Bulgaria joined us for many of the early workshops in Romania, including Yanka Tzvetanova, the PSBH National Coordinator for Bulgaria. The national coordinators and team members from neighboring countries often lend a hand when a new program is being established. This has the advantage of keeping travel costs down while capitalizing on successful regional experience. Despite any potential rivalries between neighboring countries, it is generally accepted that they face similar problems.

One of the most rewarding experiences for a facilitator is attending the follow-up workshop that takes place 3–6 months after the initial training session. During the follow-up session, which is usually a half-day, participants report on the progress of their projects. Their sense of accomplishment and pride is huge, and for me, as a facilitator, it is downright exhilarating. Sheer joy comes from empowering people to think differently, to network among themselves to maximize their chances for success, to use local resources that they probably never knew existed, and to realize that large sums of money are not needed to accomplish change.

Through the PSBH process, participants learn to take responsibility for their projects and carry them forward. After participants complete their projects, they consider where they might replicate them and what they want to accomplish next. Completing a project does not mean that the participant's responsibility for it is over. A project should be sustained or even expanded. Participants may also use the PSBH process to move in a new direction. The experience of going through the PSBH process and implementing a project changes the lives of participants forever. They will never view the world quite the same way as they did before.

The program grows as participants come back to us and ask if they can be trained as facilitators and join the team in their region. This is how we build regional teams nationwide. I had the pleasure of seeing this growth first hand, as several participants from groups I worked with seized the opportunity to become facilitators. Today, PSBH is a nationwide program in Romania, and over 700 projects have been completed.

Meanwhile, Yanka Tzvetanova invited Paul and me to help with PSBH workshops in Bulgaria. Yanka was a guiding hand for us during the early days of the Romanian program and we were only too happy to help. In March 2006, Yanka and I proposed to DHF that we hold the first workshop to deal specifically with health and social issues affecting children. That month, CHNF cosponsored the first Children's Health Initiative in Pleven, Bulgaria. CHNF and the Pleven Municipality funded 30 projects that resulted from this workshop. Topics included children's health, rehabilitation of disabled children, health promotion, and health education.

Bulgaria, like Romania, became fertile ground for PSBH projects with CHNF. While I realized early on that CHNF would be able to plug into an infrastructure of professionals to implement projects, Paul and I never imagined in our wildest dreams what *we* would accomplish by learning the PSBH methodology ourselves and how that would change *our* thinking! We also did not realize that our interaction with DHF would enable our foundations to work with PSBH participants in two Eastern European countries to do projects that we never would have thought of doing or, without partnership with DHF, would not have been possible. Thus, my second goal in this chapter is to illustrate the synergy that can be achieved when nonprofits use the PSBH methodology in cooperation with DHF. The projects described here were collaborative efforts among CHNF, the

Andrea Foundation in Romania, and the Association for Better Health in Bulgaria, DHF's partner organizations in those two countries.

Computer Clubs for Children

The first project Paul and I initiated in Romania was called Computer Clubs for Children. In 1999, a PSBH participant designed a project to prevent and reduce delinquency in teenagers by teaching boys carpentry and girls cooking and sewing. While the intention of this project was good, it struck us as being too gender specific and limited for the modern world. We wanted to expose Romanian teenagers to computers and teach them life skills that would help them get jobs. In 1999, the Romanian government included in its national agenda the creation of a computer-literate workforce to meet the challenges of a modern society. So the timing was perfect. But we got it wrong initially because we did not practice what we were teaching. We were still learning ourselves. We initially placed the program in an orphanage and hired graduate students recruited from mathematics, economics, and engineering universities as instructors. The financial burden of these salaries proved impractical and we redesigned the program using the PSBH methodology.

The second time around we got it right, and at very little cost. We moved the program into the schools where we would impact our original target population, the orphaned teenage boys and girls, as well as the general school population. Participants would learn how to access the Internet and learn word processing, spreadsheet, and presentation skills that would make them marketable employees. We approached the Ministries of Education and Child Protection, and they helped us arrange a waiver of the usual import tax for donated computers. The hardware we donated either replaced outdated computers or provided the first computers the schools ever had.

The program used "local resources" in the United States and Romania. Donors provided hardware, software, and services. From the United States, AT&T donated 250 Toshiba laptop computers, a Microsoft employee donated Windows and Office software with a matching gift from Microsoft Corporation, Symantec Corporation donated Norton Antivirus and Norton Internet Security software, and Air France allowed me to take the computers as extra luggage while waiving most of the cost. In Romania, the Romanian Education Network, a part of the Ministry of Education, and MobiFon SA, a telecommunications company, provided Internet access. The United Nations Development Program (UNDP) in Romania heard about what we were doing and partnered with us for two years; we welcomed the additional clubs the UNDP opened. Our program grew to 18 clubs in schools all around Romania.

In 2001, Yanka asked us to replicate the Computer Club program in Bulgaria and, together with the Association for Better Health, we opened a club in the Ivan Vasov School in Pleven. The school then applied to Hewlett Packard for more computers, and we received a generous donation of desktop computers. A year or two later, the school built a modern Internet communications laboratory with additional donations from the technology industry. This domino effect is another benefit of the PSBH process—participants demonstrate what they can do on a small scale, thereby allowing them to attract more support and facilitating expansion.

Over the past 10 years, many of the "graduates" of Computer Clubs for Children have gone on to work in computer-related fields for companies like Cisco Systems in Romania, whereas others secured jobs in the business world. Because of the downturn in the economy following 9/11, and the consequent decrease in donations, the program has not grown much since 2002. Amazingly, however, many of the laptop computers we provided are still in use today. We hope to revive this program as the world economy recovers.

Medical Resource Center

At the same time as we were setting up the Computer Clubs for Children, Paul and I received a request to provide medical journals to the Medical College of Dambovita. As an alternative, we donated five laptop computers to establish a Medical Resource Center. This center provides Internet access to the latest medical information for 200 physicians and students and facilitates communication with colleagues both nationally and abroad. In addition, 150 family physicians in Dambovita County are using the computers to maintain medical records on their patients. The center has also enabled the Rotary Club of Tirgoviste, located in the same building, to provide Internet access to its members and to use the computers for their community-based activities.

Dialysis Machines

The Rogosin Institute is a major provider of dialysis services in New York City. Periodically, we replace our dialysis machines with the latest technology and recycle our old equipment. In 2003, the institute, together with CHNF and the Andrea Foundation, coordinated the donation of 35 Baxter dialysis machines to the Ministry of Health in Romania. CHNF paid for the shipping. SofMedica, the Baxter distributor for Romania, cleared the donation through customs, delivered the machines to the recipient institutions identified by the Ministry of Health, and installed them. The Ministry of Health then awarded SofMedica a service contract to maintain these machines. Hospitals in Ramnicu Valcea, Slatina, Braila, Resita, and Turnu Severin are now treating patients with these machines. This donation has permitted these institutions to reduce the number of shifts required to treat their patients and to optimize the dialysis prescription for each patient. This donation was made possible in part by the infrastructure established by the Romanian PSBH program and its accessibility to the appropriate government officials.

Clinical Diagnostic Reagents

During one of my early trips to Bulgaria, Yanka and I visited a diabetes clinic as part of a series of project site visits. While we were there, the clinic ran out of glucose reagent used for determining blood glucose levels. Patients were "crashing" and there was no way to determine their blood glucose levels. One of my responsibilities at The Rogosin Institute is to run a clinical laboratory, and this site visit impelled me to help prevent this from happening in the future. A few months later I found myself sitting across the table from Peter Fitzgerald, the CEO of Randox Laboratories Ltd., a diagnostic company located in Crumlin, in Northern Ireland. I had a simple question for him: "Do you ever have short-dated reagents that you wind up throwing out?" I knew the answer would be yes. Randox defines useful shelf life as 3 months and cannot sell the reagents beyond that time. When Peter asked me with a smile, "What do you have in mind?" I said, "Would it be cheaper to dispose of those reagents or ship them to a central distribution point in, say, Bulgaria?" He simply responded, "We hate waste."

Randox ultimately became a regional resource for Bulgaria. CHNF and the Association for Better Health coordinated the donation of short-dated reagents to four regional medical centers identified by the Ministry of Health in Pleven, Stara Zagora, Varna, and Gabrovo. Gabrovo University Hospital volunteered to be the central receiving facility and delivered donations by truck at their expense to the other regional centers. This program not only made local testing at these centers possible for blood tests that formerly had to be sent out but also freed up funds for other uses. This project plugged into the DHF infrastructure in Bulgaria and was made possible by PSBH participants. The program was active from 2003 to the end of 2005. The hospital system in Bulgaria is currently undergoing extensive reorganization, which has temporarily interrupted the program. We hope to resume the program once the reorganization is complete.

Training Parents of Low Birth-Weight Children

During a PSBH workshop in Pleven in 2004, a physician proposed a project dealing with low birth weight of premature children. Almost all of these children died at home after discharge because their parents did not know how to take care of them. CHNF provided support for the physician and three nurses to train biological and adoptive parents of underweight newborns on the proper care of their babies after discharge from the intensive care unit. The project also provided follow-up care until the children reached normal weight. Parents of 70 children participated in the program, and all of the children survived. Two of the 10 children whose parents refused to participate in the program died after discharge. The project was presented at the Bulgarian National Congress in Neonatology in June 2005 and now serves as a model for neonatal care nationwide. This project was an incredible opportunity to help improve the lives of premature infants and change the standard of care in an entire country at a nominal expense! This is PSBH at its best—effecting change by example and replication.

Heating and Hot Water System for an Orphanage

Although DHF has not established a PSBH program in Moldova, without the PSBH methodology we never would have been able to accomplish the following project. The original heating system in Chisinau was the old Soviet system of steam pipes radiating out underground from the center of the city. Very little heat reached the Municipal Special Children's Orphanage during the cold months of the winter, so the orphanage had no hot water for bathing. My wife and I knew this because when our children first came home, they screamed as we lowered them into the bathtub until their feet touched the warm water, at which point they looked surprised.

Paul and I, together with Neonila Matova, the President of the Charitable Foundation Andrea in Moldova, employed the PSBH methodology to organize a project to install a modern heating and hot water system at the orphanage. Because we could not fund the project ourselves, we designed a project together with the Municipal Department of Children's Rights Protection, the mayor's office in Chisinau, and local businesses. Although Chifa Svetlana, the director of the Department of Children's Rights Protection, credits CHNF and the Charitable Foundation Andrea with being the driving force behind this project, the truth is that she and the mayor's office recruited the other partners that made the project possible. The other indispensable person was Neonila Matova, who oversaw every aspect of the purchasing and construction. As a result of this local commitment, the project evolved into a community action project, and the natural gas-fired heating and hot water system was completed in March 2005.

Conclusion

DHF's PSBH program has profoundly changed the way I view the world and how I think about humanitarian aid in general. DHF provides a methodology for problem solving that trains people to think through the problem they want to solve and to take an intelligent step-by-step approach toward a solution. It places the responsibility for action squarely on the individual. By working together with DHF and the NGOs that host PSBH in Romania and Bulgaria, CHNF has accomplished far more during the past 10 years than we ever imagined was possible. Now CHNF serves as a model for other NGOs. Almost all of our projects cost very little, but all share the common thread of empowering human potential through knowledge. Romania and Bulgaria are only 2 of over 30 countries where DHF continues to unleash human potential around the world.

20

Brazil

Daniel Becker, Kátia Edmundo, Daniella Bonatto,
Geisa Nascimento, Socorro Lima, and Wanda Guimarães

Occupying half of the South American continent, with an area of 8,514,877 sq km, Brazil has a 7,500-km Atlantic Ocean coastline and borders every South American nation except Chile and Ecuador. Its 200 million people of indigenous, African, and European heritages make Brazil a melting pot of humanity. With a median age of 29 years, it is also one of the youngest of the world's populations. Brazilian art, music, literature, and science are all vigorous and well known around the world. The Problem Solving for Better Health program has been in Brazil for almost two decades, and led by its local team, it has become a major force in helping poor communities transform themselves with regard to the health and quality of life of their residents.

The Problem Solving for Better Health® (PSBH®) program was introduced to Brazil in 1991 by the Dreyfus Health Foundation (DHF), in partnership with a group of health professionals associated with the Federal University of Rio de Janeiro (UFRJ). The initial program goal was to improve medical and/or teaching practices at locations in university hospitals and other health services.

Some of the same health professionals were then involved in a second project funded by DHF. Since 1986, the Vila Canoas Health Program has operated the Primary Healthcare Unit in Vila Canoas, a small *favela* (low-income community) of about 2,500 inhabitants in Rio de Janeiro. The unit was initially organized as a traditional health service, focused on a curative approach using medical specialists and nurse technicians. Some of these professionals had participated in PSBH workshops and were able to promote change in the unit as a result. They implemented the family health model by replacing all specialists

Daniel Becker is Chairman of the Board, Kátia Edmundo is a director, Daniella Bonatto is a project coordinator, Geisa Nascimento is a project advisor, Socorro Lima is a director, and Wanda Guimarães is General Coordinator, at the Center for Health Promotion (CEDAPS), Rio de Janeiro. CEDAPS is the Dreyfus Health Foundation's implementing partner in Brazil. Daniel Becker is also PSBH National Coordinator for Brazil and PSBH Regional Coordinator for Latin America.

with a general practitioner, a social worker, and a community health agent. The new team was trained in prevention and health promotion and utilized a comprehensive primary healthcare approach. They consulted the community about its health priorities and subsequently started several group educational activities and initiatives to improve quality of life.

The Vila Canoas team then met with several groups working with similar health models in other Brazilian states. This led to an advocacy process that presented the ideas to the Ministry of Health (MOH). In 1994, the Family Health Program (FHP) was officially launched in six municipalities, with teams composed of one doctor, one nurse, one nurse technician, and six community health agents. Each team was responsible for the health of communities with 4,000–6,000 residents. This approach soon became a success, improving health indicators where it was applied. Fifteen years later, the FHP benefits almost 100 million Brazilians in 5,000 municipalities and has decreased mortality and morbidity in poor areas. Moreover, the program is internationally recognized as the most important, innovative health initiative in Brazil in many years. DHF and PSBH have been an integral part of this historic movement.

In 1993, with the support of DHF, the UFRJ group behind Vila Canoas and the PSBH programs created its own nongovernmental organization, CEDAPS, initially known as the Center for the Development and Support of Health Programs. CEDAPS became DHF's local partner in Brazil, responsible for the implementation of the PSBH program. PSBH became CEDAPS's brand, its main methodology used in all of CEDAPS's programs. Gradually, CEDAPS became involved with health promotion, a rapidly growing area of public health. This provided the organization with a focus and a scientific framework and led to the creation of national as well as international peer groups and networks. In 2000, CEDAPS became known as the Center for Health Promotion, although it kept its original acronym since it was well known in Brazil. Under CEDAPS's coordination, PSBH became recognized in Brazil as a structured social intervention methodology in the public health and health promotion fields.

In 2004, CEDAPS created the Network of Healthy Communities, which comprised 60 community groups and grassroots organizations working together for health promotion. The people who suffered from social problems became part of the solution to the issues. The community-based interventions developed through PSBH addressed problems such as domestic, street, and school violence; lack of cultural and sports activities; HIV/AIDS and other infectious diseases; lack of hygiene and good nutrition; adolescent pregnancy; environmental issues; low self-esteem in youth; smoking; hypertension; diabetes; and limited resources for older adults.

In 2008, CEDAPS celebrated 15 years. PSBH gave CEDAPS its uniqueness through the collaborative and innovative characteristics of its methodology and, through CEDAPS, PSBH became sustainable in Brazil, where it is known as Construção Compartilhada de Soluções em Saúde (Shared Construction of Solutions in Health). PSBH/Shared Construction mobilizes people to solve social problems using available resources, a process that fosters a network of sustainable social projects in communities.

Health Promotion

Health promotion is a process that enables people to increase control over the determinants of their health and thereby improve their quality of life. Health promotion relies on five strategies to reach its goals: (1) healthy public policies—multisectoral, integrated, action-producing public policies and programs that promote health and equity; (2) health-promoting environments—interventions in communities, schools, and workplaces to make them healthier; (3) development of personal skills—expansion of knowledge and skills, and encouragement of participation by, and empowerment of, individuals to seek better health conditions; (4) support for community action—community empowerment, mobilization, and participation; and (5) restructuring of health systems—a new model of care with emphasis on prevention activities and promoting partnerships with community groups to tackle health and social problems and enhance health-promoting factors (World Health Organization, 1986).

The action of civil society organizations, such as CEDAPS, is essential for most of the aforementioned strategies. The work developed by CEDAPS is based on the belief that the community is the core of social transformation and that its people are the best resources for problem solving. Therefore, it is crucial to create opportunities to build their potential and to promote their participation and interaction with civil society and public organizations.

The PSBH program has proven to be an effective tool for health promotion. It contributes to building individual and group potential, strengthens the mobilization and participation of social players, fights immobility, and enables change in communities and organizations. PSBH/Shared Construction has enabled communities to assert their needs and obtain better resources.

Cycles of Shared Construction of Solutions in Health

The PSBH methodology is a process that includes activities such as seminars and workshops for the purpose of creating local action plans. In Brazil, this process is called a cycle. The four phases of a cycle are (1) preseminar (including identification of institutional partnerships and selection of workshop participants and issues to be addressed), (2) workshop (including diagnosis of the community and capacity building of individual or group participants in specific themes), (3) seminar (including development of action plans), and (4) follow-up (including site visits conducted by CEDAPS staff, meetings, and networking). The experiences accumulated throughout the 15 years of existence of CEDAPS and 17 years of existence of PSBH in Brazil have resulted in several different categories of cycles. Cycles may complement each other, and often two or more work together. The next few sections of this chapter describe the various cycles.

Open Cycle

The first phase of PSBH in Brazil was characterized by open cycles. These were essential for the development of a network of participants involved in local action in Rio de Janeiro and in the Santos region. Individuals representing a cross section of society, and from varied locations and professions, were selected to participate in this network for social change.

Between 1994 and 2001, 10 open cycles were conducted with a total of 281 projects developed addressing issues such as the environment, community organization, children's health, chronic diseases, the reorganization of health services, mental health, drug abuse, sexually transmitted disease (STD)/AIDS, violence, and poor education. Less than 50% of these projects were completed due to a fragmented follow-up and monitoring process. As a result, a field staff member was recruited to provide direct support, systematization, and collection of information for the duration of the projects. A database and follow-up materials were developed as well.

Territory-Based Cycle (PSBH Initiative)

The CEDAPS team launched the Problem Solving for Better Health Initiative™ (PSBHI™) program, or territory-based cycle, in Brazil using techniques and ideas from international programs like the World Health Organization's Healthy Cities and Communities. The PSBHI process includes regional mobilization, creation of a local council to co-manage the initiative, promotion of partnerships, and a full collaborative community meeting. This approach was introduced to the DHF network in several Latin American countries.

The territory-based cycle catalyzed growth within CEDAPS and PSBH in Brazil. Two regional initiatives—the Santa Cruz Initiative (SCI) and the Vila Paciência Initiative (VPI)—were developed and produced significant local change in the participating communities. The lessons learned guided several other PSBH cycles. CEDAPS became a leader in the health promotion and local development fields, collaborating with a number of international initiatives. These partnerships led to the formation of the Network of Healthy Communities, possibly the most important result of PSBH in Brazil to date.

The SCI (2000–2002) and VPI (2002–2004) resulted in a total of 104 action plans to address various issues, such as education, employment, women's health, housing, sanitation, transportation, and STD/AIDS prevention. The territory-based approach of the initiatives brings new elements into the discussion of ethics and citizenship to address social exclusion. Thus, the SCI and VPI reinforce the idea of individual and collective empowerment by enhancing the ability of local residents to promote social change.

The SCI was the first initiative with the sponsorship of DHF and the collaboration of Rio de Janeiro's City Hall. It became the pilot for Rio's Healthy City program. Its goal was to promote health and foster local development in Santa Cruz. Twenty-one action plans were completed, directly benefiting more than 3,000 people and indirectly over 8,000. Activities included lectures on STDs and contraceptive methods; improvement of pre- and postnatal care; literacy workshops; art, dance, and cooking lessons to decrease school dropout rates and violence; identification of employment opportunities and job-skills training; craft workshops and fabric painting for income generation; fundraising events for community revitalization projects, featuring local artists and authors; and events for people with disabilities.

Based on the positive results of the SCI, the local council that co-managed the initiative and CEDAPS focused their efforts on a single community, Favela do Aço, or Vila Paciência, the poorest and most violent *favela* in the region. This initiative, VPI, produced 25 action plans carried out by residents, benefiting more than 8,000 people in the community. Some actions included surveying and renovating homes with structural problems; cleaning campaigns to reduce garbage in vacant lots and to unclog the sewage system; promoting inexpensive, nutritional foods; creating a community vegetable garden; implementing weekly educational and recreational programs for children; screening for high blood pressure; and conducting STD/AIDS prevention activities (Figure 20.1).

Fifteen young residents were trained in construction, which opened new job opportunities for them. Several made improvements in their homes and found work in their community. As a group, they built a kitchen to prepare food for workers and children and sell to local businesses. Training in children's activities was provided to 16 adolescents, and all of them began volunteering in the community. Each participating adolescent bonded with the group and reported changes in their personal lives, including improved relationships with their families and children.

Theme-Based Cycle

Focusing on a specific topic, such as AIDS prevention, sexual and reproductive health, or tuberculosis (TB), theme-based cycles have proven to be valuable in the intervention process. Projects are connected by the identified health or social issue, and the workshops usually include capacity building to strengthen the ability of the participants to create effective change in their communities. Some of these projects produced publications such as the *Caderno de Melhores Praticás* (*Notebook of best practices*; Bonatto, Becker, Edmundo, & Bittencourt, 2003). Six theme-based cycles were carried out between 1999 and 2008.

Four cycles focused on STD prevention. Two of these were conducted with leaders in *favelas* to develop a plan to fight the AIDS epidemic in their communities. These cycles resulted in 51 action plans. Despite limited resources, the leaders developed creative strategies and engaged a large number of residents, increasing awareness and expanding access to information and materials in low-income communities. The involvement

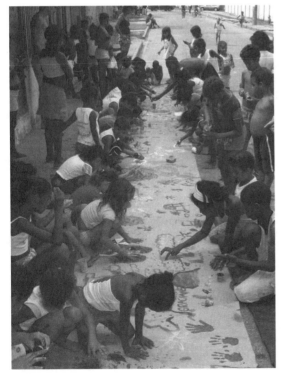

FIGURE 20.1 Children participate in a Problem Solving for Better Health project on health awareness in the *favela* Vila Paciência, Rio de Janeiro.

of community leaders in HIV prevention, creating strategies with their own ideas and resources, was the first step toward the establishment of the Network of Communities in the Fight against AIDS. This, in turn, was the initial step in the creation of the Network of Healthy Communities and the establishment of a close relationship between CEDAPS and the National HIV/AIDS program of the MOH. As a result of this experience, CEDAPS published the book *Idéias d'Agente* (*Our ideas*; Edmundo, Fonseca, & Bittencourt, 2003), describing the creative strategies utilized.

In 2008, a TB cycle promoted mobilization in the fight against the disease in low-income communities. Community organizations developed 25 action plans focused on activism, social control, discrimination, and prejudice. They concentrated on access to treatment, better housing conditions, and education. The cycle was carried out with financial support from the Stop TB Partnership, an initiative created by the World Health Organization to eliminate TB worldwide. The process included educational activities about transmission, treatment, and prevention and reached approximately 5,000 people.

The final theme-based cycle, organized in partnership with the Ford Foundation, focused on sexual and reproductive health and targeted *favelas* and outskirts of Brazilian urban centers. The cycle began in 2008 in Rio de Janeiro, Goiânia, Salvador, Belo Horizonte, and João Pessoa. Several workshops and a seminar were held, resulting in 12 action plans developed by community leaders. Eight Centers for the Promotion of Sexual and Reproductive Health were created in Rio de Janeiro. Project activities included condom distribution, workshops on sexual and reproductive health, lectures in schools, and participation in the District Health Council. More than 1,500 people directly benefited from the activities in this cycle.

Focal Cycle

Focal cycles generate action among specific social groups, such as youth or health professionals, increasing the groups' potential as agents of change. These cycles mobilize entire organizations or institutions, such as schools or health units, to improve quality, performance, and community participation. To date, the programs developed in the focal cycles have produced the highest completion rates of PSBH projects and have had a significant impact on the organizations and communities involved.

Twenty-four focal cycles occurred between 2001 and 2008, based on partnerships with public health and education programs. One of the most successful topics of these cycles is youth empowerment. The main goal is to transform youth to become a resource for the development of communities, instead of a risk group. The young developed 253 projects focusing on drug prevention, after-school tutoring, and garbage collection.

For example, the "Young Energy" project, developed in partnership with a large electricity company, Ampla, aimed to promote youth mobilization and increase the self-esteem of participants in poor territories served by the company. The youth created 69 action plans on health promotion and substance abuse prevention. Some interesting results were the increased communication between adolescents and teachers, coordination with local businesses, and high levels of participation in the projects.

Another important program was health-promoting schools, in partnership with the Municipal Secretaries of Health and Education in Rio de Janeiro. Results included demonstrated improvement in school performance; better student–teacher relationships; and more interaction among health units, schools, and communities. The programs involved 9,785 students, 863 teachers, and 4,714 families. The results of these projects led to a book, *Health promoting schools in action* (Secretaria Municipal de Saúde & CEDAPS, 2008).

Another cycle was developed to support the FHP, a massive, national, primary healthcare program serving 100 million people in Brazil. This cycle was executed in partnership with the Municipal Secretary of Health of Rio de Janeiro and resulted in 88 action plans. The goal of this cycle was to increase locally planned preventive and health promotion action in partnership with communities. Project results in the Campo Grande district of Rio included job training and employment opportunities; literacy courses; a community library; a research foundation partnership to suppress zoonoses; cleaning of vacant lots and installation of trash bins; workshops on STDs and AIDS, sexuality, and homosexuality; and increased participation in the "Theater of the Oppressed," a form of participatory theater that educates and gives voice to those living in poor conditions.

Organizational Cycle

Organizational cycles contribute to preexisting programs developed by other institutions, such as public agencies, private companies, universities, and foundations. PSBH increases participation in and ownership of the various stakeholders. These cycles strengthen the programs and partnerships, increasing the impact of both.

Two such cycles contributed to Health and Prevention in Schools, a national program created to consolidate a public policy of prevention and health promotion in schools and to promote discussions between government and civil society organizations and integration of the health-education sectors. The goal of the program is to reduce HIV, STDs, and teen pregnancy among Brazilian youth and young adults.

Yet another program in this cycle, involving the states of Goiás, Paraíba, and Minas Gerais, focused on Black women's movement organizations in partnership with the Ford Foundation. This organizational program strengthened these groups by improving their financial and technical management. Some of the outcomes included better organization management, training in public speaking, partnerships with universities, and teaching PSBH/Shared Construction methodology to other women's groups.

Interorganizational Cooperation Cycle

Interorganizational cooperation promotes the exchange of experiences between CEDAPS and partner organizations by recruiting and training facilitators in the PSBH/Shared Construction methodology. Such cooperation promotes the replication of PSBH/Shared Construction throughout Brazil, follow-up of action plans, and the dissemination of the Network of Healthy Communities.

Results

Cumulatively, more than 1,300 people have been trained in project development as a result of PSBH/Shared Construction. More than 50,000 people have benefited directly from the projects; an estimated 400,000 benefited indirectly. Projects have contributed to promoting health in various settings—schools, health units and programs, communities, and groups. The projects have produced a change in individual and collective attitudes toward participation, ownership, and responsibility. PSBH/Shared Construction has made valuable contributions to the fields of HIV/AIDS prevention; health promotion; primary healthcare; school health; grassroots institutional development; youth empowerment; and local development, in particular the creation of the Network of Healthy Communities.

Final Considerations

PSBH/Shared Construction methodology promotes the development of local solutions to local problems, utilizing the resources, knowledge, and strength of the people who suffer from the problems. This is extraordinarily powerful and carries huge potential for social change, mostly because of the indirect and intangible effect of increased self-esteem, participation, and social capital—in short, individual and collective empowerment. Individual, isolated actions do not solve all the problems, but they are a crucial start. Many of the initial project activities have led to collective community action and policy impact.

As mentioned earlier, the most important result of PSBH in Brazil is probably the creation of the Network of Healthy Communities, based on the World Health Organization's "Healthy Cities" program. On May 10, 2004, in the city of Rio de Janeiro, more than 60 communities and the CEDAPS launched this movement in a public ceremony with the presence of the directors of DHF. The goals of the network, which has a membership of over 150 communities, are to: (1) strengthen and empower each community through capacity building, action plans, and sharing of experiences and opportunities; (2) improve the ability of communities to defend their right to health and negotiate programs and healthy public policies; and (3) increase the visibility of the positive and healthy actions conducted by low-income communities to decrease the gap between *favelas* and the city. The Network of Healthy Communities has drawn national and international attention. Articles about the network have been published in book chapters and Brazilian and international public health journals.

CEDAPS acts as a support system, channeling its resources, projects, and institutional partnerships to the Network of Healthy Communities. Through PSBH, the network increases the ability of organizations to plan strategically and develop local action, helps organizations produce educational material and activities, articulates integrated actions to its members, promotes partnerships, strengthens the network to negotiate with the government and the private sector, and increases the visibility of the work and the causes of the movement.

After 17 years, the PSBH/Shared Construction methodology is recognized as a practical process of planning that contributes directly to the increase of social participation and empowerment of communities in the promotion of health, equity, and quality of life in Brazilian society. We all seek utopia—an integrated, equitable, and healthy society. As Mário Quintana (1951), a Brazilian poet, said, "If things are unreachable … there is no reason not to want them. … How sad the paths, if not for the presence of magic stars" (p. 213). The PSBH/Shared Construction of Solutions in Health program wants utopia in Brazil and will continue to work to achieve it.

References

Bonatto, D., Becker, D., Edmundo, K., & Bittencourt, D. (2003). *Caderno de melhores práticas* [Notebook of best practices]. Rio de Janeiro, Brazil: Centro de Promoção da Saúde.

Edmundo, K., Fonseca, V., & Bittencourt, D. (2003). *Idéias d'agente: Catálogo de estratégias comunitárias de prevenção das DST/AIDS* [Our ideas: Catalog of community strategies for the prevention of STD/AIDS]. Rio de Janeiro, Brazil: Centro de Promoção da Saúde.

Quintana, M. (1951). *Espelho mágico* [Magic mirror]. Porto Alegre, Brazil: Editora do Globo.

Secretaria Municipal de Saúde & Centro de Promoção da Saúde. (2008). *Escolas promotoras de saúde em ação: Construção compartilhada de soluções locais nas escolas promotoras de saúde do município do Rio de Janeiro* [Health promoting schools in action: Shared construction of local solutions in the health promoting schools of the municipality of Rio de Janeiro]. Rio de Janeiro, Brazil: Municipal Secretary of Health.

World Health Organization. (1986). Ottawa charter for health promotion. Geneva, Switzerland: Author.

21

Dominican Republic

Adelaida Oreste

The Dominican Republic occupies the eastern two-thirds of the island of Hispaniola in the Caribbean Sea and shares its western border with Haiti. It is home to 9.6 million people whose lineages reflect their history and the mixing of cultures that has taken place on the island since Christopher Columbus landed there in 1492. The Hispanic influence is strong, of course, but immigrants from East Asia, France, Italy, England, Germany, and the Middle East, as well as people who originally came as slaves from Africa, have enriched the human mix. Problem Solving for Better Health has taken root among communities across the country. With a median population age of 25 years and a desire to improve health and quality of life for all its people, the Dominican Republic has a bright future.

The first meeting between the Dreyfus Health Foundation (DHF) and the Dominican Republic Department of State for Public Health and Social Assistance (SESPAS) was held in 1998 through the auspices of the Directorate of Human Resources training program. Delia Collado, Program Coordinator for Latin America and the Caribbean at DHF, worked with me to develop a partnership between DHF and the Center for Integral Health and Development (CISADE).

Established in 1997, CISADE is a private, nonprofit organization dedicated to social work in the areas of health, education, gender equality, and community participation. The organization's mission is to design, promote, and implement health policies, strategies, and programs and address the social, economic, and cultural determinants that influence quality of life. The goal is to improve the well-being of the most vulnerable

Adelaida Oreste is President of the Center for Integral Health and Development (CISADE), the Dreyfus Health Foundation's implementing partner in the Dominican Republic. She is also Problem Solving for Better Health National Coordinator for the Dominican Republic.

populations, with a vision to become a great technical and ethical organization, building processes and centers that promote health, gender equality, and communitywide participation among the citizens of the Dominican Republic.

After meeting with DHF personnel and learning about Problem Solving for Better Health® (PSBH®), CISADE organized the first workshop presenting PSBH to various nongovernmental organizations (NGOs), health committees, and hospital directors. To implement PSBH, we formed a coordination committee of representatives from nine organizations and institutions, including NGOs, health programs, and hospitals. The workshop was held in February 1999, less than a year after our initial meeting. Health professionals, local health leaders, committee representatives, and community social program directors attended.

We conducted one PSBH workshop every year thereafter. Over 300 people participated in eight workshops, including health professionals, educators, community leaders, and adolescents. In addition, we hosted 115 trainings for specific groups: university teachers, students, doctors, and health promoters. Follow-up workshops were also held to evaluate the projects implemented.

One thousand projects were ultimately developed. Seventy percent of them were completed, with 85% of those achieving a positive impact in the communities. As a result, we have been able to develop solid, sustainable projects with various public and private leaders. In the following section I highlight one of the most successful.

Nutrition Education

"Prevention and Management of Malnutrition" was one of the most successful projects developed by CISADE in the Dominican Republic. It helped 1,765 children who had some degree of malnutrition, as well as 23 pregnant women who had serious nutritional deficiency, putting their unborn children at risk. Fifty-six elderly people also received aid, including many who are homeless and without families to care for them.

The goal of this project was to improve the nutrition of infants, children, pregnant women, and senior citizens through health education and the provision of vitamins and nutrient-fortified food. It was implemented in 2007 in marginalized neighborhoods in Villa Central, Barahona (old Batey Central, Barahona), Matamamon-La Victoria of the Municipality of Santo Domingo North, and Farallones del Mirador Sur-Ensanche La Paz. The project was initially developed to directly benefit a total of 1,765 infants, children younger than 13 years, pregnant women, and senior citizens, but ultimately approximately 8,825 people benefited either directly or indirectly.

All the children were treated for parasites before receiving vitamins. They were also weighed, measured, and photographed to establish a baseline of reference for their follow-up and management each month. The measurements and images document the improvement achieved over the course of the project.

Principal components of the project included nutrition education courses and workshops; provision of nutrient-fortified food, multivitamins, and milk; and training in basic hygiene and health. During educational meetings and workshops the project leaders placed great emphasis on the adequate management and utilization of nutrients. They also dispelled taboos and myths about certain nutrients that had caused some people to stop taking them. Eighty percent of the children's parents participated, as well as pregnant women and other mothers from the community.

During the implementation phase, the project leaders relied on the sponsorship and coordination of institutions, organizations, and individuals, including the Department of Nutrition (SESPAS); the Department of Social Assistance (SESPAS); Batey Relief-BRA Dominicana; the president of CISADE; student health promoters, known as "Guardians for Life"; the Association for the Development of Batey Central and Surrounding Areas; Primary Healthcare Units (UNAP); ANA Ima Tejeda public school; and local doctors, nurses, health promoters, and health educators. As a result of this nutrition project, approximately 900 parents have better knowledge of the importance of nutrition for normal development in their children and their families. The pregnant women involved had improved nutritional status, and 18 of them experienced a normal pregnancy without complications and delivered healthy children with normal birth weights. Further, the senior citizens received donations of milk and nutrient-fortified foods that have improved their health. This nutrition project is just one example of many successful initiatives led by CISADE in cooperation with DHF.

Conclusion

CISADE must achieve multisectoral sustainability and implementation on a broad scale to continue providing education, good nutrition, and health services to the most vulnerable people. We strive to raise awareness because no human being should suffer from malnutrition due to social, economic, or cultural inequality. Despite limited financial resources, we remain committed to helping people and their communities develop their potential to create a better quality of life, because working for health is working for life.

22

El Salvador

Ignacio Paniagua Castro and Mauricio Lozano

A country of mountains, plains, and forestland, El Salvador is bordered by Guatemala, Honduras, and the Pacific Ocean. It is the smallest country of Central America, with a land area of 21,041 sq km and a population of approximately 6 million. Active volcanoes, geological instability of the Pacific Rim, and hurricanes have played a significant role in the country's history. The lineage of El Salvador's citizens represents a mixing of the indigenous population with Spanish settlers to produce the largely homogeneous population of today. Problem Solving for Better Health entered the country just as the strife of El Salvador's 20-year civil war ended in 1992. The program has expanded to become part of, and enhanced by, the ongoing transformation of the country by the Salvadorians themselves.

In response to El Salvador's civil war (1980–1992), the Médicos Salvadoreños para la Responsabilidad Social (Salvadoran Physicians for Social Responsibility [MESARES]) was founded in 1989 to develop "a medical program to educate physicians, health workers and students, mobilizing health resources at a national level and taking active part in regional movements against small arms proliferation, misuse and the impact on human suffering" (Paniagua, Crespin, Guardado, & Mauricio, 2005, p. 198). The association is an affiliate in El Salvador of the International Physicians for the Prevention of Nuclear War. As a public health organization, MESARES "depends on data about the nature of events and the characteristics of those most susceptible" (Paniagua, Crespin, Guardado, & Mauricio, 2005, p. 192). It conducts studies to examine the effects of firearm violence in El Salvador and develop recommendations for policy change.

In 1992, Dr. Charlie Clement, an American doctor and a member of Physicians for Social Responsibility, a nonprofit organization in the United States dedicated to preventing

Ignacio Paniagua Castro is President of Salvadoran Physicians for Social Responsibility (MESARES), the Dreyfus Health Foundation's implementing partner in El Salvador, and Problem Solving for Better Health National Coordinator for El Salvador. Mauricio Lozano is Vice President of MESARES and Communications for Better Health National Coordinator for El Salvador.

nuclear war and reversing global warming, introduced MESARES to Dr. Barry H. Smith, Director of the Dreyfus Health Foundation (DHF). In 1993, DHF and MESARES launched the Problem Solving for Better Health® (PSBH®) program in El Salvador. MESARES designated SOLPROMESA, "Promise of the Sun," as the Spanish acronym for Problem Solving for Better Health (*SOL*ucionando *PRO*blemas para *ME*jor *SA*lud).

Problem Solving for Better Health in El Salvador

In El Salvador, 45–60 participants from different social and professional backgrounds attend a 3-day PSBH workshop, assisted by six facilitators and two members of the MESARES team. The participants agree to attend and participate in all workshop activities, which include lectures, small group discussions, and plenary sessions. Each participant develops an action plan and commits to implementing it. The MESARES team and local institution officers organize ongoing project support that includes site visits and follow-up meetings to review progress and obstacles encountered. The participants evaluate their own projects, and the MESARES Executive Board makes a further evaluation to determine levels of participation, progress, and impact. The board is the link between communities, workshop participants, and other institutions.

Participation is the key component of the PSBH process. Participants make a commitment to their community; by defining a local health problem they assume responsibility for implementing a solution, while seeking support and involvement from their peers, parents, community leaders, and members of local governmental and nongovernmental organizations. PSBH encourages involvement of the beneficiaries themselves and gives participants the independence to make decisions, follow up on their projects, and regularly evaluate them. Projects developed and implemented in communities have changed attitudes of community members because they have been carried out by actual residents and not external agents. Participants are especially enthusiastic about the PSBH process when they learn that they are part of a global effort to improve the health and well-being of individuals and communities.

El Balsamo

In 2002, MESARES initiated a PSBH program in the El Balsamo Microregion, an area that was open to the work of a significant number of both public and private organizations interested in local development. MESARES' mission was to recruit community residents, particularly young people, to bring about positive change through committed participation, organization, and communication with local government and nongovernment organizations looking for an effective influence on the determinants of health. MESARES included people already in leadership positions, such as teachers and officers from social, religious, and health organizations, to act as liaisons with these organizations.

The El Balsamo communities to which MESARES ultimately brought the PSBH program are municipalities in the departments of La Libertad (Colon, Comosagua, Jayaque, Sacacoyo, Talnique, Tepecoyo) and Sonsonate (Armenia). The El Balsamo Microregion is an area of 63,121 inhabitants, with 79% residing in rural areas and 21% in urban areas.

Forty-seven percent of the population lives below the poverty line, with 27% in extreme poverty. Ninety-two percent of the people living in rural homes have no drinking water or waste disposal and have difficult access to health facilities. The major economic activity in the area is agriculture, mostly seasonal coffee harvesting. The unemployment rate is 13%, and only 11% of households receive a remittance. Half the population is younger than 25 years of age, and half the young people do not attend school. Those who do, attend only for an average of 3 years, and the literacy rate is 23%. The average number of family members is 4.4 individuals, and in 31% of the homes a woman is the head of the household.

After meetings with communities in the El Balsamo region to confirm their motivation, interest, and willingness to volunteer, MESARES staff concluded that the residents' cognition was based on life experiences, practical approaches such as "learning while working," and therefore, community members were more responsive to effective action than to abstract ideas. Their concept of health was defined from a holistic view that linked it with social and economic determinants. To accomplish its mission to involve communities in improving their own well-being, MESARES would use a dynamic tool—PSBH, a methodology that acknowledges the value of the individual; promotes self-esteem; strives for excellence while using available resources; and encourages sustainable, immediate action.

MESARES realized that it would be a challenge to develop an effective, sustainable level of community participation in the El Balsamo Microregion (Figure 22.1). Some of the difficulties encountered included limited access to remote work areas; demand from the communities for urgent needs due to social and economic conditions and natural disasters; nepotism; biased political favors and political polarization; frustration linked to previous failed health projects; lack of sustainability for previous projects due to insufficient continued support and financing; and divisiveness in and disorganization of governmental and nongovernmental institutions, leading to a loss and waste of resources.

The Program

In August 2002, MESARES launched the El Balsamo program at a Problem Solving for Better Health Initiative™ workshop in the municipality of Jayaque. The goals for the region included four workshops with PSBH training for 40 adult and 150 youth leaders from five communities, and implementation of 50 Better Health projects, covering basic sanitation, nutrition, communicable disease treatment and prevention, reproductive health, management of the effects of natural disasters, and protection of the environment. In addition, 6 health professionals and 12 lay facilitators would be trained to teach the PSBH methodology, 5 potential liaisons to governmental and nongovernmental organizations would be identified, and 40 community teams would be established to develop sustainable actions. Follow-up meetings and field visits would take place for 2 years following each workshop.

Another objective was to implement a system for responding to natural disasters, specifically earthquakes, as well as addressing the issues of crime, violence, and drug use. In January and February 2001, earthquakes destroyed 8,037 houses (80% of the villages). The relief work in the Jayaque municipality after the earthquakes led MESARES to conduct a

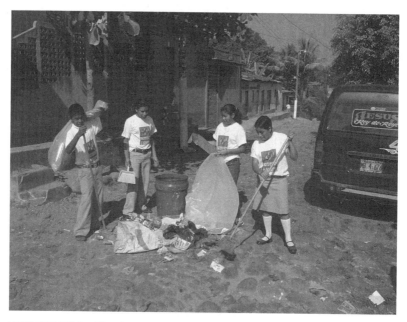

FIGURE 22.1   Youth participate in a community clean-up project in the El
Balsamo Microregion.

PSBH workshop for those affected. The follow-up activities for projects developed at the
workshop enabled the association to establish relationships with the other organizations
and local leaders working in the region. MESARES developed a plan to deal with natural disasters by involving teams of community residents to work with local officers to
achieve a safer environment and prevent crime and drug abuse. In addition, a psychologist was hired to counsel community members.

MESARES gained prestige for using the PSBH method to create orderly collaboration
among people solving chronic problems and tackling emergencies. The association was
invited to participate with a group of institutions in a joint effort to conduct a diagnosis of the social problems in the region, a study that would serve as a basis for strategic
planning for 5 years. As a result, MESARES established an alliance for local sustainable
development in the El Balsamo Microregion.

Through PSBH workshops held during the first 5 years of the program, young leaders in the El Balsamo Microregion became health promoters who have managed and led
sustainable and comprehensive local development projects for their communities using
available resources, particularly human resources. One hundred leaders younger than
20 years of age and 70 adults generated more than 100 action plans impacting health
and quality of life. Successfully completed and currently active projects have focused on
sanitation and protection of the environment, prevention of infectious diseases, mitiga-
tion of the effects of natural disasters and community safety, mental health, at-risk youth,
recreation and sports, and employment. The projects have directly benefited almost 2,000
people and have indirectly benefited more than 8,000.

MESARES strengthened project implementation by establishing Community Health
Committees in each town composed of project leaders who work together as a team

and collaborate with local organizations that can provide information, resources, and training.

Lessons Learned

Action is the best way to motivate young people to participate and work together, and young people, in turn, can motivate community members to get involved in problem solving. Lack of self-esteem, lack of time, lack of trust from adults, and fear of failure are barriers to encouraging young people to participate. With their enthusiasm, creativity, and a natural inclination to bond socially, young people can be effective by working collaboratively with adults who can provide leadership and support. When a community develops a collaborative approach to solving health and social problems, personal, political, and economic ambitions are left behind. Although the grassroots approach overcomes differences, it is necessary for leaders and local authorities to share the aims of unity and consensus as well. Frequent workshops and overemphasis of theoretical topics are not effective in training youth. Success begins with taking action immediately and including technical knowledge, motivation, leadership, and other skills, as the action requires. Many government programs include community participation as a strategy but lack a methodology to make it work. PSBH gives all people a tool and a voice, and with these, the young people of the El Balsamo Microregion have become effective resources for problem solving in their communities.

Reference

Paniagua, I., Crespin, E., Guardado, A., & Mauricio, A. (2005). Wounds caused by firearms in El Salvador, 2003–2004: Epidemiological issues. *Medicine, Conflict and Survival, 21*(3), 191–198.

23

Guyana

Aptie Sookoo

Located in the northeastern corner of South America, Guyana is bordered by Venezuela, Brazil, Suriname, and the Atlantic Ocean. With a history that included the British, it is the only English-speaking country in Latin America. Its people are a broad mix of Amerindians, Afro-Guyanese, East Indians, Chinese, and Portuguese lineages, making the country and its culture one of the most diverse in the world. Most of the population of 800,000 lives along the Atlantic coast. Agriculture and rich natural resources, such as bauxite and gold, have defined the economy. The Problem Solving for Better Health program has been pleased to be part of the nation's progress toward better health and quality of life since 1992.

Problem Solving for Better Health in Guyana

A collaborative initiative between the University of Guyana, the University of Texas Medical Branch (UTMB) at Galveston, and the Dreyfus Health Foundation (DHF) introduced Problem Solving for Better Health® (PSBH®) to Guyana in May 1992. International facilitators from Brazil, Ghana, Guyana, and the United States guided 80 participants through the PSBH process during a 3-day workshop. Of those 80 participants, 24 were from St. Lucia, Grenada, Dominica, and Anguilla; they were in Guyana to also attend a 1-month residential course, Issues in Community Health Management. The course was sponsored by UTMB, the Pan American Health Organization/World Health Organization, DHF, the Guyana Sugar Corporation, and the Guyana Mining Enterprise. The PSBH workshop was intended to (1) identify problems in critical areas of the Guyanese health system, (2) prioritize the problems, (3) develop approaches to problem resolution, and (4) share possible solutions.

Aptie Sookoo is Public Health Inspector for Hastings & Prince Edward Counties Health Unit, Ontario, Canada; he was Problem Solving for Better Health National Coordinator for Guyana from 1996 to 2002.

I became involved in PSBH as a participant at the initial workshop. At the time, I was a public health inspector employed by the Regional Democratic Council of Cuyuni/ Mazaruni (Region Seven). I was excited to participate because I felt the workshop would be an opportunity for training and acquisition of skills that would enable me to solve community health problems. At the workshop, I developed a project to address the fact that many children younger than 5 years of age were repeatedly treated at the local hospital in Bartica for diarrhea.

Geraldine Maison-Halls, the first PSBH National Coordinator for Guyana as of June 1992, and others, including Vonna Lou Caleb, a succeeding National Coordinator, provided the foundation for the expansion of the PSBH program. In July 1996, after obtaining a degree in public health, I was appointed the National Coordinator, a position I held until I immigrated to Canada in September 2002. Omar Khan succeeded me, and the current National Coordinator is Ismay Murray.

Traditionally, PSBH programs have included international facilitators along with national facilitators at workshops. This exchange provides valuable opportunities for sharing experiences with PSBH and learning how similar problems are solved in different parts of the world. While recognizing the value of international facilitators, the Guyana program focused on building the capacity of local facilitators who understood the local healthcare delivery system and were in a good position to advise project leaders on what works within Guyana.

We held a monthly facilitators' meeting at the University of Guyana to plan for the future and obtain feedback on the development of community projects. We mailed copies of the DHF newsletter *Connections* regularly, not only to program participants, facilitators, and partners, but also to all government ministries. Abstracts from completed projects on topical health issues were published in the *Health Interaction Newsletter*, a Guyanese publication of the DHF's Communications for Better Health® program.

The PSBH program in Guyana developed several partnerships with organizations that have diverse roles in the delivery of health services. The partner organizations include the Guyana Sugar Corporation; the Guyana Nurses Association; the National Insurance Scheme; the Democratic Council for Region Two (Pomeroon/Supernaam); the Department of Education for Region Three (Essequibo Islands/West Demerara); the Departments of Health for Regions Three, Four (Demerara/Mahaica Subregion), and Ten (Upper Demerara/ Berbice); the Ptolemy Reid Rehabilitation Centre; the Georgetown Public Hospital; the Guyana Sewage and Water Works; and the Guyana Responsible Parenthood Association. Many PSBH projects have been implemented in cooperation with these partners.

Local Health Projects

The PSBH approach is to identify community health problems that do not require extensive resources to solve. This means that participants have to look carefully into their communities for the solutions to those issues. Prior to a workshop, participants are asked to identify at least two problems in their community and bring these ideas to the training session. The following projects are examples of problems that were solved with very little funding.

June Bair's project, "Establishing a Referral System between Help and Shelter and the Georgetown Public Hospital," was a successful initiative that addressed issues faced by abused women. Help and Shelter, a local nongovernmental organization dedicated to preventing domestic and sexual violence and child abuse, designated a specific room at the shelter for the initial examinations of abused women as part of the project plan of action. These efforts resulted in increased privacy for the women and faster turnaround time for all referrals to the hospital. This project continues to be supported by the administration and staff of the hospital.

Mary Williams, the councilor for Region Two, and her teammate implemented the project "Control of Chigger Fleas in the Mainstay/Whyaka Community," a campaign to control chigger flea infestations with malathion, a low-toxicity, low-cost insecticide. Chigger fleas burrow into the skin, usually of the foot, causing itching followed by pain. Severe or multiple bites can lead to secondary infection, including bacteremia, tetanus, or gas gangrene. This project resulted in an increase in school attendance and a greater focus on learning as a result of less itching, pain, and infection among students.

A project that I implemented, "Assessing Diarrheal Protective Behavior in a Hinterland Community in Guyana," identified some of the misconceptions the staff at the Bartica Hospital had about how diarrhea was managed in the home. I conducted a study that found families were reusing unwashed dippers to take water from home containers for drinking. The contaminated water given to infants and children younger than 5 years of age accounted for a significant number of diarrhea cases in this age group. As a result of this project, the hospital staff instituted a health education campaign at the hospital on diarrheal disease control, emphasizing the use of clean and protected dippers. In addition, the hospital staff became more aggressive in promoting the use of oral rehydration salts as an effective means of managing childhood diarrhea in the home.

Community Health Worker Annette London's project, "Increase Childhood Immunization Among Children in Kaneville and Grove, East Bank Demerara," led to a change in the immunization schedule at the Grove Health Centre to accommodate working parents who often are not able to bring their children to the immunization clinics during the scheduled times. In addition, to deliver much-needed immunization against preventable childhood illness to as many children as possible in the two communities, the project leaders instituted a procedure for "house calls" for families that could not get to the health center at any time.

A project led by Environmental Health Assistant Royann Marques and others, "Promoting Increased Disinfection of Drinking Water at the Home Level in an Area of Grove, East Bank Demerara," resulted in a greater awareness by the community of the relationship between water quality and diarrheal episodes. The project leaders advised community members that protecting their plumbing from damage and their water from contamination were equally as important as the integrity of the water distribution system. Understanding that adults learn better by doing, the leaders proposed an interactive demonstration of treating water with sodium hypochlorite and bringing water to a rolling boil for 1 minute to make it safe for consumption. Given by healthcare providers at the Grove Health Centre, the demonstration was significant in educating the community.

Yvonne Walcott, a senior nurse, and Brynece Browne, a Ministry of Health employee, implemented the project "Improving Documentation of Nursing Notes in the Male Medical Ward at the Georgetown Public Hospital." This project influenced institutional care at the hospital by reducing the length of stay in the ward. The two project leaders instructed hospital nursing staff on the importance of taking accurate notes to enable the physicians to make sound decisions in managing the illnesses of their patients. The staff nurses soon recognized their critical role in the entire process of disease management and healing. The administration and staff at the hospital are sustaining this project.

The results of all the PSBH projects are shared with health workers who are responsible for delivering health services within a particular community. The completed project reports are available at the university of Guyana Library and at the Faculty of Health Sciences at the university. Many students review these documents as they undertake similar projects within other communities.

Conclusion

In a country such as Guyana, with a high rate of emigration and its remaining citizens often rooted in the past, with outdated practices and few means of communication, it can be difficult to maintain a consistently dynamic environment for PSBH. Indeed, poverty can consume success by limiting aspirations and frustrating good efforts. Nevertheless, PSBH participants are often surprised to learn that they can, even with limited resources, be agents of change. As one Guyanese PSBH participant explained, "PSBH repeatedly demonstrates that there is wisdom in doing something, rather than nothing at all, for a small change can be significant in improving the quality of life for many."

24

Mexico

Héctor Marroquín Segura

Mexico is located between the United States and the Central American countries of Guatemala and Belize. It is the third largest country in Latin America, after Brazil and Argentina, with a land area of 1,964,375 sq km and a population of 110 million. It is a major economic and political force, with its natural mineral resources, strong industrial base, service sector, 31 geographically and ethnically diverse states and Federal District, as well as the world's largest number of Spanish-speaking people. Mexico has a rich history that includes the Mayan and Aztec empires, Spanish colonialism, and a sometimes-turbulent but ever-strengthening independence since the 1800s. Problem Solving for Better Health, launched in San Luis Potosí in the 1990s, is now a part of Mexico's forward progress.

In Mexico and in other developing countries, the underlying causes of most disease, disability, and death are poverty, inequality, and other social disparities. Thus, these problems require changes in behavior on many levels. The close relationship between behavior and health has been explored by the World Health Organization (WHO), which estimates that almost 40% of worldwide deaths are related to the following risk factors: low prenatal and birth weight, unsafe sex, high blood pressure, smoking, alcoholism, lack of potable water, lack of sanitary facilities and hygiene, high cholesterol levels, smoke from burning solid waste in the home, iron deficiency, and high body mass index (WHO, 2002). WHO predicts that life expectancy could increase by 5–10 years if people, communities, health services, and governments make decisions to reduce these risks (WHO, 2002).

In this chapter, I describe the Mexican experience with a program that mobilizes the community to improve health education, including collaborative work between health

Héctor Marroquín Segura is a professor at Escuela de Ciencias de la Salud, Universidad del Valle de México, San Luis Potosí, and Problem Solving for Better Health National Coordinator for Mexico.

professionals and community groups who identify specific problems and health risks. The emphasis is on the use of local resources to develop better health.

The Mexican Health Promotion Program

Mexico has a long tradition of community involvement, capacity building, and empowerment to improve health. In 1983, the right to health protection became a constitutional order (México, 2000). In 1984, the General Health Law was issued to regulate and define the contents and objectives of this social right to health protection and to promote and restore the individual and collective health of Mexicans (México, 2006).

In 2006, the Health Promotion Operational Model was developed by the Directorate of Health Promotion of the Ministry of Health (Santos-Burgoa et al., 2009). The model recognizes health as a valuable commodity, a product of social evolution that emphasizes the genuine interest of the people and their consolidation in the search for better health and life. In the National Health Program 2007–2012 (México, 2007), health promotion and prevention actions focus on reducing the impact of diseases and injuries on individuals, families, communities, and society through a national health pact ("Health, A Job For All"). The pact guarantees the following: (1) to provide a Preventive Services and Health Promotion kit for individuals and families, (2) to address the causal determinants of disease burden through a socioecological model, and (3) to reform First Contact Care.

San Luis Potosí: Health Inequality

San Luis Potosí (SLP) is one of the 32 states of Mexico. It is located in the north-central part of the country and has three geographic regions: the high plateau where the capital, of the same name, is located; the central zone; and La Huasteca. SLP is made up of 58 municipalities. It has 2.4 million people of unequal geographic distribution; 43% of the population is concentrated in the metropolitan area of the capital, with the rest scattered throughout 8,000 rural communities.

SLP's economy comprises industry and services in the state capital and agriculture in the remaining municipalities. There is a great contrast between the prosperous capital city and the underdeveloped rural areas. The majority of the municipalities are highly marginalized and, as a result, there is a large labor migration to the capital and the United States.

Public services, such as water, drainage, sanitation, and highway administration, are concentrated in urban areas, and rural areas have little access to these services. Healthcare services are unequal; the causes of illness and death in urban areas are similar to those of developed countries, while those in rural areas are dominated by infectious diseases, nutritional deficiencies, and poor reproductive health. In addition, the state is facing an epidemic of obesity, with more than half of the population affected. These individuals have high diabetes and hypertension rates. Addictions, especially among youth, are also a public health problem, as are violence, accidents, and infant and maternal mortality.

San Luis Potosí Initiative

The SLP Initiative grew from a collaboration between the Dreyfus Health Foundation (DHF) and a peer group of public health professionals from the Colegio de Salud Pública de San Luis Potosí (College of Public Health of San Luis Potosí) who were interested in the health and well-being of marginalized areas. DHF has supported the school with its Problem Solving for Better Health® (PSBH®) methodology, administrative guidance, and funding for project development.

The initiative was launched in 2002 at a Problem Solving for Better Health Initiative™ (PSBHI™) workshop in the rural community of Escalerillas, SLP, and in 2003, a second workshop was held in Villa de Reyes, covering the semiurban areas of the municipality. In 2005, we initiated a joint PSBH project with SLP's Secretary of Health to benefit several state programs. Rural areas in Huasteca Potosina were the focus of projects from 2004 through 2006. All initiative projects remain active. Since the inception of the SLP Initiative, 218 project leaders have participated in a total of 11 new and follow-up PSBHI workshops and developed 193 projects, benefiting 26 local areas in various municipalities of the state. The following sections describe a sampling of these projects.

Children's Health and Physical Education

During youth, we develop habits and behavior that last our entire lives. Developing a healthy lifestyle is fundamental for physical, mental, and social health, and for the prevention of disease. It is therefore important to participate in some form of physical education in our early years.

Escalerillas is a rural community with 10,000 people, mostly children and adolescents. The residents work mainly in construction and services for the neighboring city of SLP. A high rate of emigration to the capital and the United States has contributed to acculturation, family disintegration, and risky health behavior. The only education in the community is at the preprimary and primary levels.

Janett Quistiano, a teacher at the local primary school asked the following "Good Question:" "Will a physical education program, with 120 students between the ages of 6 and 14 years, at Escalerillas Primary School, during the 2002–2003 school year, create a habit of exercise among 50% of the students?" At the start of the school year, Janett and her team of sports instructors held classes in soccer, baseball, and basketball for 125 children, who subsequently competed in various competitions and tournaments. At the end of the 10-month project, 112 children remained in the program and 78 became involved in sports activities outside the program. The soccer and basketball teams represented the school in different competitions, and 16 children were selected to participate in events at a regional level. Most important, the school incorporated the physical education project into its curriculum.

In addition, to promote the school, the project team organized sports activities during the academic year for the entire community. Parents and other residents participated enthusiastically along with the schoolchildren. At the end of the project, the local team held a marathon for children in the streets of Escalerillas, and members of the Mexican PSBH team presented the winners with trophies. The project succeeded in bringing the students, the school, and the larger community together to promote health through physical skills development, discipline, socialization, and fun.

Maternal Mortality Among Indigenous Women

Brought on by poverty, gender inequality, and poor health services—common problems among the indigenous population—maternal mortality is considered a social tragedy that leads to family disintegration and a high risk of disease and death to orphaned children. In Mexico, more than 70,000 children become orphans each year because of maternal mortality. In SLP, there have been 610 maternal deaths over the last 15 years, leaving 3,110 children orphaned. On average, there are 35 maternal deaths a year.

The indigenous population of the Huasteca region of SLP consists of the Huastecos and Nahuatl ethnic groups. Approximately 340,000 people live in small, isolated, and marginalized rural communities that have major health problems. The use of traditional medicine is a cultural practice, and although the practice includes some elements of modern medicine, there is limited access to such medicine.

The indigenous municipality of Aquismón has the highest rate of maternal mortality in SLP and nationally. In 2005, Ma. Elena Córdova developed a team of nurses and housewives, and together they trained local leaders, families of women of childbearing age, midwives, and health personnel in detecting signs of danger; making decisions for the mother's care; transferring the mother to a health service; and providing immediate, quality attention.

The team formed a local group to support pregnant women, their partners, and midwives in prenatal care, the diagnosis of obstetric risks, the importance of seeking healthcare services in case of risks, and the timely transferring of the women to the county hospital for necessary care. They trained 25 midwives and integrated a cohort of 40 pregnant women. They conducted prenatal checks to detect possible risks, found 11 women to be at medium risk, and took them to the hospital. One woman was diagnosed with severe preeclampsia and received treatment at the hospital. The team feels that this project set a precedent for recognizing the importance of prenatal care and having a plan to prevent maternal death.

Sex Education for Life

Rodolfo Zermeño's project, "Sex Education for Life," was conducted by a team of four, including two teachers, a nurse, and a psychologist, at the 21st Technical High School at Villa de Reyes between October 2003 and June 2004. The training phase of the project was implemented from October to December 2003 and consisted of an intensive course for 30 students on anatomy, human relationships, feelings, sexual behavior, sexually transmitted diseases, pregnancy, contraception, and sex myths. The promotion phase took place between April and June 2004, when the 30 students from the training phase became health promoters who taught the course to their classmates. With this innovative system of health promotion, the project team achieved its goal of increasing knowledge of human sexuality and sexual health by 70% among 760 students at the 21st Technical High School in Villa de Reyes, using talks, workshops, and dynamic activities.

Active Aging

WHO (n.d.) defines active aging as

> the process of optimizing opportunities for health, participation and security in order to enhance quality of life as people age. It applies to both individuals and population groups. Active aging allows people to realize their potential for physical, social, and mental well-being throughout the life course and to participate in society, while providing them with adequate protection, security and care when they need.

In Mexico, the ancestral culture of respect and consideration that once existed toward older adults is diminishing. Contemporary culture gives privilege to *having* instead of *being* and places greater value on young people who are productive and active, while devaluing senior citizens, who are seen as unproductive and dependent on others.

The number of people older than 60 years is increasing in SLP. The health needs of the older generation are major, more complex, and costlier than for the younger population. SLP does not have cultural, educational, recreational, or work programs, or the urban infrastructure, for the older generation. Therefore, the elderly are condemned to an aging process marked by inactivity, disease, and decreasing abilities. More than 100,000 senior citizens live in the state and do not benefit from the healthy, active-aging programs promoted by WHO.

Juan Jose Gonzalez implemented his project in an area of Ciudad de Río Verde, SLP, in 2002. Together with his team of schoolteachers and physical education instructors, he organized 10 groups of approximately 20 people older than 60 years to participate in physical and recreational activities. A total of 204 elderly people participated in walking exercises, stretching, and aerobics for 3 weekly, 2-hour sessions over a period of 6 months. A group of clinical nursing students measured their vital signs and used charts to measure their progress. Respiratory capacity was recorded, as well as cardiac and arterial tension.

By the end of the project, 186 people had completed the activities. The project improved their physical and respiratory health, and increased their circulation. Surveys indicated that the participants were pleased with the project and its results. The project is ongoing, and new groups of seniors are participating. Some of the participants from the first group are still involved.

Conclusion

There are many theories and publications about models and strategies for creating community capacity and empowerment to promote health. However, it is difficult to evaluate and implement health promotion on a local level, especially in marginalized communities. The use of modern technology for information and communication in the public health field, in addition to traditional practices, is one of the innovative strategies incorporated into current conceptions of public health. The best stimulus for community-wide participation is to work for and with communities, guiding them and giving them tools for empowerment and capacity building. In this context, the role of the health sector in supporting collaborative processes of the community should be revised and clearly established. Health workers need to understand that they are obligated to help local organizations mobilize their own resources and actively participate to benefit the health of their community.

Helena Restrepo, who spoke at the WHO Fifth Global Conference on Health Promotion, stated that the

> challenge for health promotion in developing countries is to come up with new ways to effectively support local communities. Four findings in this sense should be highlighted. Local communities have incredible creativity and a great will to survive. Development of healthy public policies at the local level is more successful than at the national level. A new epidemiological approach like 'community epidemiology' ... is a strategy tested in Latin American countries that allows for the humanization of statistical data on morbidity and mortality. Communities know which are the best choices for improving their health and quality of life, when opportunities are given to them by power structures (Restrepo, 2000).

Local communities in the globalized world today, more than ever, need support and guidance for community capacity building and empowerment to benefit health. The support of development agencies has shown the great potential for health and well-being to proliferate while working with the communities. The communities need continuous stimulation and support from public and private sources. Despite the inspiring experiences of community participation and the empowerment of marginalized groups in diverse countries, there is still an urgent need to stimulate the application of these strategies, promote the participation of development agencies, and guide leaders who have a genuine interest in the community.

Community leaders, development agencies, participating organizations, and health workers should be responsible and held accountable for community capacity building and empowerment. The successes or failures of their programs and projects should be properly documented. DHF's successful PSBH model has worked in more than 30 countries, promoting networks of small projects developed by individuals to benefit the health and welfare of their communities. Many of these small projects have been replicated and expanded and have become self-sustaining. I am pleased to acknowledge these efforts and, at the same time, document and publish the wealth of knowledge and benefits derived from my own experiences with PSBH in Mexico.

References

México. (2000). *Constitución Política de los Estados Unidos Mexicanos, Ed.* México: Porrua.

México. (2006). *Ley General de Salud, Ed.* México: Porrua.

México. (2007). *Programa Nacional de Salud 2007–2012.* México: Edición de la Secretaría de Salud.

Restrepo, H. E. (2000, June). *Incremento de la capacidad comunitaria y del empoderamiento de las comunidades para promover la salud.* Paper presented at the World Health Organization's Fifth Global Conference on Health Promotion, Mexico City, México.

Santos-Burgoa, C., Rodríguez-Cabrera, L., Rivero, L., Ochoa, J., Stanford, A., Latinovic, L., et al. (2009). Implementation of Mexico's Health Promotion Operational Model. *Preventing Chronic Disease.* Retrieved January 19, 2010, from http://74.125.113.132/search?q=cache:1b6ulpOTNC8J:www.cdc.gov/pcd/issues/2009/Jan/08_0085.htm+Mexican+Model+for+Health+Promotion&cd=6&hl=en&ct=clnk&gl=us&client=safari

World Health Organization. (n.d.). *Ageing and life course: What is "active ageing"?* Retrieved April 29, 2010, from http://www.who.int/ageing/active_ageing/en

World Health Organization. (2002). *The World Health Report 2002—Reducing risks, promoting healthy life.* Geneva, Switzerland: Author.

25

Peru

Eric Tribut and Anna Zucchetti

Located on the Pacific coast of South America, Peru borders Ecuador, Columbia, Brazil, Bolivia, and Chile. It is a country of great variety, including the rainforests of Iquitos, an arid coast, and the Andes mountains. Its history is distinguished by the centuries-long Inca empire, the Spanish conquest, and the pace and strength of the country today. Peru's population of 28.5 million is also varied, with 50% Quechua Indians, 33% mestizos (people of mixed indigenous and European descent), and 12% Europeans. This blend produces a vibrant mix of influences in the country's music, art, and literature. Led by the local team, Problem Solving for Better Health is helping poor communities near Lima unleash their potential to make changes for better health and quality of life.

Grupo GEA and SOLPROMESA

Grupo GEA (Group for Environmental Enterprises) is a private nonprofit organization, established in 1992 and based in Lima, Peru. Its institutional mission is to contribute to the economic, social, and environmental development of the communities it serves, using the country's natural and cultural resources to create fair and just relationships among societies, the economy, and the environment. Grupo GEA has participated since 2003 in the SOLPROMESA Network. SOLPROMESA, or "Promise of the Sun," (*SOL*ucionando *PRO*blemas para *ME*jor *SA*lud), is the acronym in Latin America for the Dreyfus Health Foundation's program Problem Solving for Better Health® (PSBH®). Grupo GEA understands the valuable PSBH methodology to be, in the words of the organization's former Director of Sustainable Tourism Eric Tribut, "the art of adding together individual determinations, capacities, and available resources to create trust and well-being in the communities."

Eric Tribut is an associate member of Grupo GEA and former Director of the Sustainable Tourism Program. Anna Zucchetti is Founder and Executive Director of Grupo GEA, the Dreyfus Health Foundation's implementing partner in Peru. She also is Problem Solving for Better Health's National Coordinator for Peru.

More than 200 people have participated in SOLPROMESA/PSBH workshops hosted by Grupo GEA in the communities of Lima Sur (South Lima) and Arequipa. The participants are from the coast and the mountains and include 13-year-olds to senior citizens. They are mothers, farmers, professors, students, nurses, and tour guides. They are people who began the process with skepticism and a pessimistic attitude and grew to be the ones who encouraged others to stop complaining and start taking action. To date, SOLPROMESA workshops have benefited more than 20,000 individuals. In addition, more than 120 support organizations have been involved, including educational institutions, nonprofit organizations, private companies, and government agencies.

SOLPROMESA has enabled Grupo GEA to establish an updated network of local leaders, all of whom have shown their determination with actions, not just words. Beyond the completion of their respective SOLPROMESA projects, these leaders gained trust in themselves and progressed from reaching small objectives to accomplishing big ones. SOLPROMESA has helped Grupo GEA better understand that one of the main ingredients to becoming a successful leader and motivator in the development of sustainable projects is confidence.

Today at Grupo GEA we incorporate the SOLPROMESA/PSBH methodology from the very beginning into all aspects of the capacity-building process of our community development projects. This methodology has allowed us to more effectively apply the "scale up" concept: We start with small, successful, and influential initiatives to build a solid foundation for wide-scale solutions focused on improving the quality of life in communities. We have witnessed how pioneering ideas have become a reality, and this confirms the need for our organization to continue being creative and innovative.

One way we have used the SOLPROMESA/PSBH methodology is in our youth leaders group, "Buena Voz" (Good Voice); we adapted the methodology to be implemented by adolescents and young adults, reinforcing their leadership skills through successful completion of community development projects in their own neighborhoods. To give this youth program its own identity, we changed the name SOLPROMESA to ADOPTAR SU BARRIO (Adopt Your Neighborhood). Sixty-two projects initiated in our youth workshops have benefited more than 15,000 people, mostly children and adolescents.

SOLPROMESA entrepreneurs have internalized the idea that poverty is not a social condition but a state of being. We are not poor, but we are in a state of financial poverty, and we should not allow this poverty to obscure the riches present in our available resources, riches that come to light using the SOLPROMESA/PSBH methodology. These riches are environmental and cultural, the social and creative capital of our communities, our solidarity, the energy of our young people, our responsible mothers, and the skills and aptitudes inherited from our ancestors. The utilization of these riches has been crucial to the success of the SOLPROMESA program in Peru. Today the program's social entrepreneurs, as well as its team of facilitators, are convinced, that, again in Eric Tribut's words, "if everyone wins, we win more."

The small local initiatives generated by the SOLPROMESA program in Peru are invaluable, for they have become viable businesses (agriculture, tourism, craftsmanship), they have developed leadership skills (neighborhood committee presidents, youth council leaders, community development promoters), and they have initiated stable relationships with institutions that foster community development (universities, art museums, nongovernmental organizations). We have included some of

SOLPROMESA's activities and success stories since program inception in the following section.

SOLPROMESA Activities

The first SOLPROMESA workshop in Peru was held in May 2004 in the Lurín River Valley. Fifty participants attended from the Lima Sur districts of Lurín, Punta Hermosa, Pachacamac, Cieneguilla, Villa El Salvador, and Villa María del Triunfo, along with a team of 13 national and international facilitators.

Of the 50 projects generated at the workshop, almost 75% have been completed successfully or are still active and showing good progress. The projects address issues of child and adolescent health (infant malnutrition, school dropouts, teenage pregnancy, access to vocational education, and juvenile violence); conditions of community living (unemployment and job security, deterioration of community facilities, difficulties gaining access to potable water, and contamination of sources of water for human consumption and farming); and community health and safety (inefficiency of the solid waste management systems, insufficient family and school hygiene, parasitosis and anemia, and neighborhood safety).

In 2005, the Lima Sur Initiative was launched with 39 participants from the districts of Pachacamac, Villa María del Triunfo, Lurín, Villa El Salvador, and Cieneguilla, and other districts of the Lima Sur metropolitan area. Fifty-nine young adults from five different schools in Lima Sur, members of the Buena Voz network, participated in the Adopt Your Neighborhood Initiative. All graduated from the Buena Voz Leadership Training Program, also hosted by Grupo GEA, and participated in a preselection process that took into account both their leadership levels and the individual projects they had previously completed. From these two initiatives, a total of 61 participants successfully finished their projects. Four of these projects were the result of collaborative efforts of two or more individuals.

The projects and campaigns established under the SOLPROMESA framework directly benefited 5,234 students at the schools represented by the Buena Voz participants, as well as the lives of 270 families and 362 additional adults and young people living in Lima Sur. Projects targeting students and their schools included programs for street safety, improving parent–child communication, avoiding gang membership, planting trees, and building school libraries. Projects benefiting families and uniting neighbors for change in their communities included programs for trash removal and recycling; home and street accident prevention; street vendor location; and, again, parent–child communication.

In 2007, Grupo GEA trained 21 youths from Lima Sur in project development and execution using the SOLPROMESA/PSBH methodology. Throughout the year we motivated these social leaders to work together on collective efforts, encouraging groups of two or more young people from the same neighborhood and local youth organization to participate together. Of the 21 leaders, 17 successfully finished their projects, accomplishing a total of seven social initiatives. These projects, as well as projects generated during a 2006 Adopt Your Neighborhood Initiative, benefited 350 students at various educational institutions. The projects included programs on sexuality and reproductive health, the risks of gang membership, caring for neighborhood green areas, developing a life plan, and providing cultural events and other activities for the young.

SOLPROMESA Stories

SOLPROMESA projects continue to benefit individuals and communities in Lima Sur and, since 2009, the Colca Valley in Arequipa. In the following sections we present some examples of SOLPROMESA projects that have been implemented in these areas.

Yogurt of the Valley

The enthusiasm of four young women and their desire to overcome the difficulties of developing a home business gave rise to the project "Yogurt del Valle." The women's delicious and nutritious product, made with fruits from the Lurín River Basin, is currently marketed in the districts of Pachacamac, Lurín, and Cieneguilla. After developing their project at a SOLPROMESA workshop, Karina Inga, Fatima Espino, Leonor Rojas, and Janet Gutierrez arranged to meet with food engineers at the La Molina Agrarian University to learn about cost-effective food production, processing, packaging, safety, and marketing. With growing confidence and an excellent, quality product, they went from making 5 liters to selling 200 liters a week, fulfilling a growing demand. "At first, we were doubtful. We didn't know if people were going to like our product ... we conquered our fears, we believe in our product. We are working and growing," says Janet.

Guinea Pigs for the Future

Eighteen-year-old Roger Rodriguez, motivated by Grupo GEA's SOLPROMESA workshop on business management and, supported by his high school teacher Percy Calagua, decided to take on the challenge of starting his own business. After partnering with two friends, he began his commercial venture in 2004, confident that raising guinea pigs, a staple in the Peruvian diet, would be a profitable business. The first few months were difficult, especially because Roger was the victim of a robbery and suffered the loss of half of his animals. A short time later, he had the opportunity to partner with two students from the Universidad del Pacífico (Peru) to form a new company. The three partners obtained a shed for 1,000 guinea pigs, a small packinghouse, and a security booth. SOLPROMESA had helped Roger to overcome his shyness, which had previously limited him in many ways. Today, Roger's company is considered to be one of the most successful guinea pig microenterprises in Lima Sur. His business supplies guinea pigs to large supermarket chains and various restaurants throughout Lima.

Recreation Park in Centro Poblado Rural Picapiedra

Sonia Huaman, President of the Executive Board of CPR (Rural Village Center) Picapiedra, wanted to create a space in her town designated for young children. With this idea in mind, she participated in a SOLPROMESA workshop. There, she proposed a project to adapt space in the middle of the central plaza into a play area filled with rustic children's toys, all in nontraditional, colorful shapes made from locally available wood, rope, rocks, and sand. Immediately after the workshop, Sonia began to work on her project. She rallied her neighbors, and with help from local businesses, she obtained trucks to transport the materials. She encouraged young architectural students from the Universidad Ricardo Palma to help pro bono, and in 6 months the park was ready. Today, more than 200 children a day enjoy the park.

Sustainability of SOLPROMESA

Through SOLPROMESA/PSBH, our social entrepreneurs in Peru learn skills that help them identify problems within their communities and give them the tools to solve them. They develop relationships with community organizations and improve their public speaking skills. They become leaders in their communities. These new leaders are transforming social problems into challenges and finding endless possibilities for bettering their lives and the lives of their families and neighbors. Grupo GEA aims to continue consolidating our social capital by strengthening the capacity for social entrepreneurship and youth leadership in Peru.

26

Jordan

Mahmoud M. Alkam and Darwish Badran

Jordan, which became an independent state in 1946, sits at the crossroads of more ancient and contemporary civilizations than perhaps any other country in the world. A land of 88,778 sq km and some 6 million people, Jordan shares borders with Syria, Iraq, Saudi Arabia, Israel, and the West Bank. Its three major zones include desert in the east, uplands in the center, and the Jordan Valley at the northwest end of the East African Rift System. The country is distinguished by being a constitutional, hereditary monarchy with a parliamentary form of government. Problem Solving for Better Health was established in Jordan with the Center for Educational Development at the University of Jordan, and has gained greatly by the input and involvement of the local participants.

Jordan's position at the crossroads of the Middle East is apparent as regional conflicts keep the country firmly in the eye of the international community. Jordan will have to balance its global profile with its need to combat issues at home, most specifically its population boom and the desperate need for a sustainable water supply. Four-fifths of Jordan's land is desert. The eastern part of the country is almost entirely desert, but the land near Amman, the capital, is greener and hillier. This terrain continues until the edge of the Great Rift Valley, and as the land descends to the Dead Sea, the climate gets hotter, saltier, and more arid. At the edge of the Dead Sea, the land is checkered with salt deposits, and very little grows in the area.

Jordan's population makeup is 98% Arab and 2% Circassian, Chechen, and Armenian (Index Mundi, 2010). A significant percentage of the Arab population is made up of

Mahmoud M. Alkam, now retired, was Health Professions Training Officer at the Center for Educational Development (CED), the Dreyfus Health Foundation's implementing partner in Jordan. He also is Problem Solving for Better Health and Communications for Better Health National Coordinator for Jordan. Darwish Badran is Director of the CED, University of Jordan, Amman.

Palestinians. The country is overwhelmingly Sunni Muslim (92%), but there is a close-knit Christian population (6%) that lives in concentrated areas; the rest of the population is Shia Muslim and Druze (Index Mundi, 2010). Despite an already high unemployment rate, Jordan will soon face a new challenge in providing jobs for young Jordanians— United Nations statistics indicate that 34.5% of Jordanians are less than 15 years of age (United Nations, 2009).

Another challenge faced by Jordan is being one of the world's most water-poor countries. Annual per capita water availability is only 179 cubic meters, ranking Jordan among the lowest countries in terms of water consumption, according to the United Nations Educational, Scientific and Cultural Organization (UNESCO, 2006). It has been speculated that at current levels of consumption, Jordan's water table may be severely depleted in as few as 2 decades. With the impending population boom, the demand for water will only increase. Radical water projects will be required in the future as the current sources, the Jordan and Yarmouk Rivers, are shared with other countries in the region. Jordan has not been blessed with many conventional natural resources. In addition to the lack of water, there are no large oil or gas reserves. Jordan does have significant mining activities, however, exporting both phosphates and potash.

Despite these national challenges, the average education level in Jordan remains among the highest in the region. Jordanians are respected as highly skilled workers in a number of fields, including medicine, law, and education. The national literacy rate is 92% (male, 96%; female, 88%; World Health Organization, 2010). Education remains mandatory for children until the age of 15 years. Higher education features a higher percentage of women than men, because many men drop out to work after secondary school; nonetheless, many girls drop out well before they reach university level. Education has been actively promoted throughout the country, especially with a focus on information technology (IT) development and education for women in the far reaches of the kingdom.

Healthcare in Jordan includes three components: the government sector, with agencies such as the Ministry of Health (MOH), Royal Medical Services (RMS), and public university hospitals; the private sector; and the international and charitable sector, including the United Nations Relief and Works Agency for Palestine Refugees in the Near East (UNRWA).

The MOH is responsible for all health matters in the kingdom, with areas of focus including health promotion, disease control, prevention of nutritional deficiencies, maternal and child health (MCH), school health, health of the elderly, and prevention and management of noncommunicable diseases. The MOH provides primary, secondary, and tertiary healthcare services in 32 hospitals. Primary healthcare services are mainly provided through an extensive healthcare network consisting of comprehensive health centers, primary healthcare centers, and village clinics and MCH centers. The RMS mainly provides secondary and tertiary care services. It has 10 hospitals with 1,801 beds, comprising 18.3% of hospital beds in Jordan. The RMS is responsible for providing health services and comprehensive medical insurance to military and security personnel, both active and retired staff and their dependents. Beneficiaries of the RMS also include staff of the Royal Court, Royal Jordanian Airlines, Mu'ta and Al-Bait Universities, and other national public institutions. Public university hospitals such as Jordan University Hospital and King Abdullah University Hospital (Jordan University of Science and Technology, Irbid) also provide secondary and tertiary care services.

The private sector provides clinical services at the primary, secondary, and tertiary care levels. Fifty-six private hospitals have 3,569 beds, comprising 36.3% of hospital beds in the kingdom, and there are about 2,600 private clinics nationwide.

The international and charitable sector includes UNRWA for Palestine Refugees, Caritas, and other nonprofit agencies that provide primary healthcare services. UNRWA's overall health policy focuses on the direct provision of essential health services to Palestinian refugees. The registered refugee population in Jordan in 2004 was 1.7 million; less than 20% resided in camps. The agency runs 13 primary healthcare facilities inside the refugee camps and 10 facilities outside the camps. Services include free primary healthcare at UNRWA facilities, with emphasis on family health and disease prevention and control. UNRWA also provides assistance toward the cost of secondary medical care, especially emergency and life-saving treatment, at external healthcare facilities, and basic sanitation and related environmental health services in refugee camps. UNRWA reports that refugees made more than 2.2 million outpatient visits to UNRWA facilities in 2004, meaning that each of the agency's medical officers saw an average of 102 patients daily.

Problem Solving for Better Health in Jordan

In 1992, the Center for Educational Development (CED) at the University of Jordan received correspondence from the Dreyfus Health Foundation (DHF) regarding a phenytoin (PHT) database developed by DHF. The CED is a nonprofit university institution devoted to training in and development and promotion of health services, medical education, and research. Driven by curiosity and a desire to extend our contacts to new areas and expand our access to scientific libraries in other countries, we responded to DHF's invitation to receive information on PHT. In late 1992, we received a letter from the director of DHF, Dr. Barry H. Smith, enclosing a draft document on the Problem Solving for Better Health® (PSBH®) program, explaining its philosophy, objectives, and process. The letter offered to help in the organization and implementation of the program in Jordan. CED carefully studied the program's objectives, contents, and methodology.

In order to gain further insight into the PSBH methodology, we requested that our staff attend a workshop at a site where the program was already implemented. DHF invited the CED Director and Training Officer to participate in a PSBH workshop in India, where we had an informative and enjoyable experience. In 1993, Dr. Smith visited our center, and in September we held the first PSBH workshop at the University of Jordan in Amman. A second workshop followed immediately. Most participants were doctors, nurses, and administrative personnel representing health providers in Jordan. Encouraged by positive feedback, CED decided to establish a collaborative relationship with DHF.

The PSBH program in Jordan is coordinated by CED. To date, it has been implemented in 15 cities and regions throughout the country, in collaboration with the MOH, UNRWA for Palestine Refugees, national and regional government officials, and nongovernmental organizations. The program includes individual and community sensitization; training in scientific research; and development of appropriate, alternative solutions to local health problems. One particularly successful application of PSBH in Jordan is a specific program for nurses and nursing students, Problem Solving for Better Health-Nursing™ (PSBHN™). As of January 2007, more than 31,650 people in Jordan had benefited from the PSBH and PSBHN programs (Figure 26.1).

Health and social issues addressed by PSBH and PSBHN projects in Jordan include communicable diseases (gastrointestinal disease, HIV/AIDS, sexually transmitted diseases), economic issues (skills training, income generation, occupational health, work safety), environmental health (animal/insect/pest control, waste management, water supply/quality), healthcare and health policy issues (access to health facilities and services, children's health, hospital administration), health promotion and lifestyles (dental and oral health, nutrition and malnutrition, substance abuse), mental health (psychological and psychiatric disorders, stress), noncommunicable diseases (cancer, cardiovascular disorders, diabetes, respiratory disorders), nutrition (food safety, obesity), social issues and services (crime, cultural beliefs and perceptions, domestic abuse, violence), and women's health (family planning, teenage pregnancy, prenatal, postnatal care).

All of us serving on the front line of healthcare are in a daily struggle with health problems of all sizes, types, and levels of complexity. We know that to improve the health of our people, save lives, and promote a better quality of life we must search for appropriate, practical, and relevant solutions to these problems. Solutions should be implemented using human and material resources that already exist. Quite often, the solution is simple, known, and already within our reach, but we need just a little extra help to realize and implement it. The PSBH program encourages good-hearted individuals to seek new approaches and innovative methods, using creative and critical thinking, which will assist them in solving the problems of their communities.

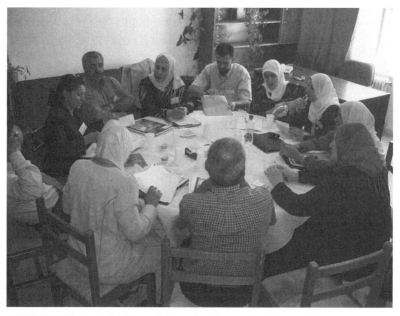

FIGURE 26.1 A Problem Solving for Better Health workshop in Jordan.

DHF's Communications for Better Health® program has added value to the PSBH experience by helping to publish project data. The *Jordan Health Digest* is a tool through which we disseminate locally relevant and useful health information to health workers, especially those in urban areas or those who have limited access to up-to-date information. We cover health topics important to medical and nursing practitioners as well as to every person interested in the improvement and promotion of health in Jordan. We are committed to helping health workers develop their competencies and to providing reading material that enhances continuing medical education.

Testimonials

Fatimeh Atieh is a vocational and technical education specialist for nursing at UNRWA Headquarters in Amman. This is her story:

> In 1994, when I returned from my maternity leave, I learned that my friend Andaleeb was working on a project developed at a PSBH workshop at the University of Jordan. She encouraged me to attend a PSBH workshop also. It was my first experience attending a workshop that was conducted in a way that differs from what we are used to, and included different levels and types of staff members. The content of the workshop was closely related to my work as a health education supervisor, and I quickly adopted its approach. I soon joined the PSBH family and began my journey as a facilitator for the program.
>
> My project was titled "Home Management of Acute Respiratory Infections for Children up to Three Years" and was implemented at Zarqa Health Center, UNRWA. In spite of the difficulties my team and I faced at that time, we were enthusiastic to complete the project and see the results. One mother who attended the project activities had a sick child. She acquired new knowledge and skills about identification of risk signs and symptoms of respiratory tract infections, implemented what she learned for her child, and immediately took the child to the hospital. We realized that many children's lives could be saved if mothers are aware of the risk signs and symptoms of respiratory tract infections, know what to do, and how to do it. This confirmed my belief that these projects are helpful. We just need to increase our commitment to provide better care and service. Upon completing the project, a flip chart on home management of acute respiratory infections was produced by UNRWA. The chart was utilized to implement health education activities for several target groups at UNRWA health centers, schools, and women's program centers.
>
> Participating in these workshops for different target groups in different areas developed my knowledge and enabled me to communicate effectively with all concerned, present ideas and thoughts in a more systematic approach, improve my English, and broaden my knowledge about the culture of my society. Working as a vocational and technical education specialist at the UNRWA headquarters and supervising nursing and paramedical courses allowed me to develop and enrich the curriculum for these courses. I introduced the PSBH methodology into the curriculum of paramedical courses, using the title "Graduation Project." Participants received two credit hours.
>
> In order to continue PSBH in Jordan, the major issue is how to approach health institutions to present the PSBH methodology and influence decision makers to

accept the program for training their staff. The program can improve quality of services in a cost-effective way. Health institutions could improve their processes and increase staff efficiency by implementing PSBH.

Andaleeb Kandah is the supervisor of health education at the Educational Development Centre, UNRWA. Here is her story:

> All the moments my friend Fatimeh and I spent together replay in my mind as a film with scenes, and in each scene we were given a sign that might have great influence on many people we met while teaching PSBH over 15 years. The program provided me with many skills and a vision to develop my career and myself. It allowed me to think of my community in terms of ownership, and I want to teach everybody the PSBH method to improve the health of our people and our community. As a result of my dedication, PSBH was incorporated into the health education course at UNRWA. The teachers appreciated the great impact PSBH had on the health of our students.

Conclusion

The objective of PSBH is to encourage people to want to be healthy, to know how to stay healthy, to do what they can individually and collectively to maintain health, and to seek help when needed. Implicit in this objective is the concept of self-care and self-reliance at the individual and collective levels. It might be wise, though, to ask what we really mean by *self-care*. Self-care is not just a matter of nonlicensed doctoring. It is a means by which people can take much greater responsibility for their own health, based on an understanding, in their own language, of what health is all about—how to protect it, how to promote it, and what to do when it goes wrong. The concept of self-help is, therefore, inseparable from the concept of self-care.

However, part of this understanding is to realize the limits of self-care so that people will have the wisdom to know when to contact the first level of the formal health system. Each country, each community, must develop self-care based on its own needs. But whatever the situation is, formal health systems will have to stimulate and guide the self-care process. This is the only way we can avoid conflicts. We must try to win over the medical, nursing, and other allied health professionals to make them understand that the advocates of self-care do not propose that it should ever replace doctors, nurses, and other health personnel in the caring process. On the contrary, self-care will demand additional patience and efforts on the part of health workers to enable people to achieve self-reliance. Health systems are not just "baskets" to accommodate consumer demands. Consumers need to assume certain responsibilities. We have found that the PSBH methodology not only encourages individuals to assume personal responsibility for their health but also fosters a collaborative and integrative approach to healthcare.

Reflecting on almost 16 years of experience in organizing and implementing the PSBH program in Jordan, at CED we feel proud and honored to be part of this global family and to have helped so many people to have better health and improved quality of life.

References

Index Mundi. (2010). *Jordan demographics profile 2010.* Retrieved May 2, 2010, from http://www.index-mundi.com/jordan/demographics_profile.html

United Nations. (2009). *Social indicators: Indicators on child and elderly populations.* Retrieved May 2, 2010, from http://unstats.un.org/unsd/demographic/products/socind/child&elderly.htm

United Nations Educational, Scientific and Cultural Organization. (2006). The state of the resource: Nature, variability and availability: Water availability. In *The 2nd UN World Water Development Report: Water: A shared responsibility, 2006* (chap. 4, pt. 2g, pp. 130–136). Retrieved April 30, 2010, from http://www.unesco.org/water/wwap/wwdr/wwdr2/table_contents.shtml

World Health Organization. (2010). *Jordan: Socioeconomic indicators.* Retrieved May 2, 2010, from http://www.emro.who.int/emrinfo/index.asp?Ctry=jor

27

Houston, Texas

Marsha Johnson Copeland and Valerie D. Jackson

With a population of approximately 2.3 million, and a greater metropolitan area of close to 6 million, Houston is the fourth largest city in the United States. The population is less than one-half White, one-third Hispanic, and one-quarter African American, providing a lively ethnic mix. Houston is a major oil and petrochemical center with a thriving high-tech industry, engineering services, and advanced medical care and research facilities. The city is characterized by pride in what has been accomplished, optimism for the future, and a "can-do" attitude known as "the Houston factor." However, as in every city in the U.S., not everyone is sharing equally in the resources that are available. Problem Solving for Better Health was introduced to the city as a tool to help make needed changes, with the belief that success in Houston can provide a model for improvement in other U.S. cities.

Problem Solving for Better Health® (PSBH®) program participants in Houston, Texas, have always believed they are part of a movement that will change the world. Through their dedication and hard work, the program, initiated by the Dreyfus Health Foundation (DHF) in 2003, has grown steadily each year. Project leaders have carried out almost 100 small-scale projects addressing a wide range of healthcare issues, including diabetes, HIV/AIDS, obesity, the nursing shortage, teen violence, poor prenatal care, and drug-related recidivism.

Many participants involved with the program have implemented their projects with little or no funding, using available resources and relying on partnerships they develop while serving their communities. These individuals tend to view their work as their

Marsha Johnson Copeland is the Problem Solving for Better Health (PSBH) National Coordinator for the United States. Valerie D. Jackson is the PSBH Program Director for Solutions for Better Living, the Dreyfus Health Foundation's implementing partner in Houston.

mission; therefore, they are not easily deterred or discouraged by challenges. Their enthusiasm and conviction inspire their peers to join the effort and, as a result, their projects continue long after initial seed funding from DHF.

Solutions for Better Living

When DHF began working in collaboration with the Houston Endowment in 2007, the endowment determined that a local DHF affiliate should be established. As a result, we developed an organization called Solutions for Better Living (SBL). SBL's mission is to identify and nurture a new cadre of leadership in Houston, including social entrepreneurs who are committed to community development. This mission is based on the belief that the bold innovation and talent needed to positively impact the most underserved areas of Houston already exist within the hearts and minds of those who live there.

People who become involved in local community service efforts are passionate about making a difference but often lack the tools or skills to effectively carry out and sustain their efforts. Most believe that they will be able to rely on grants from foundations or other organizations and do not build sustainability into their project proposals. SBL teaches them to think differently, by adopting an entrepreneurial, for-profit business approach to community service projects.

SBL teaches project leaders to operate as social entrepreneurs who identify problems and apply business principles to organize, create, and operate projects to solve those problems. Societal issues must be approached innovatively in order to make an impact. Sustaining project activities also requires a creative revenue-generating idea. Because business skills are not innate, SBL offers support and guidance to project leaders to encourage sustainable and successful ventures. This approach merges philanthropy and enterprise. Through the PSBH methodology, SBL helps community project leaders identify available resources and develop strategies to ensure the continuation of their initiatives. Project leaders must submit action plans that do not depend on grants or private donations, and they are required to generate revenue as part of the process.

In the process of encouraging project leaders to think like social entrepreneurs, the SBL management team provides educational workshops and technical assistance. The workshops include accounting and budgeting, corporate law, marketing strategies, and business plan development. These workshops are designed to provide participants with skills to further develop and expand their projects.

Problem Solving for Better Health Projects

Over the years, Veon McReynolds, a community activist, observed that a lack of physical activity by families in underserved areas of Houston led to an increase in the incidence of diabetes, heart disease, and obesity. He believed physical activity and exercise for inner city residents would be more stimulating and fun if families exercised together. In 2004, he attended a PSBH workshop and developed a project called "Tour de Hood" to provide families with an opportunity to improve their health through a monthly bicycle-riding event. In 2009, this became a weekly activity. Participants receive loaner bikes, healthy snacks, helmets, and t-shirts at no cost. Although Veon commits much of his time and personal resources to keep "Tour de Hood" operating, the event continues largely through support from the community (Figure 27.1).

At the age of 25, Lyndon Carter was involved in a car crash with a drunk driver. As a result of irreparable kidney damage, he began dialysis treatment. Refusing to give in to despair and feel sorry for himself during dialysis, Lyndon began to take an active role in his care by educating himself about kidney failure and treatment. During a 2009 PSBH workshop, Lyndon developed a project, "Making Ends Meet." As part of the project, Lyndon serves as an advocate to renal patients and provides them with information he obtained during his own treatment. His primary goal is to provide new dialysis patients with the opportunity to learn from someone who has walked in their shoes.

Through this project, Lyndon shares information commonly offered by renal social workers, who have enormous caseloads and are often unable to reach all predialysis patients. Meetings are held bimonthly at the Memorial Herman Wellness Center in southwest Houston. The first session is an informative meeting for new patients; the second session includes a test to review the information covered in Session 1, additional information, and the opportunity to speak with current dialysis patients. Lyndon recruits patients for his project by marketing through doctors and dialysis social workers, word of mouth, and referrals from the American Association of Kidney Patients and the National Kidney Foundation.

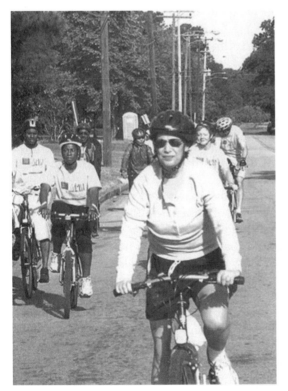

FIGURE 27.1 "Tour de Hood," a Problem Solving for Better Health project developed in the Third Ward, Houston, Texas, to promote bicycling for better health.

Lyndon hopes to be financially self-sufficient from the sale of promotional items such as hats, t-shirts, coffee mugs, and pens. He has considered negotiating contract agreements with hospitals, dialysis centers, and the National Kidney Foundation in order to conduct his project activities with their patients, employees, and members. His ultimate goal is to travel the United States and host citywide conferences for patients and healthcare workers. This venture is personal for Lyndon, and his passion radiates. Lyndon's tenacity and perseverance ensure that his project will flourish. He works daily to promote his services by appearing on television, developing a professional website, meeting with doctors and hospital administrators, and participating in forums and health fairs. Like all great entrepreneurs, Lyndon devotes many hours of hard work toward his project in order to ensure its success.

Another PSBH project leader is Linda Etuk. When meeting Linda for the first time, her twinkling eyes and smile project warmth and friendliness. She often gives hugs of encouragement to those who need them. But when Linda works on behalf of children who live in the most underserved communities of Houston, she is determined and refuses to take "no" for an answer.

In 2006, Linda experienced a parent's worst nightmare: Her oldest son, Phillip, was killed in a car accident. He had taken a leave of absence from college to work in New Orleans, Louisiana, after Hurricane Katrina and was driving home to reenroll at Texas State University. After the accident, Linda became depressed and struggled to make sense out of her life. How could Phillip, who was known for his sunny disposition and bright smile, have been taken from her and her family? An answer came in the form of a quiet revelation. Phillip, the intelligent, compassionate, and kind young man she raised, may have been gone, but the love, care, and encouragement she had given him remained. There were many other children who needed what she had to give, and she was determined to make a difference in their lives.

As a tribute to her son, Linda established the Phillip Cares Foundation to improve the lives of children in the Third Ward, the center of Houston's African American community. The area struggles with high crime rates and the economic challenges of gentrification. Although Linda had never before been to the Third Ward, Phillip attended Texas Southern University there; he had enjoyed the time he spent in the community and often spoke fondly of his experiences and the people he met there. Linda felt compelled to positively impact the community her son loved so much. She was motivated to transform the way the Third Ward was viewed by outsiders and how those living there viewed themselves, especially children and adolescents.

Linda attended a PSBH workshop in 2008. She initially wanted to develop an action plan to establish a school in the Third Ward in her son's memory, the Phillip C. Shynett Preparatory Academy. However, after the first day of the workshop she realized that a school would be a huge undertaking and should instead be part of her long-term goals; she decided to focus first on the high rate of obesity among children living in the ward.

Linda believes that improved access to healthy foods is critical to decreasing the incidence of childhood obesity in the United States. The lack of access to fresh foods in poor neighborhoods makes it difficult for children and their families to eat nutritious diets. Therefore, the mission of Linda's project, "Fruits of Their Labor," is to provide affordable access to fresh fruits and vegetables. One of the ways to obtain fresh produce is to grow it locally. As a gardening enthusiast who had kept a traditional garden in her own home for many years, Linda planted her first organic garden in the Third Ward at the Cuney

Homes housing project. Once the garden yielded a crop, her team of volunteers sold the produce to residents, at a cost that was 85% less than grocery store prices, and distributed it free to those who could not afford to pay. Linda plans to expand "Fruits of Their Labor" to include four additional sites in the Third Ward and hopes that her efforts will have a ripple effect, positively impacting the lives of generations of children and their families.

During a recent presentation in Houston, DHF's PSBH National Coordinator for the United States, Marsha Johnson Copeland, spoke about a conversation she had with Sallie Harrell. Ms. Sallie, as friends and family know her, has worked with the Houston program since 2003. Marsha asked her what she thought about using one of DHF Director Dr. Barry H. Smith's favorite Ethiopian proverbs during an upcoming presentation: "When spider webs unite, they can tie up a lion." Ms. Sallie sat back in her chair and thoughtfully repeated the phrase. She laughed and gave her approval. "You know what?" she said, "You need to use that one, because I'm telling you that sounds just like us!"

One of several PSBH projects that Ms. Sallie has implemented dealt with recidivism among drug-addicted women who had recently been released from prison. In recovery for over 15 years herself, Ms. Sallie began a peer counseling project for women who would receive little or no such support once they left prison. With some initial project funding, she offered counseling to 10 formerly incarcerated women for 1 year. To date, almost half remain drug-free and have not committed additional criminal offenses. Ms. Sallie has expanded her prison initiative to hold domestic abuse prevention meetings for women in the Third Ward. She is also instrumental in bringing other project leaders into the Third Ward, where she continues to work and build partnerships. Each time she meets someone who expresses a desire to "do something," that person either volunteers for her project or develops his or her own project.

Conclusion

Veon, Lyndon, Linda, and Ms. Sallie are examples of rising social entrepreneurs. Like so many other problem solvers in Houston and around the world, they are passionate about the work that they do in their communities and view that work as a fulfillment of their life's vision and purpose. They understand the intrinsic value of making a difference in this world, and they consistently reach out to assist and cheer on others who are trying to improve quality of life in the community. They are determined to move past gender, culture, race, and religion and are willing to work together toward the transformation of their communities. Their individual efforts touch lives. If asked, each one will tell you a story that expresses his or her desire to comfort, educate, and transform the lives of those around them. However, upon further examination one can see that they themselves have been touched, comforted, educated, and transformed through their participation in PSBH.

28

Newark, New Jersey

Wesley N. Jenkins

Just 13 km from the lower end of New York City, Newark is a city of some 300,000 people with a greater metropolitan area of over 2 million. First settled in 1666 by Puritans, the city became a center for manufacturing in 1790 and continued as such until the mid-20th century. Its industrial sector ultimately declined, as happened in many parts of the United States. By the 1950s, with urban decay increasing, the White population was moving to the suburbs, so that by the 1990s the city was three-fifths African American. All the problems of urban decay and poverty made Newark a challenging environment for change and improvement, but major progress has been made. Problem Solving for Better Health has been a part of that progress since the 1990s. Newark is another model for what can be done to improve the lives and health of U.S. citizens.

In 1999, I was invited to participate in a Problem Solving for Better Health® (PSBH®) workshop sponsored by the Dreyfus Health Foundation (DHF) and the New Community Corporation (NCC) in Newark, New Jersey. Because I was not sure what to expect, I was a little closed-minded about the experience at the beginning. At the time, I was a young community organizer working for the sister company of NCC, Babyland Family Services, Inc. As an organizer, I had some strong ideas about what my community needed. I was skeptical about the entire PSBH process.

The first day of the workshop started with an opening address from the Director of DHF, Dr. Barry H. Smith. He explained the process that we would experience for the next 2 days. All of the participants were divided into small groups with assigned facilitators. We were expected to begin creating an action plan to address the various health conditions in our community. That seemed easy because there were so many issues. We could

Wesley N. Jenkins is Executive Director of Babyland Family Services, Newark, New Jersey, and Problem Solving for Better Health Program Coordinator for New Jersey.

have addressed diabetes, heart disease, asthma—the list could have gone on and on. The PSBH process surprised me because it suggested that we think about health in a very different way.

Individuals talked about not being able to have a relationship with their grandchildren; not being able to exercise at their senior citizen centers; and children not being able to play outside because of gang violence, causing them to play video games as an alternative activity, thereby increasing obesity. These were very different issues from those I expected to hear about in a workshop addressing health problems, but the process was leading our group to have real discussions about health and the many approaches needed to address each of the identified problems.

Bringing a group of socially separated, educationally diverse, and yet community-minded participants into a nontraditional discussion about health was interesting and challenging. The more educated members of the group found it difficult to relate to the nontraditional approach taught by the facilitator. The individuals who were less educated seemed to be lost in the more academic approaches that were proposed. I was feeling caught in the middle. Yet the facilitator was skilled in refocusing our attention on our problems and possible solutions rather than the method used to solve the problems.

By the end of the first day we were all exhausted, but something had happened. We had begun to talk about our problems in a collective way—not as separate problems but as problems that when taken together equally impacted the community we all served. Several of the participants exchanged phone numbers, and some called others to help them write their "Good Questions." I was so moved by my experience that I could not wait for the next day.

The second day began with a plenary session in the morning in which Dr. Smith spoke about the concept of the "Good Question." My group had bonded as a team the day before, and we were ready to begin. Most of us had our "Good Question" ready to go. When Mrs. Thomas, an elderly woman, read her "Good Question," there was not a dry eye in the room. She desperately wanted to save her grandson from the streets and build a relationship with him. She had tried taking him to church with her, but that effort had failed. In working through this problem during her small group session, she realized that she should focus on her grandson's interest rather than hers, so she decided to take him to basketball games. In carrying out her action plan, Mrs. Thomas built a solid relationship with her grandson and became someone he turned to for encouragement and support.

Mrs. Thomas's problem may not seem like a health issue, but her project was profound and cost effective. Saving just one grandson from the streets can result in a huge savings in healthcare costs. If Mrs. Thomas could save her grandson, she could prevent him from becoming the victim of gun violence, drug addiction, or incarceration. Each of these negative circumstances impacts the cost of healthcare and puts pressure on a healthcare system that is already stretched too far. The PSBH process helps all of us rethink our bias against social projects and opens us up to new perspectives on healthcare that go beyond the traditional, recognizing that positive relationships are important for promoting health.

Next, it was my turn to work on my "Good Question." Gang violence was on the rise in the city of Newark. I was the father of two young sons, who were at risk of gang influence. My first thought was to hold a weeklong seminar to address gang violence with a group of people from around Newark. Newark is a large city, and I had a full-time job and family. After thinking about these factors, I began to narrow my focus in order to achieve the maximum amount of success. Eventually, my "Good Question" proposed an overnight "sleepover" program for 25 students from the St. Rose of Lima Youth Group in the North Ward of Newark to discuss the dangers of gang violence, with the goal of reducing gang participation by 50%. The program took place in the St. Rose of Lima gym in August 1999. The project was a success because I focused on a population to which I had access, and I monitored the results. This was the PSBH process in action.

Such was the beginning of my relationship with DHF and my interest in PSBH. Soon after attending the workshop I met with Marsha Johnson Copeland, the PSBH National Coordinator for the United States, to discuss ways to replicate the process and maximize its effectiveness in the United States. Because of my newfound enthusiasm for the PSBH process and candor about how to move it forward in my community, Marsha asked me to develop another workshop in Newark.

One of the challenges we faced in hosting the new workshop was attracting and engaging more local residents and working professionals, who sometimes have preconceived ideas and biases about community needs. In addition, a 2-day workshop was difficult for most community residents, who could not easily take the time off from work to attend. We examined various ways to keep the PSBH process moving forward while meeting the logistical needs of the population we wished to recruit. We also had to examine the tense relationship between the local host hospital and the community.

Newark and the University Hospital of the University of Medicine and Dentistry of New Jersey (UMDNJ) already faced challenges arising from the university expanding its physical presence. Community members were skeptical about having the PSBH workshop at the hospital, because, in their view, UMDNJ had displaced a community to build the hospital and medical school. This issue was at the forefront of the discussion about hosting the workshop, even though the workshop itself would ultimately serve to bring both forces together to address the health needs of the community and educate healthcare professionals about how to best provide services throughout Newark.

The PSBH process brings people on opposing sides together to find common ground. Once I understood DHF's goals and its approach to health, I was better prepared to engage others in a healthy discussion about how to solve problems in Newark. I enlisted the aid of several community leaders from various professions to recruit workshop participants, and Marsha and I met with the Vice President of Community Affairs at UMDNJ to enlist the university's help in attracting healthcare professionals to the workshop.

It was an exciting time for me as an organizer. Dr. Smith and I met with a group of doctors from UMDNJ to explain the PSBH process. At first, the physicians thought this was an opportunity to obtain funding for a particular project. After they heard the PSBH presentation, however, most were interested because they had projects that required community participation; around 15 doctors agreed to participate in the workshop. In fact, not only were they going to participate but also the university was willing to sponsor the workshop.

With one group ready, we now had to find community members to participate. They were much harder to recruit because they wanted the workshop held in the community, as opposed to the hospital, so the doctors would have to leave their comfort zone and experience the community environment. The community members certainly had some legitimate issues with what they perceived as the hospital's poor public relations in the past. However, I saw this opposition as an opportunity to begin a new discussion about healthcare delivery that centered on team effort. I convinced the community leaders to trust the process and allow us to hold the workshop at the hospital.

All the preliminary work was done in preparation for the workshop, and it was time for the big day. Facilitators attended from around the world—Brazil, El Salvador, Ghana, and the United States. We organized small groups within the workshop that included a mix of doctors, community residents with various social service backgrounds, and community activists. Participant discussions got off to a slow start, but by the end of the day there were fireworks. The participants had discussed issues that included the treatment of patients in the emergency room, hospital policies, and the lack of community involvement in community-based health initiatives. At the end of the first session, representatives from each small group reported on the participants' progress defining their projects. The consensus was that the participants needed more time, because the teamwork process was still taking place. That was a good sign to me because it meant the groups were engaged in meaningful dialogue about their differences and possible common ground.

Something was changing. Less disagreement was taking place and more unity was beginning to occur within the groups. Doctors were listening to community leaders and community leaders were listening to doctors and other healthcare professionals. It was remarkable. They were actually working together. This was the power of PSBH.

The next morning, I paced back and forth; I worried that some participants would feel apprehensive about implementing a project on their own and would not appear for the second day of the workshop. I was shocked and amazed that all but two individuals returned. The day began with a discussion of the "Good Questions" generated. Most participants had developed their "Good Questions," and the interesting fact was that they had worked on them collectively. What a difference from the beginning of the workshop!

One significant success of this PSBH effort in Newark was that a solution to an existing, yet struggling, immunization program ultimately benefited approximately 10,000 children. The immunization van had been going into Newark communities at 9:00 A.M. on weekdays, but few residents showed up to be vaccinated. When the director of the program stated this issue in his workshop group, a community resident responded, "Do you think all Black and Latino people don't work?" The question was shocking to the doctor because he thought the problem was simply that the community did not understand the importance of immunization for its children. The outcome from this discussion was twofold: Two individuals from different perspectives came to an understanding through PSBH methodology, and the number of vaccinated children increased by 80% as a result of changing the time and day the van visited communities. In addition, this problem was resolved at no cost. The PSBH process is such an important tool, not only for clarifying misconceptions about approaches to healthcare delivery within communities but also for developing needed programs and assuring that resources are used properly for community benefit.

After completing the workshop and evaluating the success of the projects, I recruited another group of participants to discuss the possibility of expanding the workshop to Irvington, New Jersey, where we could repeat the process with Irvington General Hospital. DHF; Babyland Family Services; and the newly elected mayor of Irvington, The Honorable Wayne Smith, collaborated to host the workshop. The building of this coalition introduced DHF to a new partner and resources from the local government.

The prospect of working with the government was exciting, because this collaboration would be the first time in the United States that local government and DHF worked together on a PSBH initiative. DHF had attempted this partnership approach in other communities across the country but always encountered a bureaucrat who did not quite understand what PSBH could do for the health and welfare of his or her constituents. Finally, we found someone who was community-minded enough to work with us in bringing PSBH to a broader population, with the government playing a key role.

After Dr. Smith and I met with Mayor Smith, the mayor agreed to financially support what had become the Essex County Health Initiative. The coalition began recruiting residents from across Essex County, including Newark and Livingston, to participate in the workshop. The mayor spoke about PSBH at town hall meetings, and community residents became involved. To think that someone was asking for their opinions about what was needed in their communities—wow, what a concept! At one of the meetings a resident asked, "What's the catch?" It was an understandable question, because before DHF's arrival no foundation had ever engaged the local residents in solving their own problems. The Irvington workshop ultimately generated approximately 100 participants, more than any previous PSBH workshop in the United States.

Since the success of the PSBH programs in Newark and Irvington, I have continued to foster relationships with local community leaders to spread the philosophy of PSBH. The process is an extremely useful tool for challenging individuals to come together to solve health issues. The most powerful aspect of PSBH is its capacity to enlighten, inspire, encourage, and motivate the most ordinary persons to achieve extraordinary results in their communities. During my many discussions with Dr. Smith, I came to realize that PSBH is a radical approach and one that I love because it puts unlikely heroes in places where they can effect change, one project at a time.

29

Mississippi Delta

The Mississippi Delta lies just below Memphis, Tennessee, and extends south approximately 200 miles to Vicksburg, Mississippi. The Delta is 60 miles wide, bounded on the east by the Yazoo River and on the west by the Mississippi River. It is an alluvial plain, rather than a true delta, created by flooding over thousands of years that has given the area some of the richest soil in the world. The Delta has contributed much to U.S. culture through its blues music, literary tradition, and religious faith. It has a strong, resilient people, predominantly of African American descent. The Delta also has some of the worst poverty and health problems in the United States. Problem Solving for Better Health is in the Delta to help unleash the potential of the people there to create a model of change for rural America.

Problem Solving for Better Health in the Mississippi Delta

Julian D. Miller and Marsha Johnson Copeland

Life in the Mississippi Delta appears to be all about numbers—economic indicators, poverty and jobless rates, and other measures of social and community well-being. The numbers in the Delta are dismal; they are some of the worst in the United States, comparable with—and sometimes worse than—those of countries in the developing world. Poverty levels in the Delta are significantly higher than the national average (20% in the Delta vs. 13% nationwide); the Delta has the highest obesity rate in the United States, leading the nation in deaths resulting from cardiovascular disease, with a rate more than 30% above the national average; the highest stroke death rates in the nation are also in the Delta region, and Mississippi is at the bottom of the list of states with regard to income (Bloom & Bowser, 2008). Demographers have said that in order for life expectancy in the

Julian D. Miller is Problem Solving for Better Health (PSBH) Program Coordinator in the Mississippi Delta. Marsha Johnson Copeland is PSBH National Coordinator for the United States.

Delta region to be equivalent to the average U.S. life expectancy, it would take a 135% increase in income (Bloom & Bowser, 2008). The Delta has been at the bottom looking up for a very long time. The region's story is one of grinding poverty, destitution, and utter hopelessness caused by a crippling legacy of slavery, racism, and deep social and economic injustice.

The Delta's dismal numbers, however, do not tell the full story. Known for its unique culture and heritage, rich history, and warm and inviting atmosphere, the Delta inspired some of the most popular music in the world, including jazz; rock and roll; and the blues, which traces its roots to Clarksdale, Mississippi. This music emanated from the struggles of destitution and social injustice endured by Black sharecroppers and tenant farmers from the 1860s through the 1940s. Despite these struggles, hard work, family, faith, and a solid core of positive values fueled the Delta's communities. The opportunities for the region to remake, renew, and rebuild itself arise from the values that have enabled the people to endure the social and economic problems in the Delta. So while the numbers say the Delta is at the bottom, the numbers have it wrong. The essential goodness of the people makes them stronger and more determined to climb to the top, so, quite possibly, the bottom may be the best place to be after all. The citizens of the Delta possess an enduring spirit and tenacity and therefore are more than capable of creating positive change.

History of Problem Solving for Better Health in the Delta

The Dreyfus Health Foundation (DHF) launched its Problem Solving for Better Health® (PSBH®) program in the Delta's Coahoma County in 2003. Over the years, PSBH participants have achieved significant success in identifying solutions to health problems that affect the well-being of individuals living in the region. Approximately 80 quality-of-life, economic, health, and educational projects have been developed and completed. At least 20 of these projects are ongoing and have taken root as established and integral parts of community life. Through partnerships with academic institutions, hospitals and clinics, local government agencies, nonprofit organizations, and numerous individuals, DHF has created a network committed to the development of better health and economic opportunity in the Delta. This interdisciplinary network works collaboratively to promote health and economic development in the Delta.

The ultimate goal is the development of a self-maintaining, self-replicating process of transformation among the people of the Delta. Individual efforts have already coalesced in some communities, providing evidence of a significant community transformation.

A Personal View

Julian D. Miller

My own life story in the Delta has been a blend of tragedy and triumph. I was born on June 14, 1985, in Clarksdale, a small, impoverished, rural Mississippi Delta town. The day before, doctors had told my mother with certainty that I would be stillborn. But I was born a healthy seven pounds, five ounces. When I was 18 months old I was diagnosed with a crippling bone condition that turned my feet inward. I had to wear braces on my legs, and doctors said there was a 70% chance that I would be permanently disabled. However, the braces corrected the condition shortly after my second birthday; I have been walking normally ever since.

I was raised in a small town of about 300 people where more than 50% of my community lived in poverty. The town has an annual budget of 17,000 USD a year, collects only 700 USD in property taxes, and the school district has one of the worst performance rates in the state (the state itself being at the bottom of the nation in educational performance). Despite the circumstances, I progressed through the local school system and was admitted to Harvard University, earning a bachelor's degree in government in 3 years. Following graduation I decided to go back home and work as a local coordinator for DHF's PSBH program in the Delta.

My experience growing up in the Mississippi Delta has taught me that true success is accomplished through adversity, and failure exists only when one does not learn from— and become better because of—that adversity. I see successes every day in my work with community projects and my interactions with people in the Delta.

Problem Solving for Better Health Projects

Lose Weight, Feel Great!

Through my work with DHF, I reconnected with my first grade teacher, Sister Teresa Shields, a member of the Sisters of the Holy Names of Jesus and Mary. Sister Teresa works in Jonestown, Mississippi, with Sister Kay Burton and other nuns in the town. Sister Kay runs the Durocher House, which offers educational programs such as volunteer training, general educational development and after-school tutoring, and piano and carpentry lessons. Sister Teresa directs a similar institution, the Jonestown Family Center. Established in 1992, the center has grown to include the Montessori Children's House, a toddler playgroup, and a health club. The center also offers special events and trips aimed at cultural development.

In the 1980s, Sister Teresa and Sister Kay were among several hundred nuns who came from as far away as Washington state to settle in small rural towns of the Delta. Jonestown, a community of approximately 50 Whites and 1,600 Blacks, might appear grim to an outsider. Almost half of the adults lack a high school diploma and are unemployed. Consistent with other isolated Delta towns, there is no public transportation in Jonestown, and almost one third of the households do not own a car. However, the nuns and their colleagues do not focus on the numbers. They are focused on overcoming differences and affirming hope in the face of despair. They have accessed available resources and leveraged them to create innovative partnerships to address the challenges.

Until 2007, Sister Manette Durand, a nurse practitioner, was the only healthcare provider in Jonestown. In 2004, she attended a PSBH workshop and developed a project to address the overweight adolescent females living in the town. "Lose Weight, Feel Great!" initially began as a diet and exercise program for 15 sedentary, overweight adolescents. What started in a small, renovated shed with a single set of free weights has evolved into a full-fledged fitness center. Sister Teresa also attended a PSBH workshop and built on

Sister Manette's success; in collaboration with several community partners, she started the Jonestown Health and Fitness Club, which has been operating since 2005 and has a membership of 500.

Alligator Aggies

Mechelle Wallace also attended a PSBH workshop, where she developed a community garden project in Alligator, Mississippi, appropriately named "Alligator Aggies." Originally from Minnesota, Mechelle came to the Delta as an AmeriCorps Volunteers in Service to America member and pursued a master's degree in community development at Delta State University (DSU). Upon moving to Alligator, Mechelle and her husband decided to clear the land around their house to plant a large vegetable garden. Following the PSBH workshop, Mechelle's goal was to turn the land into a community garden for Alligator residents.

The first year, the garden produced an abundance of vegetables, which succeeded in motivating community members to plant their own vegetable gardens for even greater access to healthy food. Mechelle was able to obtain grants to sustain the garden, including funding to build a greenhouse. The greenhouse enables Mechelle and the community gardeners to grow produce and sell it year round at the farmers' market in Cleveland, Mississippi.

Mechelle has a vision for what she wants the future of "Alligator Aggies" to be. While she already provides gardening activities for local students as part of her project, she is seeking partnerships with local school districts to establish the community garden as a sustainable, after-school learning program.

New Delta Rising—Mississippi Delta Initiative

Building on 5 years of successful activity, a new PSBH effort, DHF's New Delta Rising—Mississippi Delta Initiative, has been created. The initiative focuses on the Delta's 11 core counties: Quitman, Humphreys, Bolivar, Coahoma, Tallahatchie, Leflore, Sunflower, Sharkey, Issaquena, Tunica, and Holmes, and has the potential to become a model for rural development in the United States. The New Delta Rising rally in fall 2009 officially launched the initiative. The event was an unprecedented opportunity for those who live and work in the Delta to assert their vision for change and to become part of the solution. New Delta Rising focuses on the principle that success stems from coordinated, multisectoral efforts with the people themselves, their families, and their communities as the critical agents of change.

Conclusion

The people of the Delta are united by their rich heritage, deep humanity, and common struggle to create better lives for themselves and their children. Their commitment to change, their ideas, and their hard work are already sparking a movement to benefit lives in the region. The progress to date provides clear evidence of what is possible. PSBH is just one piece of the ongoing broader effort for positive change in the Delta. We believe that the people of Mississippi, many of whom are leading or participating in these community initiatives, can set an example and standard for what the rest of the United States can and must achieve.

Problem Solving for Better Health-Nursing in Mississippi

Pamela Hoyt-Hudson

Because nurses are on the front line of healthcare, they need to become part of the solution when addressing community health problems and workforce issues. Several Mississippi nurses had already participated in the community-based PSBH program prior to 2003 and implemented projects to solve local problems. Dean Lizabeth Carlson at Delta State University School of Nursing (DSU SON), for example, attended the very first PSBH workshop held in Clarksdale, Mississippi. She was determined to decrease the nursing student dropout rate at DSU SON. It was this project that eventually led to a partnership between the DHF and DSU SON to address local nursing workforce issues in the Mississippi Delta as part of Partners Investing in Nursing's Future (PIN), a national initiative funded by the Robert Wood Johnson Foundation (RWJF).

Partners Investing in Nursing's Future

Judith Woodruff

The current and future shortage of appropriately educated and culturally competent nurses in the United States threatens the safety and morale of the nursing workforce, increases healthcare costs, compromises patient safety and outcomes, and ultimately diminishes the ability of dedicated health professionals to provide the best care and services for their communities. This shortage will affect virtually every sector of society. Surmounting these challenges requires innovative strategies, collaborative partnerships, and a long-term investment on the part of individual communities. The nursing shortage will not be solved with a one-size-fits-all national, top-down approach; only a network of interventions and practices can sustain impact.

PIN, a unique, collaborative initiative of the RWJF and the Northwest Health Foundation (NWHF), addresses nursing issues at the community level through funding partnerships with local and regional foundations. This initial investment of funds creates a financial incentive for local and regional communities to develop tailored solutions to nursing workforce issues.

One of the most important outcomes for the PIN program is ensuring strong partnerships at the local and state levels, so that the funded projects can move forward beyond the life of the grants. The program focuses on increasing the racial, ethnic, and gender

---

Judith Woodruff is Program Director of Health Workforce, Northwest Health Foundation, and Program Director for Partners Investing in Nursing's Future.

diversity of the nursing workforce, providing better access to care, including greater patient choice and satisfaction, and improving patient–nurse communication.

In the first year of the PIN program, Mississippi was the only state to receive two grants, and both were focused on developing the African American nurses in the Delta. The grants aimed to recruit and support nursing students through graduation, employ and retain them in the Delta community as practicing registered nurses, and find new ways to bolster the nursing faculty in the region. The PIN program funded DHF, in partnership with DSU SON, to improve the retention and progression of minority nursing students in the Delta area, where attrition in the baccalaureate program had been as high as 54%. The PIN grant enabled DHF and DSU to strengthen existing efforts to develop and retain a diverse nursing workforce in the state using DHF's PSBH model. As part of the DHF PIN project, members of the Eliza Pillars Registered Nurses of Mississippi, a professional organization for African American nurses, worked directly with individual students as mentors, helping them to understand quality of life and healthcare opportunities in the region. The PIN project also engaged practicing nurses and students in developing solutions to local health and social problems.

The following section describes both of the PIN grants awarded in Mississippi, to DHF and to the Mississippi Hospital Association Health, Research and Educational Foundation (MHA-F). It highlights the successes resulting from DHF's Problem Solving for Better Health-Nursing™ (PSBHN™) initiative and the partnerships established throughout the region between individuals, organizations, and projects. The ability to create expanded capacity statewide through a network of small and large projects that interrelate and that share technical and human resources has become increasingly important to ensure sustainability of impact in Mississippi.

Partners Investing in Nursing's Future in Mississippi

Frances C. Henderson

When the request for proposals came out on behalf of the RWJF PIN Program in 2005, the International Nursing Program Coordinator at DHF, Pamela Hoyt-Hudson, contacted Dr. Lizabeth Carlson, Dean of DSU SON, to discuss the possibility of submitting a grant proposal to address nursing workforce issues in the Delta region of Mississippi. Dean Carlson had already participated in the community-based PSBH program led by DHF, was familiar with the PSBH methodology, and had implemented several projects. Hoyt-Hudson then worked with several nursing colleagues, including Dr. Joyce Fitzpatrick and me, to develop the proposal to meet the local need as outlined by Dean Carlson. As a result of their combined efforts, DHF, in partnership with DSU SON, received a grant in the first cohort of 10 national PIN partners in 2006.

The PIN project developed from one of Dean Carlson's successful PSBH projects. Alarmed by the high number of first semester dropouts at DSU SON, Dean Carlson had attended a DHF PSBH community-based workshop to take action and address this problem. Dean

---

Frances C. Henderson served as a nursing consultant to the Dreyfus Health Foundation on the Partners Investing in Nursing's Future project and Problem Solving for Better Health-Nursing initiatives.

Carlson's solution was a camp for minority nursing students, predominately African Americans, to teach them skills they need to succeed in the nursing program at DSU and improve the rate of program progression, especially through the first semester. She designed a 2-week camp that included study and math skills sessions, time management lessons, a nurse shadowing opportunity, and an introduction to the culture of the Delta. Although it was a relatively small project, the camp was highly successful. As a result, Dean Carlson was determined to scale up her idea to improve the rates of program progression, not just through the first semester but also through the entire program. This was the impetus for the PIN proposal titled "Minority Nurse Mentoring in the Mississippi Delta."

Minority Nurse Mentoring in the Mississippi Delta

First Component

The DHF Delta PIN project had four components. The first component of the PIN project involved a series of focus groups. For this part of the project, my "Good Question" was "How can focus group interviews; cultural diversity workshops; and exploration of culture, history, and heritage provide guidance for addressing the shortage of African American nurses in the Mississippi Delta?" Her objective was to obtain input from the local community on the reasons for the problem in order to help the community develop a plan to address it.

Because the problem is the shortage of African American nurses in the Delta, Dean Carlson and I identified nurses, nursing faculty, and African American nursing students as the key people to comprise the focus groups. The focus groups included 8–10 people in homogeneous groupings, so that, for example, students comprised a focus group separate from faculty, and faculty at each of the two schools of nursing participated in separate groups. Eight focus groups were conducted in Cleveland and Clarksdale, Mississippi, during October and November 2006. Four focus groups comprised nurses from area hospitals: Delta Regional Medical Center, Greenwood Leflore Hospital, Bolivar Medical Center, and Northwest Mississippi Regional Medical Center. Two groups were African American nursing students enrolled at DSU and Coahoma Community College (CCC), and two were faculty at those schools. There were 76 focus group participants: 40 nurses, 20 students, and 16 faculty members. Six questions were asked of each focus group:

- Question 1: What are characteristics of persons who should enter a nursing career in the Mississippi Delta Region?
- Question 2: What strategies or approaches should be used in recruiting students into a nursing career in the Mississippi Delta?
- Question 3: What are some approaches or strategies that are needed to keep students in the nursing program and help them to be successful?
- Question 4: What supports do new nursing graduates need to work as nurses in the Mississippi Delta?
- Question 5: What would prevent nurses from staying in the Mississippi Delta to practice nursing?
- Question 6: What support is necessary in Delta communities to build and sustain a nursing workforce that mirrors the community population?

Second Component

The second component of the PIN project addressed an issue that emerged from the focus groups: the need to expand strategies for exploring and valuing cultural diversity and to build a sustainable nursing workforce that mirrors the community's population in the Mississippi Delta, the majority of which is African American. To address this, the focus group participants, along with senior students at DSU, were invited to participate in a 3-hour forum at DSU on "Exploring and Valuing Cultural Diversity." Participants were expected to (1) explore their knowledge of the language of culture, (2) explore their level of comfort when engaged in interactions with persons whose race/culture is different from theirs, (3) assess intent and meanings of messages sent and received in interactions between persons of different races/cultures, (4) explore rationale for valuing cultural diversity, (5) identify messages that communicate the valuing of cultural diversity, and (6) generate strategies that demonstrate the value of cultural diversity.

Forum activities included a pre-assessment and post-assessment of participants' knowledge and experience with each objective, a 14-item assessment of the language of cultural diversity, and discussion of a homework assignment designed to help participants explore their level of comfort when engaged in interactions with persons of different races/cultures. The assignment was to think of an interaction where you applied successful strategies for dealing with a situation where racial and/or cultural differences were apparent factors. Participants answered the following three questions: (1) What rationale supported your behaviors? (2) Are you satisfied with your interaction? (3) If you are not satisfied with your interaction, how would you have handled it differently?

The pre-assessment based on the objectives gave participants an opportunity to rate their level of knowledge and experience with the forum expectations prior to their participation. Participants then shared answers in a group setting; by the end of the experience of sharing answers, participants were laughing at themselves and were visibly engaged in the process. The carryover of this mood into the discussion of the homework assignment helped some participants to feel secure enough to share their own personal stories of interactions. On the post-assessment results based on the objectives, participants' ratings of their level of knowledge and experience were noticeably higher than on the pre-assessment. The forum was a success in that it helped participants to explore the reality of cultural diversity and determine how they communicate and demonstrate their valuing of cultural diversity in their everyday lives.

Third Component

The third component of the PIN project emphasized minority nurse mentoring; it was initiated by Dr. Sonja R. Fuqua, a member of the Eliza Pillars Registered Nurses, who has a career in nursing practice, education, and management. Dr. Fuqua coordinated the mentoring program as part of the overall goal of retaining African American nursing students at DSU. To begin, there were several focus groups at area hospitals and with nursing students and nursing faculty to determine what they thought a mentoring relationship should be. The information was compiled and mentors were identified. A mentoring relationship workshop was held for those African American nurses who expressed an interest in participating in the program. During the workshop, participants discussed what a mentoring relationship would be like: the expectations, strengths, and weaknesses of the mentors and how they could offer available resources to the students. Once the mentor and the mentee had established a relationship, they were to meet monthly, at a minimum. Dr. Fuqua asked the mentors to keep a log of their contacts and report that information for the purpose of maintaining records.

Hospitals and other workplaces benefit when students are mentored, remain in the nursing program, and pass the boards. Among the barriers to increasing the number of minorities in nursing are the lack of a systematic mentoring infrastructure and the paucity of minority nursing faculty. The "Good Question" that emerged from the focus groups related to mentoring was "Will mentoring African American nursing students at DSU increase their retention and graduation rates, as well as their passage rate of the nursing licensure examination, and influence them to remain in the Delta after graduation?" To address this question, three objectives were formulated: (1) increase retention of minority nursing students by 50%; (2) increase by 50% the number of minority students who pass the nursing licensure examination on the first testing; and (3) increase by 50% the number of minority students who intend to remain in the Delta area after graduation.

In terms of outcomes, all three objectives were met over a 2-year period when compared with the previous 2 years. In 2006, three African American students graduated and two passed the licensure examination on the first testing. In 2008, 10 mentored African American students graduated, 5 of whom passed the licensure examination on the first testing (the remaining 5 passed on subsequent testing), and all 10 remained in the area to work as nurses. While mentoring was not the only factor in these outcomes, it was a key factor.

Fourth Component

The fourth component of the PIN project included a PSBHN workshop, and the projects that were implemented as a result. The workshop was held in January 2006; nursing faculty from DSU and CCC participated, as well as several Chief Nursing Officers (CNOs) from local hospitals in the Mississippi Delta. Stemming from their participation, three faculty groups from DSU SON designed and received funding for three projects with the goal of addressing the nursing shortage. The projects developed were S.U.P.P.O.R.T. (Support, Understanding Provided by Parents/Others Reality Training); R.E.A.D.Y. (Professional Roles in Nursing/Education in Nursing/Assertiveness and Accountability in Nursing/Determination and Desires in Nursing/Why do you want to be a Nurse?); and S.M.A.R.T. (Student Mentoring Achieves Retention and Transition).

Another result of the workshop was the "Camp Coahoma" project, developed by Dr. Evelyn Smith, the former Director of the Associate Degree Nursing Program at CCC. The CCC RN program did not have a structured orientation or retention component. The attrition rate was high for the first class. In response, Dr. Smith developed the Nursing Student Tracking and Retention (N-STAR) program, which mobilized the faculty and the student body to take action. The project became part of the orientation program for new nursing students/registration at CCC.

Rebecca Edwards, CNO at Greenwood Leflore Hospital, also attended the PSBHN workshop and developed a project proposal to decrease turnover rates at the hospital.

Her target audience was initially 25 nurse managers. Because one of the principles of the PSBHN program is optimizing available resources, DHF consulted the Mississippi Office of Nursing Workforce (ONW), the implementing institution of the other PIN grant in Mississippi, to see if there was potential for collaboration on Ms. Edwards's project. ONW agreed to lead a series of "leadership/management trainings," not only for Greenwood Leflore but also for all seven area hospitals in the Mississippi Delta, because ONW already had successful modules available and could easily tap its network of nurse leaders in the state as potential guest speakers for the series. This was an unexpected and very positive outcome of Ms. Edwards's project, which ultimately led to further collaboration between DHF and ONW after the leadership series.

Mississippi Critical Nursing Faculty Shortage Initiative

The other PIN program grant in Mississippi in 2006 was awarded to MHA-F, and ONW served as the implementing partner for the project. Wanda M. Jones, a registered nurse who is Executive Director of the Mississippi ONW, and Debbie Logan, another registered nurse who is a project director for the Mississippi ONW, developed the project. Among ONW's organizational goals are (1) creating a statewide database of nursing supply and demand statistics, (2) providing workforce data and analysis to assist in the development of nursing workforce policy, (3) identifying continuing education needs of the nursing workforce, and (4) expanding partnerships between nursing education and practice-related organizations and the community.

ONW's PIN project was titled "Mississippi Critical Nursing Faculty Shortage Initiative." The purpose of the project was to address one of the root problems contributing to the nursing shortage—the nursing faculty shortage. The goal was to develop a comprehensive approach to recruit and retain nurse faculty who reflect the ethnicity of the state population. The four specific project goals were to (1) develop an innovative, accelerated educational path to a faculty career; (2) develop an evidence-based image and recruitment campaign to showcase the nurse educator role; (3) develop multiple adjunct faculty roles with more formal relationships between education and practice; and (4) improve the educational and clinical workplace climates.

To assess workplace environments, a pilot project was conducted with two of the state's nursing programs. Faculty members completed a survey to assess a series of variables related to organizational culture and job satisfaction. Subsequently, the majority of Mississippi schools of nursing participated in the survey, enabling the development of a detailed database on recurring themes and factors related to faculty retention, satisfaction, and commitment. Further, in August 2008 the project launched a website, iTeachNursingMS, which features helpful resources for new faculty or nurses interested in pursuing a teaching career. Other project accomplishments include developing and implementing a "Saving Nurses Saves Lives" public service campaign that contributed to significant increases in the state nursing faculty salary scale; providing information to hospitals, schools of nursing, and other stakeholders on the shortage of nurses and nursing faculty; and expanding and strengthening partnerships between schools of nursing and hospitals. Jones and Logan are proud of all of these achievements and their implications for the future of nursing education and practice in Mississippi.

Conclusion

How do we overcome nursing workforce issues statewide in Mississippi? The key ingredients are working together locally and regionally, developing solutions that are relevant to existing conditions on the ground, and learning to successfully leverage multiple funding sources. The common thread through all of these projects is the power of partnerships. The planning, implementation, and evaluation of each project demonstrate the value of collaborating and networking to unleash this power. Long-standing and ever-evolving Mississippi partnerships, energized by the concept of local solutions to local problems, are beginning to make a sustainable difference in the health status and quality of life in the Delta by increasing the number of nurses in the workforce. DHF, DSU, MHA-F, and ONW are grateful to the PIN program, NWHF, and RWJ for their collaborative spirit that has led to many more successful partnerships, in Mississippi and beyond.

Retaining Talent in Mississippi

Arthur G. Cosby and Tonya T. Neaves

For the last few years, several of us at the Social Science Research Center (SSRC) of Mississippi State University have been investigating the geographic health of the United States under the rubric of *Healthy and Unhealthy Places*. At the foundation of this research has been the identification of regions, such as the Mississippi Delta, whose overall health is so profoundly different from the rest of the nation that it merits a more focused analysis and, perhaps, tailored interventions. "Understanding the connections between location and relation is key to understanding the meaning of place" (Neaves, Feierabend, Butts, & Weiskopf, 2008, p. 10). It has, therefore, become exceedingly important for social researchers to not only answer questions of *where* but also attempt to answer questions of *why there* (Campbell, 2001; De Blij & Alexander, 2000).

We have based our research on the straightforward assumption that, on average, people live longer in healthy places and, correspondingly, die earlier in unhealthy ones. Because we are using the information about death in the United States as the determinant of unhealthy places, death statistics are essential in identifying the health status of locations (Fitzpatrick & LaGory, 2000). Of the available data sets that the National Center for Health Statistics (NCHS) maintains, the Compressed Mortality File (CMF) has county-based mortality statistics for over 80 million deaths that have occurred in the United States between 1968 and 2006 (NCHS, 2000, 2007, 2009). With these data we have identified regions of the nation with disparate health outcomes, including the Black Belt, Appalachia, and the Mississippi Delta.

The confluence of poverty, poor education, and racial discrimination, overlaid with historical and cultural influences, has limited the availability of human capital in these regions, and in the health arena, there are too few doctors and nurses. It is often difficult

Arthur G. Cosby is William L. Giles Distinguished Professor and Director of the Social Science Research Center (SSRC), Mississippi State University. Tonya T. Neaves is a Research Fellow and Project Coordinator at the SSRC.

to retain the ones who are currently there and perhaps even more difficult to recruit new medical professionals to the regions. The remainder of this section focuses on the challenge of developing innovations that aim to recruit talent to the Mississippi Delta and retain it there.

Part I: The Meaning of Health

Measuring Rural Health

The demographic history of the United States has been a transition from a primarily rural, agrarian-based community to an urban, service-based society. As a result, the rural–urban paradigm has shaped the way in which many Americans think about and respond to place (Eberhardt et al., 2001; Ricketts, 1999). Over the past century, many governmental platforms and much scientific literature have outlined health policy for a rural lifestyle (Clifford & Brannon, 1985). This has been especially evident with the establishment of the National Rural Health Association and the Office of Rural Health Policy as well as with the publications of the *Journal of Rural Health* and *Rural Healthy People 2010*. However, "an understanding of rural America's future should be rooted in knowledge of the complexity and diversity of existing rural society rather than reliance on misconceptions or myths about" rurality (Cosby, 2008; Gamm, Hutchison, Dabney, & Dorsey, 2003; U.S. Department of Agriculture, 2010). It may, therefore, be more important to consider a policy platform based on healthy and unhealthy places rather than on rural and urban places.

The availability of health outcome data at appropriate geographic levels, the utilization of spatial statistics, and advances in spatial technologies and visualization techniques allow researchers to think in new ways about place and health (Cossman, Cosby, James, & Jackson-Belli, 2002; Cossman, Cossman, Jackson-Belli, & Cosby, 2003). The CMF contains an immense amount of information, including number of deaths, crude death rates, and age-adjusted death rates, all of which can be searched by place of residence, age group, race, gender, year of death, and underlying cause(s) of death. Utilizing the CMF data as an affixed record of deaths allows researchers to examine specific geographic areas of where there are high death rates (Ingram & Franco, 2006).

Unhealthy Places

Our investigation showed that, from a national perspective, counties with high death rates were neither evenly spread geographically across the United States nor of a random pattern. Instead, there were readily discernable clusters of unhealthy counties with much higher mortality than others (Cosby, 2007; Cosby et al., 2008; J. L. Cossman et al., 2007; Cossman et al., 2003; Cossman, Cossman, Reavis, & Cosby, 2007; Kawachi, Kennedy, Lochner, & Prothrow-Smith, 1997; Murray et al., 2006; Satcher et al., 2005). Though these concentrations of mortality had been recognized by others previously, our healthy and unhealthy approach somewhat differed by focusing on the clusters as "places" that could be fundamentally different in a broad range of social and cultural influences. Most important, the unhealthy clusters are readily recognizable regions, places with names that also have distinct historical and cultural identities. In more familiar terms, our unhealthy places are approximately the regions that we know as the agricultural-based Black Belt, Appalachia, and the Mississippi Delta.

Part II: Living and Working in the Mississippi Delta

About the Delta

The Delta is a land dominated by a rich, storied history and a slow-growing, agricultural economy (Cosby, Brackin, Mason, & McCulloch, 1992). More specifically, the Delta is heavily embedded with the legacy of a plantation society—where there is a "stark orientation to the past," where "high culture sits beside grinding poverty," and where there is a "noticeable racial divide and consciousness" (Austin, 2006).

The Mississippi Delta is a series of counties easily recognized by their physical elements, where the land is relatively flat, with rich, fertile soil ideal for growing a variety of crops. Beyond physical similarities, however, some counties are included as part of the region for their historical and cultural commonalities as well as socioeconomic indicators shared with some of the more traditional counties (Austin, 2006; Neaves et al., 2008).

Over the past three decades, the Mississippi Delta has drawn attention because of its dissipating population and, more important, its persistent and ailing socioeconomic conditions—circumstances that have been shown to perpetuate each other and, consequently, have led to major disparities in health outcomes (Cosby & Bowser, 2008; Mirvis, Chang, & Cosby, 2008). There are two dominant explanations for underlying causes of health disparities in the Delta. One explanation centers on the social determinants of health resulting from poor education; sustained poverty; and, most important, prolonged racial discrimination. Second, access to healthcare presents a challenge, due to the geographic remoteness of the region, limited transportation, and the special challenges these represent for disadvantaged populations.

The Image of the Delta and Residential Choices

The Mississippi Delta is more than a statistical aggregation of counties. It is a place with a distinctive history, culture, and name—a place that is part of our nation's psyche. Indeed, many Americans are conscious of the poverty, poor education, and racial discrimination in the Delta, and this awareness is a double-edged sword for the region (Williams & Jackson, 2005). Many people outside the Mississippi Delta have a great desire "to help." For decades, numerous committed individuals and foundations have given generously, both their time and money, in efforts to improve the region. The national consciousness of conditions in the Delta, however, also cuts in the other direction. The Mississippi Delta is broadly viewed as a place with limited opportunities and possibilities, and, consequently, is a place that has a special problem with attracting new and retaining existing talent.

Mississippi is rarely considered a favorable location for career advancement or lifestyle amenities. The implications of this are far reaching. Students from other areas across the country seldom choose to relocate in Mississippi, while students from Mississippi will often select to leave the state. It is much easier to attract or recruit a Mississippi graduate to California or New York than it is to attract or recruit a California or New York graduate to Mississippi. But students in Mississippi, like students elsewhere, often prefer locations near their own homes, families, and schools, and these choices suggest a major source of talent for the state. Mississippi, and in particular the Mississippi Delta, must capitalize on attracting and retaining graduates from within the state. The institutions of higher learning in states such as Mississippi are incredibly important to their state's future because they contain the most promising and reliable source of talent.

Of course, residential preferences vary greatly within a state. Some regions of Mississippi have more success attracting talent, whereas some others, such as the Mississippi Delta, have more challenges. One might ask, "What value would an information system that identifies the potential flow of talent within Mississippi have for regions like the Delta, which struggles to attract such talent?" In fact, the most challenged places could be the greatest beneficiaries of such an information system.

Attracting Talent to the Delta

Practically all professions and disciplines face challenges in attracting talent to the Mississippi Delta. Shortages of doctors, nurses, and other healthcare professionals are persistent problems for most communities in the region. Many Delta communities have limited healthcare capacity and are located at significant distances from medical centers in Memphis, Tennessee, and Jackson, Mississippi. Moreover, distance to healthcare is a qualitatively more difficult challenge for the disadvantaged. Lack of convenient and reliable transportation is a major healthcare constraint. Identifying the relatively few university and college graduates who might have a preference for pursuing their profession in the Mississippi Delta could be like finding several golden needles in a single haystack.

Imagine that we have an information system tracking the residential preferences of every graduating student at Mississippi's universities and colleges. This is a talent pool that is well over 10,000 individuals with expertise in most disciplines and professions. Many of these graduating students will identify more than one location within Mississippi as a potentially desirable place to pursue their career. Since these students have multiple options, the *potential flow* of human capital, or of talent, is far greater than the number of students. Such an information system could be constructed so that representatives from locations throughout the state would know which graduates with which degrees had to have expressed preferences for their region, and such information would assist every business and organization in Mississippi to identify and recruit talent. The information system could also impact the recruitment of new businesses to the region by representing the "best information available" about the university and college-level talent available for their enterprises. Additionally, the knowledge would be incredibly important in developing informed decisions about business expansion and diversification.

Even relatively small businesses can benefit from information about potential talent flows. As an example, a large casino industry has developed in Tunica County in the northern portion of the Mississippi Delta. The number of casino employees actually exceeds the population of the county, and gaming revenue from the casinos often exceeds 1 billion USD per year. Imagine a one-person accounting firm in Tunica prior to the arrival of the casinos. When the casinos came, the accountant's business rapidly expanded with the growth of the gaming industry to the point that a one-person firm could no longer effectively operate within the new business demands. The accountant then would face the dilemma to either cap the practice or to expand the firm by hiring additional accountants. One critical issue facing the accountant would be the availability of attracting accounting talent to a practice in a small, rural Mississippi Delta community. If there were an information system in place that could identify the accounting graduates who indicated a preference for Tunica County as one place to pursue their profession, the accountant would then be in a better position to make an informed decision. Such an information system is profoundly important for a state like Mississippi that suffers from barriers to attracting talent from outside the state.

Discussion

Improving the talent of the Mississippi Delta is an essential part of any comprehensive strategy for improving the region. Several years ago, we had the good fortune to become acquainted with DHF and its programs within the Mississippi Delta region. We were especially interested in the nursing workforce initiative being led by Pamela Hoyt-Hudson, the International Nursing Program Coordinator for DHF, which applies the PSBHN approach to the training and retention of nursing students in the Delta. The selection of nurses was the most strategic point of intervention to improve the healthcare workforce in the region. There are many schools of nursing in the Delta whose graduates would presumably be likely to practice their profession in the region. The PSBHN programs focused on (1) recruitment to nursing programs; (2) higher graduation rates; and (3) placements within the region. Furthermore, expanding the nurse workforce in the Delta helps address the dearth of primary healthcare, especially because there are more nurses than available doctors.

The PSBHN program focuses on developing and utilizing the resources within the Mississippi Delta to improve the region's healthcare workforce. However, PSBHN did not have a component designed specifically to attract nursing talent from outside the region. We at the SSRC hope to harness information technology to give distressed regions such as the Delta an improved capacity to attract and retain talent. We began by exploring the following line of reasoning: The United States is a very open and mobile society. It is a society that allows a relatively free flow of talent based in large part upon individual preferences and perceptions of opportunities. Our open society grants considerable latitude to individuals in their aspirations and choices for education, occupation, marriage, and reproduction. Can we utilize our knowledge about human capital and how it flows as part of a regional development approach? In addition to these life cycle choices, Americans also have a great deal of freedom in choosing their residence—the place they prefer to live and work. Can we exploit an understanding of residential preferences to our advantage?

By partnering with DHF in the PSBHN programs we can add an additional dimension, recruitment from outside the Mississippi Delta, to the overall effort. To that end, a group of SSRC scientists with support from the Delta Health Alliance initiated a project called "Development of an Interactive Web-Based System for the Use and Assessment of Human Capital among Health and Other Professionals in Mississippi." The goals of the project were to (1) develop a Web-based instrument that measures community/geographic relocation preferences of college students pursing health-related professions, (2) administer the instrument to samples of students at Mississippi institutions of higher learning, (3) assess the potential flow of human capital (health professionals) to various locations within the Mississippi Delta, and (4) draft a summary report that assesses the potential for developing a talent-to-location information system and outlines the necessary sequence of activities. This was essentially a pilot test of the concept's feasibility in the Mississippi environment.

Implications

The pilot test with Mississippi nursing students pointed to a number of challenges with our approach to assessing and possibly influencing the flow of human capital. Foremost among these was the complexity of the students' residential choices. The students were making multiple choices with varying degrees of certainty. Their choices also were qualitatively different in their geographic reference. Some students gave choices that were geographic points or locations, such as Jackson, Mississippi. Others' choices, however, tended to be more broadly defined in terms of buffers, regions, or even distances from a specific place. To capture such different ways of relating one's residential preferences, we developed an interactive Web-based survey with maps. This approach had a number of advantages in that it not only managed the complexity of students' responses but also provided a method of data collection that would easily scale up to include multiple professions and disciplines and multiple university and college sites.

We are now at the stage of implementing a more comprehensive application of the survey with a broader range of nursing schools within the state. Fortunately, DHF has secured a grant from the W. K. Kellogg Foundation to support PSBHN programs designed to enhance the Mississippi Delta nursing workforce, and our group has been invited to join the effort by expanding the scope of the survey project. This work began in early 2010 and is programmed for a 1-year trial period. In addition to developing and applying approaches to collecting information about residential preferences of nursing students, this year's project addresses how this information can be used to enhance recruitment. We plan to work closely with the existing leaders in the state for nursing workforce issues, primarily the Mississippi ONW. This approach will be an additional tool for ONW to use in their workforce development. Success would mean increasing the talent pool of nurses in the Delta and institutionalizing the approach by transferring the management, operation, and oversight of the data system to the ONW.

Community Development

John J. Green and Sarah J. Leonard

Within the community development literature there is a focus on "models of practice," including self-help, technical assistance, and conflict approaches (Christenson, 1989;

John J. Green is Director of the Institute for Community-Based Research and Associate Professor of Sociology and Community Development, Delta State University. Sarah J. Leonard is an Assistant Director for the College Board Advanced Placement Program.

Green & Haines, 2008; Green, 2008; Hardina, 2002). These models are often augmented by a fourth approach that is participatory and empowerment oriented (Chambers, 1997; Freire, 1972; Gaventa, 1980; Selener, 1997). This section describes the successes and challenges encountered in DHF's PSBH and PSBHN programs using the participatory and empowerment-oriented approach to program evaluation. We will review the PSBH model, present how the model has been utilized in the Delta region, and then share insights from our involvement with the programs. The analysis draws from our participation in, and evaluation of, PSBH efforts.

Dreyfus Health Foundation and Problem Solving for Better Health

DHF fills an important gap by providing much-needed resources for community development. The Mississippi Delta has long been a priority area for resources from major foundations, which have helped to augment state and federal government funding. Nonprofits, faith-based organizations, and public institutions in the Delta have collectively received millions of dollars in grant monies to support their development initiatives. Like these other funders, DHF has demonstrated an interest in investing in projects in the Delta, specifically in the Clarksdale, Mississippi, vicinity. DHF takes a different approach than many other foundations. Rather than awarding large grants to organizations, DHF empowers individuals and small-scale groups through training and providing microgrants to address the issues in their communities that concern them and for which they are willing to take ownership.

Review of Problem Solving for Better Health

Problem Solving for Better Health Initiatives

DHF introduced the PSBH model in the Mississippi Delta in 2003, holding a series of workshops; as of fall 2008, DHF had documented 70 projects from the Delta region. Beginning in fall 2005, the DSU Institute for Community-Based Research conducted an evaluation of these PSBH projects in the Delta region, first with a qualitative assessment. A quantitative assessment followed in spring 2006.

The evaluation started with the compilation of project information sheets provided by DHF. This information was used to select a purposive sample ensuring that a variety of projects and perspectives were represented in the evaluation. We conducted interviews with project participants and identified 12 participants whose projects had been funded during the first 2 years that DHF hosted PSBH workshops in the Delta. We invited these grantees to participate in our evaluation and all agreed.

Evaluation questions were grouped into multiple categories, including personal and organizational background, information about the project, human capital and networks, effective and ineffective features of the project, outcomes, recommendations, and next steps. Each interview was audio recorded and typically lasted 30–45 minutes. Online respondents were emailed the list of questions and given 2 weeks to reply. Following the interviews, tapes were transcribed, and then transcripts and notes were entered into a qualitative data analysis program. Data were coded by themes that emerged from the interviews.

As a follow-up to the qualitative interviews, we constructed a questionnaire to collect quantitative data. The questionnaire addressed topics similar to those discussed in the interviews and incorporated additional ideas that emerged during the course of analyzing interview data. The sample for the survey was drawn from all PSBH grant recipients in the Delta program area. Questionnaires were mailed to 49 project participants, with 29 returned, for a 60% response rate.

Here we provide a summary of the evaluation results. PSBH projects designed and implemented in the Delta addressed a wide array of issues, but most of them shared a similar emphasis on education. Participants believed there was a need for, and value in, educating others through development of materials, sharing information, participatory interaction, and workshops. The interviewees indicated pride in their accomplishments and offered examples of how the populations served had enjoyed and benefited from the projects. "The biggest outcome is expanding [the] horizons for a few youth [in the community]. I know it's broadened their horizons because they've seen this whole other environment that they never knew existed, and here it is right in their own backyard," one participant explained. Many also felt they had created and expanded beneficial networks through their involvement with DHF/PSBH and within their own communities.

Of course, participants faced challenges with their projects as well. These included limited involvement from the wider community, issues with funding, and concerns over the future sustainability of their projects. Small-scale projects appear to work well in effecting change for targeted groups of people, but their long-term viability often hinges on involvement and buy-in from other community members as well, who can provide resources and support.

Participants also indicated a need for further training and capacity development in the areas of project evaluation and sustainability. Both of these topics are important for community development initiatives to be effective and achieve greater continuity. One participant keenly observed:

> There are so many of us who are on the ground floor [and] don't have that process. We [have] this idea, and we think if we do some activities [we can make an impact], but we can't tell who benefited. I think we've done some wonderful things with very little resources, but we have to learn a way to articulate that to others who may have resources in order to catch up and keep up.

The importance of evaluation is intertwined with sustainability in this sense, in that it allows project leaders to better understand the full impact of their projects, while at the same time providing concrete evidence of success to potential supporters.

Problem Solving for Better Health-Nursing

Because of our role with the PSBH program evaluation we were asked to also lead the evaluation for DHF's PSBHN Mississippi initiative that was part of the PIN national program. DHF's Mississippi Delta PIN project was developed to address local nursing workforce issues. One aspect of the PIN project was the utilization of the PSBH model whereby nursing faculty and hospital staff developed projects to improve student retention in nursing school, especially among minorities, and retain nurses on the job in the Delta.

Evaluation of the PIN project involved multiple methods of data collection and analysis, such as document review, analysis of nursing school performance data, and surveys of students, faculty, and other participants. Interviews were conducted with project participants, including representatives from the program, as well as those people affiliated with other PIN projects with which the DSU SON/DHF partners had developed networks (i.e., organizations in Jackson, Mississippi, and Montana). Participants included project directors, project coordinators, and PSBHN workshop participants who received grants from DHF to implement their projects. We conducted a total of 12 telephone interviews and compiled the notes from these into partial transcripts.

Overall, participants reported enthusiasm for their involvement in the PIN effort, and they expressed general satisfaction with the process and outcomes. Several of the interviewees commented on having since expanded relationships developed through the projects, and said that they have generated innovative practices for addressing the nursing shortage in the region. Resources made available through PIN and PSBHN enabled them to think outside of the box and try out new ideas on a small, feasible scale.

Participants mentioned a wide variety of successes as well as challenges. The overarching theme in their reflections revolved around the importance of relationships and collaborative problem solving. The interviewees felt that networking and partnership development were important components of PIN, extending beyond the immediate goals of the original initiative. Structuring projects in a way that encourages or even requires some level of collaboration appears to be useful for addressing challenges and developing innovative solutions.

Interview respondents described several successful outcomes from the PIN project, such as providing tools and services, demonstrating improvements in retention and licensure examination passage, buy-in and commitment to the projects, benefits of using the PSBH model, and collaboration. Providing needed tools and services to students and the existing nursing workforce was one aspect of the projects that participants felt was particularly successful. These tools included mentoring services, leadership seminars, and orientation and information for students' family members. Students are now more aware of the expectations in nursing school, faculty better understand issues students face (specifically African American students), and families of nursing students have greater knowledge about what students must confront in nursing school.

The main objective of all of these tools and services was to reduce student attrition and improve students' first-time pass rates on the state licensing examination, and participants achieved success in both areas. According to the interview respondents, nursing school retention rates have substantially improved as a result of the PIN project, and this claim was substantiated by official DSU SON data. As for passing the board examinations, all mentored students passed their boards, but not necessarily on the first try, which is important to both nursing students and nursing schools.

Overall, respondents were pleased not only with their project outcomes but also with the process. Several felt that the PSBHN process increased participant commitment and buy-in among nursing faculty, students, and nurses in the Delta. Using the PSBH model also allowed participants to develop innovative ideas to address challenges. PSBHN was found useful in helping people to conceptualize their projects and mobilize people to participate. Furthermore, they mentioned the model in terms of supporting success. As a participant explained:

> One of the things that intrigued me about using PSBH for the PIN project is that because they are low-cost interventions they're sustainable, and we indeed are

continuing all three of our projects. … Retention of nursing students is a major problem across the nation. Having a retention rate of 50% is not unusual, and to be able to do something for less than 1,000 USD that addresses that, is huge.

Another respondent commented that participants who had gone through the PSBHN training "have indicated to us that they use those skills on an ongoing basis." This demonstrates that the model may be applicable in a variety of settings and that the skills learned in the PSBHN workshop are transferable to other projects and situations.

Although participants generally regarded their participation in the PIN project enthusiastically, they did encounter challenges along the way. One interviewee felt the greatest challenge was managing competing priorities. A further challenge participants confronted was ensuring open communication between schools and clinical sites where students are placed. Building relationships with clinical placement sites such as hospitals, providing mentoring and support services while students are in school, and offering leadership workshops for nurse managers are all ways of ensuring that expectations are clearly communicated.

Successes and Lessons Learned

In this section, we summarize lessons learned from evaluation of both the PSBH and PSBHN (hereafter referred to simply as PSBH) efforts in the Delta. The goal is to move from the specific projects to a more abstract level of analysis concerning the PSBH approach to community development initiatives.

Successes

Projects that have the goal of improving health and quality of life could be considered too difficult to achieve. However, respondents in the evaluation described their projects as successfully achieving change in their communities. Sometimes they noted that changes were small, influencing only a few individuals, but they felt the impact was meaningful and had positive results. Other participants appreciated the local control that the PSBH model afforded. For instance, one interviewee talked about how participatory local decision making can influence the design of the project. The grassroots nature of the DHF projects has allowed participants to implement projects that address specific local needs. In this way, participants have a more vested interest in, and ownership of, the projects.

In addition to positive reflections about their projects, respondents' feelings about the DHF were often positive as well. Many spoke of DHF as being the catalyst for their projects; one described how DHF facilitates emotional well-being: "The Real Progress is the Spiritual Progress." This individual appreciated that DHF understands that to help and to enable are two different things and that the real value of the PSBH process is when a person commits to, and completes, his or her own project. This demonstrates how DHF and the PSBH model present a unique and innovative approach focused on empowering individuals and instigating community change.

One of the benefits resulting from these projects for most respondents was the development and/or expansion of their personal networks through their involvement with DHF. Networks developed as a result of the PSBH workshops and involvement with DHF provided a way for participants to bridge the gap in funding, since PSBH grant recipients typically receive only small microgrants for their projects. Respondents described the resources they were able to obtain as a result of their networks, including equipment, technical assistance, meeting space, and new collaborations. Participants commented that the partnerships developed through the projects had established the potential for additional collaboration in the future. Relationships among community-based organizations, colleges/universities, and hospitals, for example, were strengthened, enabling the development of new initiatives.

Lessons Learned

An important aspect of evaluation is learning more about what works well and what could be improved in a project or program. From the results of these evaluations, we have identified three primary lessons learned.

The first lesson is that PSBH workshop participants would benefit from additional technical assistance. For many participants, the workshop was their first exposure to proposal writing and, for some, their first foray into community development. They had wonderful ideas, enthusiasm, and passion but were often unsure of how to begin or what to do once their projects were operational. Several interview respondents commented that they would benefit from training in how to evaluate a project or ensure project sustainability beyond the life of a PSBH grant. Providing technical assistance would not only benefit the projects but also establish a foundation of skills and knowledge upon which participants could build in the future. By providing technical assistance, DHF could contribute to an even greater sense of self-efficacy and empowerment.

Another lesson identified from these evaluations concern the power and potential of networks. Collaboration is an integral component in the PSBH process, because participants are required to identify and attempt to utilize existing resources in their communities. This almost always means working with others to find and access those resources. Many interview respondents felt they had created and expanded beneficial networks through their involvement with DHF and the PSBH programs.

Relevance of Problem Solving for Better Health to the Practice of Community Development

The prevailing models of community development practice are ideal types used to classify, characterize, and distinguish between approaches to social change. These are helpful heuristic tools, but on the ground strategies and techniques typically overlap within and between community development programs. Elements of each model are likely used in any actual effort toward social change. The PSBH model demonstrates such real-world complexities, and evaluation offers insights for better understanding and utilizing models of practice.

In a few short years, DHF has helped to stimulate community development in the Mississippi Delta region by introducing a model of practice that synthesizes traditional approaches and combines them with participatory and empowerment leanings. Through the PSBH model, people have been trained, plans have been developed for community change, and people have implemented their plans. Community members interacted, learned from one another, and established broader networks.

On the surface, it may seem odd that a foundation based in New York facilitates participatory community development in the Mississippi Delta. However, through DHF's workshops and microfunding program, individuals in the Delta have defined situations of concern to them and their communities, identified solutions, and taken action to improve people's lives and build better places to live. They have also networked and shared their ideas with others in their communities, state, region, and beyond. Yet it takes considerable time, energy, resources, and commitment to make this approach work.

Participatory and empowerment-oriented models of community development, like PSBH, may not give explicit attention to it, but technical assistance is critical for building capacity for self-directed action. According to PSBH participants, there is a need for greater attention to technical assistance, especially in terms of evaluation and achieving organizational sustainability. From a participatory standpoint this may seem like a functional and technocratic approach to community development, but individuals and organizations desire to build and improve their capacities to pursue change.

In addition, leadership is a crucial dimension of all community development work. Through PSBH, many local Delta people have been given the opportunity to take on leadership roles as initiators of projects. A smaller number of these individuals have continued to work with DHF and with each other to promote and build on the PSBH model. There has been some difficulty achieving continuity in leadership at the Delta regional level, leaving a void. Also, no formal leadership network has been developed from the diffuse group of projects and project leaders. This has prevented the regular sharing of ideas and resources and scaling up of ideas.

Engaging diverse community members, both individuals and organizations, in social change efforts is a time-intensive process. As with most development initiatives, it seems relatively easy for educated, middle-class people to participate. Given the history of exclusion and the compounded stress of everyday life in the Delta region, developing relationships with people in less secure socioeconomic positions takes extra effort.

Small-scale projects with even limited levels of funding are important for achieving short-term wins, creating organizational and project buy-in, building skills, and developing networks to scale up existing efforts. Addressing the bigger picture, however, is important in order to achieve more comprehensive community change. There is a balancing act required. Small projects appear more doable, but they may not result in structural changes. Larger efforts have the potential for greater impact, but they often seem less achievable given resource constraints. To see longer term impacts and fundamental changes will require learning what works, what does not, and advocating for more broadly based development policy changes. This necessitates ongoing evaluation of projects, sharing of information, and advocacy.

References

Austin, S. D. W. (2006). *The transformation of plantation politics: Black politics, concentrated poverty, and social capital in the Mississippi Delta.* Albany: State University of New York Press.

Bloom, D. E., & Bowser, D. M. (2008). The population health and income nexus in the Mississippi Delta River region and beyond. *Journal of Health and Human Services Administration, 31*(1), 105–123.

Campbell, J. (2001). *Map use and analysis* (4th ed.). New York: McGraw-Hill.

Chambers, R. (1997). *Whose reality counts? Putting the first last.* London: Intermediate Technology Publications.

Christenson, J. A. (1989). Themes of community development. In J. A. Christenson & J. W. Robinson, Jr. (Eds.), *Community development in perspective* (pp. 26–47). Ames: Iowa State University Press.

Clifford, W. B., & Brannon, Y. S. (1985). Rural differentials in mortality. *Rural Sociology, 50,* 210–224.

Cosby, A., Hitt, H., Cossman, R., Cossman, J., Feieraband, N., Thornton-Neaves, T., et al. (2007). *Mapping at-risk populations: "Rural health" vs. "unhealthy places" as a dominant geographic variable.* Presentation for the U.S. Department of Health and Human Services, Centers for Disease Control and Prevention, at the 11th Biennial CDC and ATSDR Symposium on Statistical Methods, Atlanta, GA, April 18, 2007.

Cosby, A. G. (2008). The future of rural America. In G. A. Goreham (Ed.), *Encyclopedia of rural America* (2nd ed.). New York: Grey House Publishing.

Cosby, A. G., & Bowser, D. A. (2008). The health of the Delta: A story of increasing disparities. *Journal of Health and Human Services Administration, 31*(1), 58–71.

Cosby, A. G., Brackin, M. W., Mason, T., & McCulloch, E. (1992). *A social and economic portrait of the Mississippi Delta.* Starkville: Mississippi State University, Social Science Research Center.

Cosby, A. G., Neaves, T. T., Cossman, R., Cossman, J., James, W., Feierabend, N., et al. (2008). Preliminary evidence for an emerging non-metropolitan mortality penalty in the United States. *American Journal of Public Health, 98*(8), 1470–1472.

Cossman, J. L., Cossman, R. E., James, W. L., Campbell, C., Blanchard, T., & Cosby. A. (2007). Persistent clusters of mortality in the U.S. *American Journal of Public Health, 97*(12), 2148–2150.

Cossman, R. E., Cosby, A. G., James, W., & Jackson-Belli, R. (2002). Healthy and unhealthy places in America: Are these really spatial clusters? In *Proceedings of the 22nd Annual ESRI International User Conference.* Published as a CD and retrieved October 21, 2009, from http://gis.esri.com/library/userconf/proc02/abstracts/a1064.html

Cossman, R. E., Cossman, J. L., Jackson-Belli, R., & Cosby, A. G. (2003). Mapping high or low mortality places across time in the United States: A research note on a health visualization and analysis project. *Health & Place, 9*(4), 361–369.

Cossman, R. E., Cossman, J. L., Reavis, R., & Cosby, A. G. (2007). Reconsidering the rural–urban continuum in rural health research: A test of stable relationships using mortality as a health measure. *Population Research and Policy Review, 47*(4), 459–476.

De Blij, H. J., & Alexander, A. B. (2000). *Culture, society, and space* (7th ed.). Hoboken, NJ: John Wiley and Sons.

Eberhardt, M. S., Ingram, D. D., Makuc, D. M., Pamuk, E., Freid, V., Harper, S., et al. (2001). *Urban and rural health chartbook. Health, United States, 2001.* Hyattsville, MD: National Center for Health Statistics.

Fitzpatrick, K., & LaGory, M. (2000). *Unhealthy places: The ecology of risk in the urban landscape.* New York: Routledge.

Freire, P. (1972). *Pedagogy of the oppressed.* New York: Penguin Books.

Gamm, L. D., Hutchison, L. L., Dabney, B., & Dorsey, A. (2003). *Rural healthy people 2010: A companion document to healthy people 2010* (Vol. 1). College Station: Texas A & M University System Health Science Center, School of Rural Public Health, Southwest Rural Health Research Center. Retrieved July 17, 2007, from http://sp.srph.tamhsc.edu/centers/Moved_rhp2010/Volume1.pdf

Gaventa, J. (1980). *Power and powerlessness: Quiescence and rebellion in an Appalachian valley.* Urbana: University of Illinois Press.

Green, G., & Haines, A. (2008). *Asset building and community development.* Thousand Oaks, CA: Sage Publications.

Green, J. (2008). Community development as social movement: A contribution to models of practice. *Community Development, 39*(1), 50–62.

Hardina, D. (2002). *Analytical skills for community practice.* Irvington, NY: Columbia University Press.

Ingram, D. D., & Franco, S. (2006). *2006 NCHS urban–rural classification scheme for counties.* Hyattsville, MD: National Center for Health Statistics. Retrieved October 27, 2009, from http://wonder.cdc.gov/wonder/help/cmf/urbanization-methodology.html

Kawachi, I., Kennedy, B. P., Lochner, K., & Prothrow-Smith, D. (1997). Social capital, income, inequality and mortality. *American Journal of Public Health, 87,* 1491–1498.

Mirvis, D. M., Chang, C. F., & Cosby, A. G. (2008). Health as an economic engine: Evidence for the importance of health in economic development. *Journal of Health and Human Services Administration, 31*(1), 30–57.

Murray, C., Kulkarni, S., Michaud, C., Tomijima, N., Bulzacchelli, M., Iandiorio, T., et al. (2006). Eight Americas: Investigating mortality disparities across races, counties, and race-counties in the United States. *Public Library of Science Medicine, 3*, 1513–1524.

National Center for Health Statistics. (2000). Compressed Mortality File, 1968–1988 (machine readable data file and documentation, CD-ROM Series 20, No. 2A). Hyattsville, MD: National Center for Health Statistics.

National Center for Health Statistics. (2007). Compressed Mortality File, 1989–1998 (machine readable data file and documentation, CD-ROM Series 20, No. 2E). Hyattsville, MD: National Center for Health Statistics.

National Center for Health Statistics. (2009). Compressed Mortality File, 1999–2006 (machine readable data file and documentation, CD-ROM Series 20, No. 2J). Hyattsville, MD: National Center for Health Statistics.

Neaves, T. T., Feierabend, N., Butts, C., & Weiskopf, W. (2008). A portrait of the Delta: Enduring hope and despair. *Journal of Health and Human Services Administration, 31* (1), 10–29.

Ricketts, T. C. III. (1999). *Rural health in the United States.* New York: Oxford University Press.

Satcher, D., Fryer, G. E., Jr., McCann, J., Troutman, A., Woolf, S., & Rust, G. (2005). What if we were equal? A comparison of the Black-White mortality gap in 1960 and 2000. *Health Affairs, 24*(2), 459–464.

Selener, D. (1997). *Participatory action research and social change.* Ithaca, NY: Cornell University Press.

U.S. Department of Agriculture. (2010). *Measuring rurality.* Washington, DC: Economic Research Service. Retrieved January 17, 2010, from http://www.ers.usda.gov/Briefing/Rurality

Williams, D. R., & Jackson, P. B. (2005). Social sources of racial disparities in health. *Health Affairs, 24*(2), 325–334.

III

Other Models for Addressing Global Health

Introduction

Joyce J. Fitzpatrick

Efforts to address global health issues have led to a wide range of models, programs, and initiatives, many of which have been implemented on a multinational level. Solutions to healthcare problems require a multidimensional approach, for economic, social, cultural, physiological, and psychological dimensions all contribute to health and wellness, at an individual level as well as at a community level.

In Section III, other models for addressing global health issues are presented. They are similar in their broad goals to enhance health and welfare for large numbers of individuals, particularly in underserved areas, and to expand the healthcare workforce. Yet the models are different in their approaches. The strongest characteristic linking these models is the focus on community-based development to affect change. Each of these models has the potential to stand alone or be connected to the Problem Solving for Better Health® (PSBH®) model. They are included here because they represent innovative methods for addressing a wide range of healthcare problems.

In Chapter 30, Garson and Engelhard describe a model for introducing new members into the health workforce, Grand-Aides™, older persons who can be trained to extend the work of physicians and nurses. The authors recognize that the supply of professional healthcare workers is woefully inadequate throughout the world. This new care model is akin to current training programs for community health outreach workers. However, this model capitalizes on the members of society that have the longest experience with everyday health problems, provides additional specific healthcare training for them, and empowers them as members of an interdisciplinary team to make a significant contribution to the health and welfare of the communities in which they live. The proposed Grand-Aides corps has already been implemented in tandem with the PSBH model in the United States and China. Several other pilot programs are in the planning stages and evaluation criteria have been developed to determine the outcomes of care.

Chapter 31 includes the work of a large interdisciplinary team active in three countries in Africa—Rwanda, South Africa, and Zambia—in partnership with the Division of Global Health Equity at the Brigham and Women's Hospital in Boston. The U.S.

colleagues have focused their energies on developing nursing partnerships in these three African countries, building on advanced practice and research expertise developed in the United States. Importantly, the program development, while focused primarily on nurses, includes recognition that any model of healthcare must be interdisciplinary to achieve success.

The Carter Center, based in Atlanta, Georgia, provides the foundational support for the Ethiopia Public Health Training Initiative (EPHTI) described by Murray and Terrazas in Chapter 32. As in the previous two chapters in this section, with the EPHTI there is an investment in workforce development in order to meet the healthcare needs of developing communities. These authors add important lessons learned from their long-term (beginning in 1997) involvement in Ethiopia. Key to the successes they describe are the relationships that have been developed across programs and countries, relationships built on trust, communication, and transparency as well as shared goals for improving health.

Bloom and Cafiero, in Chapter 33, describe a detailed implementation model to ensure the success of public health programs. They contend that success requires action at the individual, organization, and systems levels and recognition of the contributions of stakeholders at all levels. Bloom and Cafiero detailed three other dimensions that are crucial for program success: leveraging available resources, cultural sensitivity, and pilot testing before major program implementation. Further, they provide a checklist that can be used to evaluate programs or to guide in program development.

Finally, in Chapter 34, Ahn and Tyer-Viola introduce another "big picture" variable into the formula for addressing healthcare issues. They contend that corporations have a social responsibility to address global health, and offer a process by which corporations can assess their own contributions. While many persons would agree that corporate philanthropy should make an important contribution to health, Ahn and Tyer-Viola address the societal responsibilities of the corporation to the health of employees, families, consumers, shareholders, suppliers, and communities. In conclusion, they contend that all corporations have the ability to contribute to improvements in global health and are well positioned to do so.

There are several important messages embedded in these innovative model descriptions. First, there is much energy and goodwill to be harnessed to accomplish common healthcare goals. Second, the resources are limited, but gains can be derived synergistically through development of program linkages. Third, no country is free from healthcare challenges today. The inequities in healthcare access and delivery exist in developed and developing countries. And while the solutions for addressing the problems must be local, there are advantages to sharing approaches so that we learn from each other and build on the strengths of the alternative programs. Multiple models and programs can maximize the positive outcomes for all involved.

30

Grandparents as a Global Health Resource

Arthur Garson, Jr., and Carolyn L. Engelhard

In the United States, we have a shortage of approximately 2.4 million nurses and physicians (Kirch & Vernon, 2008), creating an acute problem with access to healthcare, defined as the ability of a potential patient to see an appropriate practitioner at the right time. Professional societies, hospital associations, government agencies, and research centers in the United States have issued several reports over the past 8 years citing medical and nursing shortages (American Association of Colleges of Nursing, 2010; Iglehart, 2008). Although the magnitude of the problem has been disputed, the demographic imperative is indisputable. The "baby boomers" will turn 65 years old in 2010, and by 2030 the number of Americans older than age 65 will double and represent one in five Americans (Kirch & Vernon, 2008). A recent study projected that total ambulatory care visits for adult Americans will increase 29% between 2005 and 2025 (Kirch & Vernon, 2008). Older adults seek care from their physicians almost three times a year on average, twice the rate of those younger than the age of 65 (Kirch & Vernon, 2008). In the face of this increasing demand, combined with the trend toward earlier retirement among practicing physicians (Garson, Mick, Cabral-Daniels, & Harp, 2005) and the growing numbers of young physicians who want more control over their time, the supply of practitioners is not projected to keep up (Kirch & Vernon, 2008). If there are too few physicians and nurses, can we use them more wisely by being more efficient in the delivery of healthcare services?

In the big picture, given the trends, even with minor improvement around the edges, all signs point to physician shortages getting worse before they get better, particularly for those medical specialties that provide primary care for an aging population. Despite the growing demand for them, fewer physicians are becoming generalists. By 2025, the nation will be short 35,000–44,000 adult care generalists (Colwill & Kruse, 2008). These trends will continue if medicine delivery is not altered.

The trends are the same the world over, even without the "bulge" of the baby boomers in other countries. The world's people are getting older, and many have chronic diseases. We need people to address the increasing healthcare demand.

Arthur Garson, Jr., is Executive Vice President and Provost of the University of Virginia. Carolyn L. Engelhard is an assistant professor and Health Policy Analyst in the Department of Public Health Sciences at the University of Virginia School of Medicine.

Changing the Care Model

Perhaps the most important way to change the care model is to change demand, beginning with the patient. Ever since the advent of antibiotics, patients have gone to the physician's office with common colds, seeking medications they likely did not need. Now, with greater degrees of sophistication and greater degrees of access to the Internet, potential patients are bombarded with information and advertisements about healthcare for themselves and their families.

Patient-induced demand, however, also creates opportunities. For example, the creation of educational materials for patients specific to their conditions helps educate patients about when they need to be seen by a health professional and can provide information about prevention ways to stay healthy, and techniques to improve medication compliance. At the University of Virginia we developed a questionnaire asking individuals how they want to receive such health information. They responded that they each want their health information provided in a different way, some through the Internet, some straight from a physician, some using more oral or written communication, and so on (Cohn et al. 2006).

Moving from designing educational materials to tailoring the information on the basis of patient preferences will encourage patients to assume a greater role in their own care. Recent studies suggest that when patients are better informed of medical treatment choices under a shared decision-making model, they often choose less invasive care, leading to a decrease in the overall care provision by as much as 40%–60% (Dartmouth Atlas Project, 2007).

Who Should Care for the Patient?

In a conversation between two of the chairs of family medicine departments at renowned U.S. medical schools, one remarked, "Fifty percent of my patients could be taken care of by a good grandparent." The other added, "And 80% of the rest could be taken care of by a good nurse." The point is everyone does not need a physician for every condition.

We need to change the entire paradigm of who cares for the patient, from a single physician to an entire team of caregivers, beginning with the patient. Patients need to be educated as much as possible to be able to care for themselves. Once patients are able to self-manage their health, they can link up with virtual teams of providers through electronic health records. Known as "task shifting," this type of team-based concept has been popularized by the World Health Organization and is defined as "a process of delegation whereby specific tasks are moved, where appropriate, to less specialized health workers" (World Health Organization, 2007).

Examples of task shifting in the United States include training grandparents to provide immunizations in Washington, DC; training workers for AIDS in hospice; and training high school–educated individuals to become community health workers on Indian reservations (Takach, 2008). Community health workers are not a substitute for medical and health professionals but instead assist healthcare practitioners in improving the health status of populations, for example, by making home visits. The authors of one study stated that lay advisors are the "ideal first contact persons, screeners of problems, referrers to community resources, and healers of certain ailments" (Hinton, Downey, Lisovicz, Mayfield-Johnson, & White-Johnson, 2005).

In order for task shifting to work, one person in the team must be the "trusted advisor" or quarterback that provides the center of the "medical home." Previous studies have suggested that the presence of a team "champion" is consistently associated with team effectiveness because he or she provides motivation and encouragement and acquires the resources for the team to succeed (Shortell et al., 2004). While the idea of having a single individual oversee coordination of the team's care may seem the most efficient, in truth, these individuals cannot be on call 24/7, so backups must also be identified. To encourage consistency across team workers, the care delivered must, to a certain extent, adhere to standardized protocols. This will be especially important for community health workers who, although trained, would receive less formal training than health professionals and so would need stricter guidelines to follow in the field.

In following healthcare protocols, community health workers need to recognize that not all individual patients will "fit" the more generalized protocol, and when that happens, the community care worker should refer the patient quickly to the medical team. This ability to admit "I don't know what is going on" is vital to the success of any of these community care teams. How to deal with uncertainty is, as a rule, a more explicit part of the training of nurses than physicians, but in this task-shifting model such questioning, followed by the ability to take action, is required from every team member at every level. To accomplish this, squabbles among different types of health-care providers must stop. Physicians will also need to become more actively involved in team-based quality improvement, something that has been a major barrier to past quality improvement initiatives (Shortell et al., 2004). No longer can nurses, generalist, or specialist physicians claim to do things better than other types of providers. Competition should not be among members of a team but rather among *teams* to provide the best care.

How Would the New Care Model Work?

The intent of this model is to employ "Grand-Aides™" (usually grandparents but also others with similar skills for caring) as community care workers in primarily underserved areas. Given current demographics, the elderly are living longer and want to be active. In fact, activity is likely to stave off both mental and physical illness. Employing the elderly as community care workers, therefore, simultaneously benefits the grandparents and their communities.

The "Acute Care Grandparent" would be the diagnostic and treatment grandparent. She or he would have a defined geographic area (in a city, five blocks, or in a rural area, several miles) covering approximately 50 families. Given the need for 24/7 coverage, at least two grandparents would trade shifts in each area. Using the task-shifting model, the intent is that these grandparents visit every home in the area, make themselves known, and let the residents know how to reach them when needed. Then, the grandparents intervene when acute illness arises. The grandparents will be able to answer questions such as "What do I do with my child's fever?", "What is this rash?", and "Do I need to go to the doctor or an emergency room?" All grandparents would carry a mini-computer with a camera, which will allow access to protocols, enable data entry about the patients, and provide rapid access to a more experienced provider who can receive photographs or video from the on-site grandparent.

Because each grandparent would provide health-related advice directly to underserved patients and parents, the grandparents would require training by healthcare workers, most likely nurses. Initially, all encounters would need to be supervised via phone and the computer, but a grandparent, after passing several tests and reviews of cases, may "graduate" to calling for only complex cases. Ongoing review by the supervisory nurse would occur for every case once per month. In the United States, at least, the grandparents involved would require the same kind of liability protection given to the medical professionals on the care team.

In addition to the grandparents, the team would include a supervisory nurse who would manage a number of grandparents, provide advice to the grandparents and, upon referral from the grandparents, deal with somewhat more complex generalist problems. Next in the line of providing services might be a nurse practitioner or physician's assistant who can deliver care as an independent practitioner. Finally, a general physician would receive referrals from either the grandparent or the nurse to deal with complex issues and provide necessary referrals to specialists.

In addition to the generalists there would also be a specialty team, with a nurse and specialist physician. They may take referrals directly from patients or members of the generalist team. A specialty nurse or nurse practitioner may deal with some requests for specialty services independently or refer them to the specialty physician.

A second kind of grandparent, the "Chronic Care Grandparent," would work with the specialty team. He or she would have a geographic area and make home visits similar to the Acute Care Grandparent. But the Chronic Care Grandparent serves as more of a health coach than someone who provides information about how to access care, and part of his or her job would be to monitor and support medication adherence. With support for ongoing medical care, the expectation is that the number of visits to specialty physicians will decrease. Medicare patients require a certain amount of socialization, which prompts multiple physician visits, and to that end, the visits by the Chronic Care Grandparent should reduce the frequency of physician visits. A third, preventive care function could be incorporated into the other two functions.

Reaction

As with any system change, some will favor the grandparent task-shifting model and some will oppose it. Those who are likely to be in favor are the underserved potential patients who currently lack continuous coordinated primary and specialty care. A series of pilot tests for the "Acute Care Grandparent," including a health assessment of the relevant population, will be important initially. Measured outcomes will include a demonstration of improved health for that population, as well as a reduction in visits to physicians, clinics, and emergency departments (and a corresponding reduction in costs). Additional measures of success for the "Chronic Care Grandparent" could be improvement in medication adherence, improvement in keeping appointments with physicians, and a decrease in unnecessary physician visits.

However, not everyone will appreciate this newly configured team-based system. For example, there might be patients who feel that they are hemmed in by a required system of referrals, but at any time patients may self-refer to any level of the system. It is hoped, though, that with improved convenience and better care at a more local level, patients will consult the grandparents first, nurses second, and physicians third. It is also possible that some primary care physicians will oppose the system. At present, the range of patients seen by primary care physicians varies from the entirely well to the slightly ill to the severely ill. If such a system works, primary care physicians will largely see only sick patients, intensifying their workload. The same would be true of specialists. This is especially significant if the predictions about physician shortages come true.

Finally, those called upon to pay for such a system (i.e., the outreach for, identification of, and training of grandparents) will expect an evaluation of the program that demonstrates, at the very least, an improvement in health. Ideally, the evaluation would also show a reduction in health disparities, as well as lowered overall costs. Previous research findings (Hinton et al., 2005) suggest that these goals are possible.

Implications for Training

The implications for training lay health workers and nonphysician healthcare practitioners in a community-based team model of care are far reaching and may be controversial. Because there are new rules for people at every level of the team, new scopes of practice will need to be determined and agreed upon by various licensed bodies. These groups will have to set standards for the training required to be called an "Acute Care Grandparent" or "Chronic Care Grandparent," as well as for initial and continued testing. A similar type of training and certification process is taking place in Massachusetts, where the Department of Public Health has been working to build a network of community health workers (Takach, 2008).

Meanwhile, the nurses who are on the teams will have to have a different scope of practice because they will be making decisions as independent practitioners. The role of physician assistants will also be expanded because they could be practicing independently. In our current system, members of the workforce up the hierarchical ladder typically have the greatest problems with an increase in scope of practice of those below them. For example, physicians have traditionally argued against increased scope of practice for nurse practitioners, just as nurse practitioners have argued against increased scope of practice for nurses. It may be, in turn, that nurses or other healthcare workers will argue against any scope of practice for the grandparents.

Progress in adopting this new kind of care system will likely come from two directions: (1) When the demonstration pilot studies with patient groups are successful, patients will demand the more convenient lay services, and (2) if the societal demand for physicians and nurse practitioners continues as expected, the waiting lines for physicians and nurse practitioners will lead to increased patient dissatisfaction and put pressure on the current healthcare system to be more responsive to patient needs.

Once the model is developed and training is underway, curricula must be developed to teach what these new team-based practitioners need to know. This is something that is rarely, if ever, done: starting from scratch with a curriculum for each member of the healthcare workforce. This involves assessing how much and what kind of basic science is required for practitioners at all levels and what kind of clinical training is necessary. For every person in the healthcare workforce, training to work in teams will be essential and will involve interprofessional teaching for all members of the healthcare workforce team. As part of this training, the "what to do when I don't know what to do" training will become essential, because much of the work done by the grandparents and nurses will be protocol driven. Different training durations with modules of specific competencies could be required for those who want to enter academic medicine or, once the training paradigms are developed, the current regulations requiring 4 years of undergraduate work prior to starting graduate and professional work in the health professions might be changed. Questions of how to proceed with the training are empirically answerable by researching different methods of teaching, their necessary duration, and their effect on practice outcome in terms of capability and also patient satisfaction. To speed up the process, the training of nurses could be shortened, and a large group of grandparents could probably be trained within 6–12 months.

As we move forward toward a new paradigm of patient care and health professional training, the needed size of the workforce must be projected and continuously updated. Incentives such as free tuition and debt forgiveness may help recruit needed practitioners, particularly in underserved areas. How will we know if the model works? We will know it works by piloting elements of the model: (1) training patients in prevention and guidelines; (2) creating a Grand-Aides corps; (3) aggressively promoting teams; (4) training for and assigning work according to the true skills needed for the service, with increasing complexity in decision making from the Grand-Aide™ to the physician; and (5) removing regulatory and financial barriers.

Next Steps to a Healthier World

The Dreyfus Health Foundation is initiating pilots of the Grand-Aides model in rural Virginia; downtown Houston, Texas; rural Shanghai, and urban Baotou, Inner Mongolia. The reactions around the world have been encouraging. Access to healthcare is a problem that exists worldwide. One of the major obstacles to providing access is a shortage of healthcare practitioners in underserved areas. Although increasing the supply of physicians is necessary, we should consider changing the entire model of care to leverage capabilities of every member of the healthcare workforce. By including capable individuals, such as grandparents, in the healthcare workforce, and improving patient education tools, we can potentially reach more people and improve their health. Our ultimate goal, after all, is a healthy world.

References

American Association of Colleges of Nursing. (2010). *Nursing shortage fact sheet*. Washington, DC: Author.

Cohn W. F., Pannone A., Schubart, J., Lyman, J., Kinzie, M., Broshek, D. K., et al. (2006). *Tailored educational approaches for consumer health (TECH): A model system for addressing health communication*. AMIA 2006 symposium proceedings, 894. Retrieved August 4, 2010, from http://www.ncbi.nlm.nih.gov/pmc/articles/PMC1839357/pdf/AMIA2006_089.

Colwill, J. M., & Kruse, R. L. (2008). Will generalist physician supply meet demands of an increasing and aging population? *Health Affairs, 27*(3), w232–w241.

Dartmouth Atlas Project. (2007). Preference-sensitive care. Retrieved November 1, 2008, from http://www.dartmouthatlas.org/topics/preference_sensitive.pdf

Garson, A., Mick, S. S., Cabral-Daniels, R., & Harp. W. L. (2005). Virginia statewide physician workforce study: Current supply and future projections. Commonwealth of Virginia, VDH Office of Health Policy and Planning, cited in 2005 Annual Report. Retrieved July 6, 2009, from http://leg2.state.va.us/dls/h%26sdocs.nsf/4d54200d7e28716385256ec1004f3130/6b16b31e29d4b83985256f1c0051fb30?OpenDocument

Hinton, A., Downey, J., Lisovicz, N., Mayfield-Johnson, S., & White-Johnson, F. (2005). The community health advisor program and the deep south network for cancer control: Health promotion programs for volunteer community health advisors. *Family Community Health, 28*(1), 20–27.

Iglehart, J. K. (2008). Grassroots activism and the pursuit of an expanded physician supply. *New England Journal of Medicine, 358*(16), 1741–1749.

Kirch, D. G., & Vernon, D. J. (2008). Confronting the complexity of the physician workforce equation. *Journal of the American Medical Association, 299*(22), 2680–2682.

Shortell, S. M., Marsteller, J. A., Lin, M., Pearson, M. L., Wu, S. Y., Mendel, P., et al. (2004). The role of perceived team effectiveness in improving chronic illness care. *Medical Care, 42*(11), 1040–1048.

Takach, M. (2008). Community health centers and health reform: Highlights from a national academy for state health policy forum. Retrieved November 1, 2008, from http://www.nashp.org/Files/health_centers_forum.pdf

World Health Organization. (2007). *Taking stock: Task shifting to tackle health worker shortages.* Retrieved November 1, 2008, from http://www.who.int/healthsystems/task_shifting/TTR_tackle.pdf

31

Global Health Partnerships

Patrice K. Nicholas, Inge B. Corless, Sheila M. Davis, Lynda Tyer-Viola,
Stephanie Ahmed, Egidia Rugwizangoga, Thomas P. Nicholas,
Sheryl M. Zang, and Ana Viamonte-Ros

This chapter focuses on the establishment and advancement of global health partnerships to address the Millennium Development Goals (MDGs) in Rwanda, South Africa, and Zambia. In 2000, 189 countries of the United Nations agreed on the MDGs, with the support of the International Monetary Fund, World Bank, Organization for Economic Co-Operation and Development, and the G7 and G20 countries. The goals are to eradicate extreme poverty and hunger; achieve universal primary education; promote gender equality and empower women; reduce child mortality; improve maternal health; combat HIV/AIDS, malaria, and other diseases; ensure environmental sustainability; and establish global partnerships. In our work in Rwanda, South Africa, and Zambia, the MDGs are linked to our global nursing efforts.

Program Description

The Division of Global Health Equity (DGHE; formerly known as the Division of Social Medicine and Health Inequalities) at the Brigham and Women's Hospital (BWH) in Boston, Massachusetts, was founded in September of 2001. Through a multidisciplinary approach, the division aims to improve medical care in the world's poorest areas.

The DGHE fosters the support and coordination of training, research, and service to reduce disparities in disease burden and improve treatment outcomes at home and

Patrice K. Nicholas is Director of Global Health and Academic Partnerships in the Division of Global Health Equity and the Center for Nursing Excellence, Brigham and Women's Hospital, and a professor at the MGH Institute of Health Professions School of Nursing. Inge B. Corless is a professor and Sheila M. Davis an adult nurse practitioner at the MGH Institute of Health Professions School of Nursing. Lynda Tyer-Viola is a senior advisor in the Division of Global Health & Human Rights, MGH, and an assistant professor at the MGH Institute of Health Professions School of Nursing. Stephanie Ahmed is Director of Clinical Operations at Dovetail Health, Needham, Massachusetts. Egidia Rugwizangoga is a registered nurse in the Surgical Unit, Brigham and Women's Hospital. Thomas P. Nicholas is in the Department of Patient Care Services, Brigham and Women's Hospital. Sheryl M. Zang is Clinical Associate Professor of Nursing at SUNY Downstate Medical Center, Brooklyn, New York. Ana Viamonte-Ros is Secretary of Health and State Surgeon General, Department of Health, Florida.

abroad. The division focuses on infectious diseases (e.g., HIV and tuberculosis [TB]), noninfectious diseases (e.g., coronary artery disease, diabetes, addiction), and other health problems. With the DGHE's inception came the establishment of clinical training and fellowships for BWH physicians to share their expertise in Haiti, Malawi, Peru, Russia, and the United States (through a Boston-based HIV program). The program has since expanded to include locations in Lesotho and Rwanda. In collaboration with the DGHE, a Director of Global Nursing and Academic Partnerships was appointed and the BWH Global Nursing Program and Global Nurse Fellowship were initiated.

Rwanda

In September 2008, our first Fellow, a certified nurse midwife, went to Rwanda to develop the role of global nursing in the field of women's health, in concert with Partners in Health (PIH), a nonprofit organization with extensive clinical field rotations located in Rwinkwavu, Rwanda. The Fellow used the PIH STAR methodology (Service, Training, Advocacy, and Research), which consists of five fundamental principles:

- Access to primary healthcare is foundational.
- Free healthcare and education are essential; thus no user fees are sought.
- Community partnerships are necessary at all levels of assessment, design, implementation, and evaluation of programs.
- Addressing basic social and economic needs is essential to health.
- Serving the poor through the public sector is crucial; thus, while nongovernmental organizations (NGOs) have an important role, strengthening and complementing the existing public health infrastructure is the goal.

An example of an innovative solution to local health problems through the global nursing program is the infusion of advanced-practice nursing knowledge in Rwanda where it did not yet exist. Historically, nursing education programs in Rwanda were diploma/certificate based. In 2005, the Rwandan government upgraded nursing education by eliminating all lower-level schools and creating five priority schools for nursing and midwifery that opened in January 2007. The introduction of a nurse midwife has brought knowledge from our successful nurse midwifery practice at BWH, which offers prenatal care through our community health settings and labor, birth, and recovery care in our inpatient settings.

Our global nursing program has developed advanced-practice nursing in the community, hospital, and academic settings in Boston and has translated this application of nurse midwifery practice to Rwanda at Rwinkwavu Hospital. Pre- and postnatal care have been improved in Rwanda as a result of this fellowship through the global nursing program.

South Africa

This section describes the work of Sibusiso, a nonprofit organization started in 2003 by Sheila Davis and Christopher Shaw, two Boston-area nurses. The organization's founders were committed to providing assistance in the field in a more expeditious manner than is typical for large academic programs and NGOs. Sibusiso's mission is to foster and support HIV/AIDS care and treatment projects, encourage community development initiatives and raise awareness about HIV/AIDS, provide education and training programs, and collaborate with in-country partners. Sibusiso has three main programs: a rural village healthcare program and an urban township children's feeding program, both in South Africa, and a Boston-based bridging outreach program. The goal of the two programs in South Africa is to respond to the identified needs of local NGOs by partnering with them and providing financial support, program development, and technical assistance.

Rural Village Healthcare Program

In 2004, Sibusiso partnered with the Mahlungulu Foundation, a South African NGO established by Dr. Sarah Mahlungulu, a faculty member teaching at the University of KwaZulu–Natal (UKZN) School of Nursing. The foundation focuses its activities on the rural village of Numlaco in the Mbizana municipality in the Eastern Cape area of South Africa. Dr. Mahlungulu and community leaders struggled to provide healthcare to this area and requested assistance for their small nurse-run clinic (known as the Mahlungulu Clinic or Numlaco Clinic) and other community development projects. The collaboration between these two nurse-founded NGOs was initiated with that request.

This area of Numlaco is severely impoverished—87% of the people have a household net income of 250 USD per month. It also has a high prevalence rate of HIV (42%), and TB rates exceeding 46%. The first two projects that Sibusiso developed with the Mahlungulu Foundation were the home-based care (HBC) project (including the nurse-run clinic) and the community garden.

The HBC program began with 10 women trained by Dr. Mahlungulu in basic nursing skills. These community health workers provide basic home care to the sickest members of the community and receive small stipends for their work. They are affiliated with the Mahlungulu Clinic, which is staffed by a nurse, junior nurse, and HIV counselor. The clinic provides nursing and medical care and services for men and women of all ages with diabetes, skin infections, burns, hypertension, sexually transmitted infections, opportunistic infections (related to HIV/AIDS), TB, gastrointestinal infections, respiratory ailments, and myriad other diagnoses.

The junior nurse and HIV counselor at the clinic offer voluntary counseling and testing (VCT) for HIV/AIDS. The clinic staff does not prescribe or initiate antiretroviral treatment (ART) or treatment for TB but refers patients to the Department of Health (DOH) Clinic where they can receive these treatments. The Mahlungulu Clinic prepares people for ART by assessing readiness and educating them about medication adherence and side effects.

The clinic's services are extended by HBC workers who primarily identify individuals in the community who require treatment and follow-up with individuals who were seen at the clinic and need further assistance at home. They also provide education and follow-up to members of the community who were seen at the DOH clinic. The HBC workers play a key role in identifying needs in the community and provide counseling in homes to increase the number of people receiving VCT. Finally, HBC workers assist with logistical and supportive services, including help with social relief such as food parcels. They identify individuals most in need, provide nutrition education, and bring vegetables grown in the clinic's garden to them.

The Mahlungulu Clinic offers additional services to the local community through a health educator and community awareness programs. The health educator provides daily education in the clinic as well as to the surrounding community at meetings and local churches. She also works with local students in the six surrounding schools to provide health and wellness information once a week. Topics include HIV/AIDS, pulmonary TB, and health promotion.

Sibusiso and the Mahlungulu Foundation are committed to extending healthcare to this rural village. In 2004, the nurse-run clinic was open only 1 or 2 days a week and provided only basic nursing care with limited medication. In 2008, the clinic began operating 5 days a week, providing expanded services through a grant from Pangaea Global AIDS Foundation. Sibusiso and the Mahlungulu Foundation have worked in collaboration with the district health system and government clinics to expand services. In order to avoid incurring the large costs of providing antiretroviral (ARV) medication, patients are screened at the Mahlungulu Clinic and referred by the clinic nurse to an area district hospital that provides treatment. Once on ARV medication, the patients return to the clinic and are followed up for adherence support and symptom management.

The Numlaco village leaders identified hunger and starvation as critical problems for the village. Sibusiso addressed these issues in their second project, Gardens from Lynne (in memory of a friend of one of Sibusiso's founders), which the community developed with them. Sibusiso volunteers built a fence, tilled the land, and planted the seeds and have funded the full-time gardener, garden maintenance, and water since 2004. The HBC workers distribute vegetables from the garden to the poorest in the community, and the Mahlungulu Foundation distributes food parcels on a quarterly basis. Sibusiso supplements the funding to provide even more families with food.

Urban Township Orphan Feeding Program

Imbali is a community located in the shadow of Edendale Hospital in Pietermaritzburg, South Africa, where HIV prevalence is estimated to be as high as 47% and poverty and unemployment are the norm. In 2006, a soup kitchen operated in a local hall, providing food for the neediest children in Imbali. However, in November 2006 the program lost its support, causing the children to go hungry. Through donations, the Izimbali Zesizwe program was able to provide food and a safe site for the children to gather and participate in positive activities. These include after-school tutoring, assessment, referral for medical care, educational workshops on positive living, HIV/AIDS awareness and prevention, HIV treatment, and TB treatment. Since early 2007, Izimbali Zesizwe has grown to serve 51 children a hot, nutritious breakfast and supper every day.

Bridging Program

Early in the development of Sibusiso, some of the unfulfilled needs of the immigrant sub-Saharan African population in the metropolitan Boston area became apparent, leading to the development of a domestic arm of Sibusiso. With funding from a U.S. pharmaceutical company, the bridging program was established in 2006. The program partners with Boston-area governmental, nongovernmental, and community-based organizations and healthcare institutions to provide HIV/AIDS education, contacts with community resources, and healthcare access to sub-Saharan immigrant populations living in Boston.

Apart from providing support and education to the sub-Saharan African community in Massachusetts, the program aims to develop, implement, and evaluate an African faith-based education and empowerment pilot program. Another aim is to engage and empower faith-based community leaders to educate the sub-Saharan African faith community; decrease the stigma associated with HIV/AIDS and Hepatitis B; and enhance community mobilization for testing, counseling, and referrals.

South Africa and Fulbright Scholarships for Nurses

The Fulbright Scholarship programs include senior scholar and student scholar awards and are administered by the U.S. Department of State Bureau of Educational and Cultural Affairs in cooperation with the Council for International Exchange of Scholars. The Fulbright program was designed to create mutual understanding between the United States and other countries and to examine political, economic, social, and cultural institutions, as well as link global and public health issues (http://www.cies.org).

The UKZN School of Nursing has hosted two Fulbright Scholars in nursing, with a third scholar to offer expertise at UKZN next year. During her Fulbright experience, Patrice Nicholas taught the HIV/AIDS courses at UKZN, guided master's and doctoral degree students in their research, served on doctoral dissertation reviews, and participated in faculty colloquia. She was also invited to teach and provide clinical care at two area hospitals, St. Mary's and McCord Hospitals, and at two area hospices. The clinical education included teaching community-based caregivers through a program at the U.S. Consulate in Durban, providing nursing education on ARV medication at two hospitals, and conducting HIV symptom management research.

In South Africa, challenges often exist in retaining nurses because of challenges of migration to resource-rich countries where salaries, security, and opportunities for families are better (Kingma, 2007). The Fulbright program offers the possibility of supporting a sustainable nursing workforce in South Africa and other countries and developing what Kingma (2006) identified as *brain circulation,* whereby countries with many resources share nurses with countries that have limited resources. In countries torn by political unrest and war, the loss of nurses represents further vulnerability for a population, contributing to morbidity, mortality, and public health woes.

Possibilities for solutions include the development of robust partnerships that share nursing resources across global locations. Nursing education programs offer opportunities to teach through distance learning and provide international experiences for nurses in both resource-limited and resource-rich countries.

Zambia

Today, worldwide, there are more than 529,000 maternal deaths annually, with 99% of these occurring in low- and middle-income countries (Ronsmans, Graham, & Lancet Maternal

Survival Series Steering Group, 2006; World Health Organization, 2008). Sub-Saharan Africa has the highest maternal mortality in the world; 900 women die for every 100,000 live births (United Nations, 2008). For those children who survive childbirth, surviving early childhood without disease or mortality is a challenge. Fortunately, many low-cost interventions have been shown to improve maternal and child health (see Lancet series on Maternal and Neonatal Survival). The challenge is getting these interventions to those most in need.

In October 2005, the Honorable Maureen Mwanawasa, the former First Lady of Zambia, visited Harvard University. Soon after, members of the Harvard Humanitarian Initiative responded to the First Lady's request to evaluate the possibility of a shared partnership with the Government of Zambia. Members of the Emergency Medical Services and Lynda Tyer-Viola, a maternal child health specialist, traveled to Zambia to meet with public health activists, including opposition leaders, faith-based organizations, and the cooperating partners of the funding nations. The collective goal was to describe why the large number of health programs and finances were not improving maternity services and how best to move forward. The participants agreed on the critical need to create more emphasis on the availability of emergency obstetrical care (EmOC).

The ensuing assessment revealed that the basic capacity and infrastructure of the system lacked support. None of the health centers could perform the six basic signal EmOC functions determined by the WHO and the United Nations Population Fund: (1) administer parenteral antibiotics, (2) administer parenteral oxytocics, (3) administer parenteral anticonvulsants, (4) perform manual removal of placenta, (5) perform removal of retained products, and (6) perform assisted vaginal delivery (vacuum procedure). Only five of the nine hospitals had the capacity to conduct comprehensive EmOC that includes the ability to perform a cesarean section and provide blood transfusions. Further, infrastructure to support these services was lacking—only 61% of the health centers had electricity, and only 36% had running water. This assessment created the basis for developing an integrated program for EmOC in the rural provinces in Zambia.

Midwife care, supplemented by enrolled and registered nurses or environmental health workers, is the model of care for maternity services in Zambia. There are no obstetricians at the health centers and limited access to them at many district hospitals. Clinical officers and medical workers who are not physicians support the midwives in various settings. Enrolled or registered midwives receive basic nursing preparation and additional midwife training for 1 or 2 years. They are then posted by the government to health centers. The training for midwives is rigorous and consists of 40–50 hours a week of labor and delivery practice and clinical evaluation over a 3-month period at a tertiary or district hospital. In the assessment of district midwife practice, 88% of rural midwives believed they could identify problems at delivery, yet only 73% felt they could treat these problems. Unfortunately, the midwives do not receive adequate experience managing complications and providing emergency care in the field.

The perceptions of the community were not as positive as those of the healthcare workers. Fifty-eight percent of participating women believed the health center staff were not trained to handle difficult deliveries, and 50% felt the health centers did not have the supplies or drugs to provide the necessary care. This belief of a knowledge gap and lack of confidence in care, partnered with poor infrastructure, provided the focus for work on problems and solutions that would directly affect Zambian obstetrical care. The needs assessment showed a clear thirst for knowledge, enthusiasm to learn new skills, and a commitment to be part of a team to improve the lives of Zambian families.

After critical review and reflection, and with government support, the road map and budget developed to improve maternal child health included the establishment of an EmOC development program—the Maternal Infant Health Initiative (MIHI). A privately funded entity, MIHI has undertaken the following activities, among others:

- Development and dissemination of a program to train healthcare providers in EmOC. Subsequently, a national program was adopted; as an MOH initiative it will continue to receive funding and support for future evaluation. Refresher education offerings continue at the point of care.
- Implementation of a model of mentoring and support in the Kapiri Mposhi district. Several months out of the year a team of U.S. medical and nursing care providers and educators live in the district to work with the midwives and clinical officers to improve daily care and responses to emergencies. Their role is to provide in-the-moment support with new knowledge and reflection in action.
- Construction of an operating theater at the Kapiri Mposhi District Hospital. This small satellite theater will have the capacity for cesarean sections and limited procedures by the Medical Licensures. Training on obstetrical anesthesia and theater nursing care is ongoing.
- Training and support of the use of the six basic functions of neonatal care at every delivery. The sustained use of these actions for each delivery and a place designated within the delivery area to support this activity has resulted in increased attention to stabilization of the newborn at birth.
- Construction of a new birthing center with electricity and running water at the remote village of Nkole. The District Health Management team is providing improved access and marketing for use of the center.
- Introduction of a limited obstetrical ultrasound program to improve the quality of antenatal care and to attract women to use skilled birth attendants at delivery. Over a 2-week period repeated three times a year, the midwives are trained to diagnose a pregnancy, determine placenta location, and determine position and gestation. The primary goal of this program is the use of technology to improve identification of women at risk during pregnancy. The hypothesis is that women who have been identified as having a risk factor will use skilled care at delivery. A secondary hypothesis is that women who have skilled antenatal care and are provided with health education and information on the health of their fetuses will seek out quality care for delivery.
- Partnerships with other health organizations, such as Venture Strategies from the University of California School of Public Health at Berkeley to build political will and traction regarding basic health package needs for women. In April 2008, the drug misoprostol was registered for use in Zambia. This highly effective, low-cost medication can be administered under any conditions to treat postpartum hemorrhage. A national pilot program is under way to introduce this medication throughout the country.
- Establishment of a partnership with the University Teaching Hospital School of Nursing and Midwifery in Lusaka, Zambia, as an educational exchange of innovative teaching methods such as simulation and knowledge development for best practice.

The goal of MIHI is to scale up the model of EmOC mentoring and education in each district in the Central Province and to continue to improve the infrastructure for delivery of obstetrical services. Demonstrating the effects of focused care at the community level to the large donor agencies may shift the current funding focus on solo initiatives to a wider focus on the continuum of care. The goal is to infuse evidence and energy at the point of care and see its effect ripple within the community. The method is focusing on the needs of a community one family at a time.

Conclusion

This chapter focuses on three resource-limited countries—Rwanda, South Africa, and Zambia—that have pilot nursing projects and mature opportunities for partnerships to support global nursing efforts. The programs include interdisciplinary efforts and linkages across several organizations including hospitals, community-based organizations, academic settings, and NGOs. The concepts of *brain drain, brain gain,* and *brain circulation* served as the framework for these efforts, primarily aimed at containing the loss of nurses from resource-limited countries to resource-rich countries. Efforts to support global nursing through exchanges have proven successful.

References

Kingma, M. (2006). *Nurses on the move: Migration and the global health care economy.* Ithaca, NY: Cornell University Press.

Kingma, M. (2007). Nurses on the move: A global overview. *Health Services Research, 42,* 1281–1298.

Ronsmans, C., Graham, W. J., & Lancet Maternal Survival Series Steering Group. (2006). Maternal mortality: Who, when, where, and why. *The Lancet, 368,* 1189–2000.

United Nations. (2008). *The millennium development goals report 2008.* New York: Author.

World Health Organization. (2008). *The world health report 2008—Primary healthcare (now more than ever).* Geneva, Switzerland: Author.

32

The Carter Center's Ethiopia Public Health Training Initiative

Joyce P. Murray and Shelly B. Terrazas

Poverty, migration, wars, pestilence, epidemics, drought conditions, lack of and inadequate healthcare services, and shortage of healthcare providers are all factors influencing global health today. As HIV/AIDS progressed, the killer pandemic began affecting the health of the developing *and* developed world in ways never seen before. Consequently, there was a shift in resource prioritization and funding, along with the attention of public health experts such as Dr. William Foege, who led the public health strategy that resulted in the eradication of smallpox (Paulson, 2008). Thus, with the advent of HIV/AIDS, along with growing problems from other staggering diseases, the healthcare paradigm has transitioned from international health, which focuses on epidemics and intergovernmental relationships, to global health, which places priority on the health needs of the human race as a whole.

The World Health Report 2006 identified the shortage of health professionals as the greatest threat to global health (World Health Organization, n.d.). Major universities and schools have begun focusing on global and international education by providing support for faculty and students studying global health. By increasing the quality of professional education, and the numbers of primary healthcare providers, Ethiopia is demonstrating a workable, grassroots approach to counteracting some of the negative effects of modern globalization on healthcare delivery in resource-poor countries.

Background

In early 1989, after years of turmoil and internal political conflict, the Socialist government in Ethiopia fell. Meles Zenawi, the current Prime Minister, founded the Federal Democratic Republic of Ethiopia. The healthcare system was in shambles, and primary healthcare services (PHCS) were essentially nonexistent, especially in vast rural areas.

Joyce P. Murray is a professor at the Nell Hodgson Woodruff School of Nursing, Emory University, and Shelly B. Terrazas is Assistant Director of the Mental Health Liberia Program, The Carter Center. Joyce P. Murray is Director and Shelly B. Terrazas is Assistant Director of the Ethiopia Public Health Training Initiative.

The Ethiopian Public Health Training Initiative (EPHTI) of The Carter Center was an idea first formed in late 1991 between Prime Minister Zenawi and former U.S. President Jimmy Carter. Prime Minister Zenawi and the new Ethiopian government asked The Carter Center for assistance to improve health services for Ethiopians, especially the underserved rural populations.

The Ethiopian Public Health Training Initiative

It was not until 1997, with limited funding, that Prime Minister Zenawi and former President Carter's idea for Ethiopian healthcare education took root. With the agreement of the Ethiopian Minister of Health and Minister of Education, the initiative began with a planning session designed for Ethiopian health sciences faculty and policy makers to take the lead in setting priorities and taking ownership of the initiative. These initial planning sessions established three major goals for the project:

1. Develop health learning materials (HLMs), such as modules, manuals, and lecture notes, that are appropriate for Ethiopia;
2. Provide workshops and in-service training for university health science educators, known as "Staff Strengthening," so that the staff who train health workers are well equipped to pass along their knowledge;
3. Enhance the teaching and learning environment of the university health science classrooms where students learn basic professional skills.

These goals continue to serve as the basic structure for activities of the EPHTI today, with the addition of student training goals set by the Ethiopian government.

Developing Health Learning Materials

Until 2002, the progress of EPHTI was slow because of limited funding. Faculty from five Ethiopian universities met in workshops periodically and focused on selecting topics for HLMs, training, consultations, and planning ways to accomplish the program's major goals. In these early workshops, the first HLMs the faculty produced consisted of teaching modules on the top five health problems in Ethiopia at the time. These topics were malaria, pneumonia in children younger than 5 years, diarrheal diseases, expanded programs on immunization, and sexually transmitted infections (STIs). The modules were structured to educate and prepare the primary healthcare teams, and include a pretest, background information for all professions, four satellite modules tailored to the specific professions, and a posttest. With this structure, the modules were intended to provide Ethiopian-written and context-specific information for all members of the primary health center team. As an added benefit, because the training was done all together, the separate categories of professionals could integrate their work.

An unexpected outcome of this process was the building of relationships among the universities of the EPHTI network. Through the collective writing of the HLMs, faculty members within the schools had the opportunity to visit other university campuses and understand the common bond of the difficulties faced by each university.

Staff Strengthening

When major funding was awarded to The Carter Center by the United States Agency for International Development (USAID), the core activities of EPHTI were accelerated between 2000 and 2002. USAID funding supported the development of both Ethiopia and Atlanta offices and staff to work with the Ministers of Education and Health, universities, and other partners. With this significant funding, the second major goal of EPHTI, staff strengthening, could be addressed. Staff strengthening entailed the need to improve the skills of the faculty in the networked universities, because they were often new to their roles and inexperienced in basic teaching methods. Because of the problem of brain drain faced by Ethiopia and other resource-poor nations, most seasoned health science faculty no longer teach in their own country. To address the problem, EPHTI organized "major workshops," held periodically to plan the activities needed to strengthen teaching staff. Participants consisted of faculty from the universities, consultants, experts in selected fields, government representatives, and staff from the Atlanta and Ethiopia offices.

The planning of staff-strengthening activities in these early workshops focused on the need for development in specific skills and topics (writing in English, reproductive health, basic education). The first staff-strengthening initiatives began in 2001 with 1- to 2-week courses that selected faculty from each of the five partnering universities attended. These workshops included "Teaching & Learning Methodology and Pedagogy," "English Writing," and "Reproductive Health." The workshops were a huge success because they provided exposure to the topics that the faculty participants needed to improve their effectiveness in the classroom.

The workshops were conducted by international experts in each topic, identified by EPHTI or local consultants. To maximize the positive effect of this collective transfer of knowledge, the participants of each workshop returned to their home institutions after the "primary" workshop and taught their colleagues in subsequent "cascade" workshops on the topics they just learned. Cascade workshops were conducted by senior faculty with teaching experience who had attended a national workshop. Leading the cascade workshops allowed these senior faculty to practice their new skills with their colleagues. The following section is a further description of the workshops presented to the faculty of the EPHTI to strengthen their teaching, writing skills, and knowledge in selected areas.

Teaching and Learning Methodology and Pedagogy

Early in the initiative, faculties in the rural universities of Ethiopia lacked preparation to teach in higher education and/or health fields. Only a few teachers had any training in education and teaching methodologies. The educational environment was poor, with limited teaching aids, technology, and trained faculty. New graduates in primary health-care were hired immediately after graduation to teach in the universities. Senior faculty in the rural universities with teaching experience but no formal training recognized this as an issue and requested workshops to strengthen teaching skills.

International consultants developed and implemented the workshops. These consultants, from Emory University's Nell Hodgson Woodruff School of Nursing, in Atlanta, Georgia, were experienced educators with backgrounds in nursing education, transcultural nursing, and family nurse practice. Approximately 65 Ethiopian health professional faculty members received training each summer from 2002 to 2008. To date, 13 national workshops have been held for 484 faculty participants. As university student enrollments increased, universities decided to develop and implement cascade workshops on their own campuses. This rapidly increased the number of faculty with some preparation in the basics of teaching and learning. Cascade workshops are scheduled to occur twice a year in each of the member universities. Approximately 1,400 participants have benefited from EPHTI cascade workshops in the last 5 years.

Writing Workshops

In 2002, the African Medical and Research Foundation in Nairobi, Kenya, developed a 13-day workshop focused on writing skills for Ethiopian medical/health personnel. Writing skills are essential to the development of quality HLMs. In particular, proper documentation, referencing, and cross-referencing skills are needed to develop accurate and current materials because HLMs are used as texts and references. To assist in preventing misuse of references and information, international experts taught the faculty developing the HLMs the standardization of bibliographies, indexes, and copyrights.

Drought Response

Five Ethiopian universities, including Addis Ababa University, Debub University (now known as Hawassa University), the University of Gondar, Alemaya University (now known as Haramaya University), and Jimma University, cooperated with EPHTI to support a drought response program. With key stakeholders in Ethiopia, EPHTI developed a plan for incorporating service learning and using the time and skills of the students within the initiative. This offered an opportunity to further strengthen the teaching capacities of the faculty and broaden the experiences of students as they provided care and services to their fellow Ethiopians.

Approximately 2,191 health science students and 350 university instructors and staff were involved in curative, preventative, rehabilitative, and nutrition service activities. In almost every drought-affected area, students cared for groups with communicable diseases, nutritional disorders, diarrhea, malaria, HIV/AIDS, and other health problems. The accomplishments of the health science students include the construction of 428 latrines, 71 water sources, and 594 waste disposal pits. A total of 374,549 people received health education, 2,266 people were trained, and 3,270 children were treated at feeding centers.

Through the drought response program of EPHTI, the initiative successfully used service learning as a way to address the health-related needs of drought-stricken communities. Moreover, the program incorporated service learning teaching methods as an effective mechanism to strengthen teaching staff skills and bolster the preservice education of health professionals in Ethiopia (Downes, Murray, & Brownsberger, 2007).

Health Extension Program

Since 1970, Ethiopia has worked to develop equitable access to healthcare services with limited achievements. Currently, the country is implementing a 20-year Health Sector

Development Plan aimed at universal coverage. A project of the Ministry of Health (MOH), the Health Extension program is an innovative, community-based program that focuses on creating a healthy living environment by increasing health awareness and making essential preventive health services available at the rural village level. Two salaried health extension workers (HEWs), who are trained for a year at Technical and Vocational Training and Education Centers, are being sent to rural villages. Sixteen health extension packages categorized into three major areas were developed to guide the curriculum and training of these HEWs, including disease prevention and control, family health services, and hygiene and environmental sanitation.

Accelerated Health Officer Training Program

In 2005, the Ethiopian MOH began pursuing additional ways to increase access to quality healthcare, particularly to rural and vulnerable populations. Based on the premise that strengthening routine health services mitigates the effect of emergencies and prevents some of their serious consequences, the MOH is taking steps to strengthen the healthcare system. Healthcare services are delivered through a four-tier system that consists of a primary health center with satellite health posts, district hospitals, regional hospitals, and specialized referral hospitals. The health facilities are inadequate in quantity and quality of services provided. Hospitals are concentrated in urban areas. The poor quality is directly related to the weak health infrastructure, insufficient supply of consumable and nonconsumable medical equipment, and the shortage of skilled human resources/health providers.

The Ethiopian government has built 600 new health centers over recent years in order to better distribute healthcare among the rural areas of the country, but there is a lack of qualified personnel to work in these health centers. Thus, the MOH devised a program named the Accelerated Health Officer Training Program (AHOTP).

As the team leader and key healthcare provider in the health centers, health officers are considered critical to an effective healthcare system as the link between health centers, HEWs, communities, *woreda* (district) health offices, and hospitals. During the past 5 years, EPHTI has made significant progress toward its goals of developing HLMs, strengthening staff competencies, enhancing learning environments on campus, and improving practical field experiences and health center training. The progress shown under the initiative has demonstrated a successful approach from which the AHOTP will benefit, in terms of improvement and lessons learned. The continuation of EPHTI provides the structures and support for the implementation of the AHOTP.

The expected results of the AHOTP are to graduate approximately 5,000 health officers by 2011; place adequate numbers of health officers in *woreda* health offices, and in old and new health centers; and improve the health service indicators in order to meet the Millennium Development Goals. These goals are to reduce child mortality; improve maternal health; and combat HIV/AIDS, malaria, and other diseases.

The AHOTP uses 21 training hospitals that are affiliated with the seven universities of the EPHTI network. The practical training of the AHOTP students is conducted at these training hospitals, whereas their first year of theoretical training is conducted in classrooms at the universities. In order to facilitate the training at this large number of hospitals, EPHTI renovated the 21 hospitals to ensure they each had the needed classroom and library space to train the influx of students from the program. EPHTI also provides consumable supplies for AHOTP training, such as latex gloves, stethoscopes, and bandages.

Conclusion

Challenges

While EPHTI experienced success in meeting its objectives and establishing previously unheard-of networks of communication and collegial relationships among the seven universities with which it works, the initiative also experienced challenges along the way. One such challenge continues to be the lack of longitudinal data on health status in the areas of Ethiopia where students exposed to the program currently work. The rates of certain health indicators were not collected in a baseline study at the start of the EPHTI program, and thus today it is hard to measure the long-term, community-based effect on health status of the population that is served by EPHTI-graduated students.

Another challenge faced by the program is a lack of funding to meet all the identified needs of students and staff in the universities. There are always more textbooks, teaching aids, and computers that are deemed useful for the educational programs of the universities; however, funding is limited.

Finally, another major challenge to the Initiative is brain drain throughout the country. Educated health professionals, as in other sub-Saharan nations, depart the country in droves in search of more pay elsewhere. Consequently, the teaching staff at universities are young and often inexperienced, and the need to retain Ethiopian-trained medical professionals is a reality. Motivations for highly educated health professionals to stay in the country and serve in remote and rural areas are difficult to come by, and the subsequent faculty shortages in the AHOTP program are testament to the problems of brain drain as well as the lack of sufficient funds to pay an already-overworked teaching staff to take on more duties.

Sustainability

Many international projects are implemented without consideration of how to sustain the project when funds are depleted. In the early development of EPHTI, one issue of concern was sustainability of the project after funding sources were exhausted. Several issues were related to the three goals of EPHTI. HLMs will require updating and the development of new materials. Faculty will continue to need opportunities to improve teaching and learning skills and to update their knowledge in many health areas, such as HIV/AIDS and reproductive health.

One solution to this issue is to fully incorporate EPHTI into the Ethiopian government after foreign assistance has been depleted. Because the training of Ethiopian health professionals is a priority of the government, making EPHTI a department of the Ministries of Health or Education makes sense for sustainability. EPHTI has always been an Ethiopian "owned" project, and the logical next step toward securing the sustainability of this groundbreaking endeavor is to institutionalize the concept and administration of the initiative into the government realm.

Replication

Although the EPHTI has focused on Ethiopia since it began in 1997, the process of working with partner universities to train a corps of healthcare workers was designed so that it could be replicated in other countries. Given the achievements of EPHTI, former President Carter and The Carter Center wanted to explore the possibility of replicating Public Health Training Initiatives in other African countries. One of the long-term goals of this initiative is the expansion of the methodology to other countries in need of public health infrastructure.

In mid-February 2007, the EPHTI network and its activities were on display in the first EPHTI Replication Conference, held in Addis Ababa and Debre Zeit, Ethiopia. Seventeen ministers of health, education, science, and technology from 10 African countries joined former President Carter for the conference in the Ethiopian capital. Also in attendance were Ethiopian Regional Health Bureau representatives, university presidents and representatives, donors such as USAID, The Packard Foundation, partner organizations, consultants, and staff from the Addis Ababa and Atlanta offices of The Carter Center. Participants heard EPHTI's story through a series of presentations and discussions. Over the 3-day conference, attendees learned about EPHTI's background, the current status of many projects, and future directions.

As a model for preservice health education, EPHTI is highly adaptable and customizable to other resource-poor nations' circumstances. The HLMs of the initiative are written by Ethiopians for Ethiopians, and within the context of locally available situations and solutions, and the same could be accomplished in other countries. The unique networking and communication structures that EPHTI has formed would serve any country well because it builds its health education infrastructure from the ground up, top down, and inside out.

Lessons Learned and Future Directions

Building capacity in educational institutions in a country recovering from the fall of a Socialist government and struggling with poverty is challenging and difficult, yet seeing progress and the commitment of institutions and individuals was extremely rewarding. There were many lessons learned from the experience that are worth sharing because they were essential to the success of the project. Key lessons learned include, but are not limited to, appreciating the value of:

1. Building positive working relationships among health science faculty from seven universities;
2. Using decision-making approaches that assure participation in decisions;
3. Listening to all audiences (government, university administrations, faculty, clinical staff, students);
4. Continuously searching for funds to support the project;
5. Recognizing accomplishments with opportunities to socialize and travel to other universities to learn about different teaching/learning environments and problems faced;
6. Learning about and respecting the individuality, culture, and the strengths of participants.

These are only a few of the major lessons learned. The rewards of working on a long-term project that result in long-lasting change and improvement in healthcare and in lifelong colleagues and friends cannot be measured.

References

Downes, E., Murray, J. P., & Brownsberger, S. L. (2007). The use of service learning in drought response by universities. *Ethiopia Nursing Outlook, 55,* 224–231.

Paulson, T. (2008). But what is global health, exactly? And why does it matter? *Pacific Lutheran University Campus Voice,* pp. 1–10. Retrieved October 31, 2008, from http://news.plu.edu/node/2384

World Health Organization. (n.d.). *The world health report 2006—Working together for health—Moving forward together.* Retrieved October 31, 2008, from http://www.who.int/whr/2006/overview/en/index2.html

33

Implementation of Public Health Interventions

David E. Bloom and Elizabeth Cafiero

In recent decades, the world has witnessed remarkable achievements in the realm of global health. For example, since 1950, life expectancy has risen by two decades and infant mortality has declined by more than two thirds. But improvements such as these mask a set of wide and growing disparities that characterize global health today. For example, while life expectancy exceeds 80 years in 15 countries, it remains under 60 years in 39 countries (United Nations Department of Economic and Social Affairs Population Division [UNDESA], 2009). Infant mortality and maternal mortality today vary by factors of 52 and 2,100 across countries (United Nations Development Programme, 2007; UNDESA, 2009).

The focus of this chapter is on implementation, by which we mean those activities aimed at translating a specific policy or programmatic concept into actual practice. Implementation involves refining and extending the policy or program design and executing it in conjunction with the development of detailed budgets, timelines, backup plans, and strategic partnerships, and the management of myriad vendors, consultants, staff, clients, and other stakeholders. The prospects for successful implementation are enhanced by making implementation an integral part of the policy or program design process. Implementation is often complex, and poor implementation is as likely to lead to intervention failures as ill-conceived designs.

Implementation as a Component of Public Health Intervention

To better understand implementation, it is useful to consider it in the broader context of public health intervention. We do this by outlining a seven-phase framework that describes the process of developing and delivering a policy or program:

David E. Bloom is Chairman and Clarence James Gamble Professor of Economics and Demography in the Department of Global Health and Population, Harvard School of Public Health. Elizabeth Cafiero is a research assistant in the department.

1. *Identifying and measuring the health problem.* This phase involves defining the target health problem and gathering and analyzing data on its scale and its geographic and demographic scope.
2. *Understanding the determinants of the health problem.* This phase requires an understanding of the causal pathways through which the targeted health problem develops.
3. *Devising interventions to address the health problem.* There are several ways to categorize actions aimed at addressing a health problem. For example, interventions may be broadly divided into medical, nonmedical health, and nonhealth interventions. Alternatively, interventions may be aimed at either prevention or treatment of a health problem or the care of those affected. Interventions can also be categorized functionally according to whether they endeavor to affect health outcomes by focusing on provision of information, alteration of financial incentives, or direct regulation of behavior.
4. *Choosing among the possible interventions (priority setting).* In this phase, program planners evaluate the pros and cons of different intervention options (or combinations thereof) and select which, if any, to implement. Decisions are based on a set of criteria that may include costs, benefits, equity, time, or political priorities. Several tools are available to aid priority setting, such as cost-effectiveness analysis or benefit–cost analysis.
5. *Implementation planning.* Implementation typically begins with a detailed planning exercise in which the resources needed for the chosen intervention, and the nature and timing of their precise uses, are specified. This phase ideally includes a plan for evaluating performance. Characteristics of successful planning include anticipating potential problems, devising solutions to those problems, and involving stakeholders so they feel some ownership of the process and outcomes.
6. *Implementing solutions.* This is the execution phase of the intervention process. Implementation involves piloting the intervention, bringing it to scale, reviewing and adjusting the model, and taking actions to promote sustainability. It is a critical phase of the intervention cycle because interventions are routinely undermined by implementation failures, even in the presence of appropriate designs and resources.
7. *Evaluating the impact of the intervention.* Evaluation is the final key element of the health intervention cycle. It includes assessing health and other impacts of the intervention and the extent to which the intervention proceeded according to plan. Evaluations are typically more compelling and meaningful if the evaluation methods are specified before the implementation phase and if the evaluation is conducted independently of the implementing agent.

As a practical matter, the phases of the intervention process are not strictly sequential. Instead, program planners may move back and forth between stages as programs are developed, uncertainty is resolved, and the nature of problems change. In addition, the phases of the process are not necessarily independent of each other. For example, the generation of new knowledge about implementation will improve the ability to design policies and programs and set priorities to meet public health goals. Likewise, interventions are often designed in response to a particular health problem, without analyzing the full range of complexities involved. As a result, when proceeding to implementation, program officials often encounter challenges in the field they did not anticipate while sitting in the planning office. For these reasons, integrated thinking about design and implementation is desirable.

Implementation in Practice

To appreciate the complex nature of implementation, we sketch a hypothetical case that concerns the introduction of a new childhood vaccination into a national routine immunization schedule. We start by assuming the existence of a vaccine that health policymakers have decided to adopt. At this stage, implementation planning activities are key. They focus on the regulatory framework, including licensing the vaccine and gaining approval of the appropriate national bodies and channels of influence to introduce the vaccine into the routine immunization schedule. Health planners, manufacturers, and insurers need to determine pricing of the vaccine, potential subsidies, and integration with insurance schemes.

To initiate the program, resources need to be allocated and supplies procured in advance of expected delivery of the vaccine. The logistics of distribution also need to be arranged before program launch. This involves establishing the supply chain, accounting for refrigeration or other cold chain requirements, purchasing vehicles and supplies, and developing protocols for disposal of waste products.

In a national vaccination program, uptake matters, especially to gain benefits associated with herd immunity. This requires education of the target population, parents, health providers, and other stakeholders, including plans for dealing with antivaccine groups and vaccine side effects and adverse reactions. It also requires specific strategies to reach different population groups, taking into account, for example, linguistic, cultural, religious, economic, and political heterogeneity. Strategies to promote program acceptance and adoption among health workers are also crucial.

Surveillance is also essential to program implementation. Linking the delivery of the new vaccine to an existing surveillance system allows for the determination of vaccine effectiveness, follow-up of children who do not receive the full vaccine course. It is also necessary to make sure immunizing agents are not counterfeit and to monitor them for spoilage due to normal expiration or improper storage.

Implementation also involves activities aimed at sustainability of the program. Periodic renewal of political will and financial support is essential for the vaccination to be available to future generations of children. Plans for immunization need to align with current medical standards of practice and may require regular updating. Ongoing training of health workers is crucial for maintaining program quality, especially in facilities with high employee turnover.

This example demonstrates some of the many considerations involved in adding a new vaccine to a nation's routine immunization program. Problems in one or several of these domains may significantly impede the introduction of the new vaccine to the target population.

What Implementation Requires: Elements of Success and Failure

To be successful, implementation requires a distinct set of actions at various levels. Individual practitioners must incorporate behavioral changes into their daily practice.

Implementation at the organizational level involves the establishment or modification of structural factors to support the assimilation of new methods or norms of practice into the organization's operations. At the systems level, the formal and informal networks to which individuals or organizations belong play a role in the dissemination and adoption of new information and practices.

Although a great deal about implementation is context specific, there are several common elements that practitioners can consider to aid the successful implementation of public health interventions. Later, we highlight considerations that are particularly relevant to those interested in implementing the Problem Solving for Better Health® (PSBH®) methodology.

Involvement of Stakeholders

Local knowledge is a crucial input to the design and implementation of interventions. Stakeholders often possess knowledge that can help to identify potential barriers, assess local capacities, and inform the customization of interventions to the local context. The most natural way to unleash the benefits of this knowledge reserve is to involve stakeholders in the process of program design and implementation. Once programs are launched in the field, stakeholder participation furthers the acceptance, ownership, and sustainability of programs. By having a real role, rather than a *pro forma* one, those who are responsible for program implementation as well as end users of a program will have a stake in achieving a successful outcome.

An example that highlights the importance of stakeholder involvement is the case of sugar fortification with vitamin A in Guatemala (Mora, Dary, Chinchilla, & Arroyave, 2000). In the 1960s, scientists gathered and analyzed data on the prevalence of vitamin A deficiency (VAD) in Guatemala. Technology and legislation mandating the fortification of sugar with vitamin A soon followed. Although the intervention produced short-term success, sugar producer compliance tailed off and VAD quickly returned to preintervention levels. As Mora et al. (2000) explained intervention planning was undertaken without the involvement of sugar producers. The fortification program was seen by the politically powerful, well-organized producers as an unwelcome intrusion of the government into private sector activity, and they did not adhere to the new regulations in subsequent harvests.

Leveraging Available Resources

Limited financial resources, inadequate material resources, and underperforming human resources are a major hindrance to implementation (Taegtmeyer & Chebet, 2002). However, it is sometimes possible to effect change by using limited intervention budgets to catalyze the engagement of incremental local resources (Guldbrandsson, 2008–2009). One way to do this is by identifying the resources that exist in the target community, a process that can be aided through community asset mapping (Bartholomew, Parcel, Kok, & Gottlieb, 2006; Beaulieu, 2002).

Once community resources are identified, program planners can explore their optimal uses. For example, community members may be able to receive training to perform a distinct set of tasks in certain contexts in order to substitute for clinical healthcare professionals; these community members are often referred to as lay health workers, community health workers, health promoters, or outreach workers. A well-documented success story here is Bangladesh's experience using lay outreach workers to distribute family planning supplies, information, and encouragement. These lay outreach workers, called Family Welfare Assistants (FWAs), provided a link between women in rural villages and the government health services. Analyses have demonstrated the contribution of FWAs to fertility decline in Bangladesh between 1970 and 2004 (Levine & The What Works Working Group, 2007). Studies of immunization programs also demonstrate that catalyzing community members' capacities as volunteers is a successful method for implementing programs when the existing health workforce cannot meet demand (Prinja, Gupta, Singh, & Jumar, 2010).

Cultural Sensitivity

Another important consideration for successful implementation is cultural relevance and sensitivity. To be effective, programs need to be specifically designed for the cultural context in which they will unfold (Bartholomew et al., 2006; Smylie et al., 2004).

A family planning program in rural Afghanistan demonstrates the importance of employing culturally appropriate implementation strategies (Huber, Saeedi, & Samadi, 2008; Sato, 2007). The program was a combination of two projects aimed at increasing contraceptive use and spacing of births among rural Afghan women. Program planners engaged in dialogue with community leaders and conducted surveys and focus groups with the target population to understand their views and beliefs about family planning. In order for the implementation strategies to reflect cultural realities, the program needed to take into account the fact that the Afghan population is predominantly Muslim. To this end, the program provided scientifically accurate information on contraception along with quotations from the Quran on birth spacing. The mullahs (religious leaders) approved the program's messages and, in some cases, served as community health workers. The mullahs were particularly effective in communicating the messages to men in the community. As a result of a combination of strategies, developed in conjunction with religious leaders, that were appropriate to the cultural context, the program significantly increased contraceptive use in the target areas.

The Importance of Pilot Testing

Small pilot studies are beneficial in identifying program weaknesses and allowing program planners to adjust program components before full-scale implementation (van Teijlingen & Hundley, 2001). During the pilot testing phase, practitioners can learn from program shortcomings without risking total program failure. Several tools are available for evaluating a pilot program, including focus groups, in-depth interviews, and questionnaires.

The importance of pilot testing is evidenced by the experience of the Partners for Life Program (PFLP) carried out in six counties in the Mississippi Delta (Boyd & Windsor, 2003). The program was aimed at improving diet among low-income pregnant women by offering nutrition education in the home over an 8-week period. All program methods were pilot tested in one county, and an independent evaluation was conducted to identify program strengths and weaknesses along three dimensions: recruitment and retention, short-term impact on nutrition and dietary behavior, and user-friendliness of the program. Using a combination of quantitative and qualitative evaluation methods, investigators identified clear program successes, as well as major challenges with the program design, particularly with regard to client retention and project timeline. The pilot program was able to retain only about half of the women recruited to participate. Further evaluation revealed that the length of the program and the number of educational sessions were viewed as burdensome. The evaluation also revealed that housing relocation contributed significantly to program attrition.

In order to overcome these weaknesses and avoid the same pitfalls when expanding the program throughout the six-county region, program designers proposed changes to the model. Piloting PFLP in one county saved program resources from being wasted by identifying and addressing implementation obstacles before the program was deployed throughout a larger area.

A Tool for Implementation

Evidence and experience demonstrate that integrating implementation and design may improve the success of public health interventions. We propose a simple tool to practitioners as they undertake the challenge of implementation (Table 33.1). The tool

TABLE 33.1 *Implementation Checklist*

Program Design and Planning

1. Are all relevant stakeholders identified and involved?
2. Have stakeholders demonstrated their support for the program?
3. Has the target population expressed and identified its needs?
4. Does the intervention identify capacities available to the project at the community, municipality, state, or federal level?
5. Are appropriate human, financial, and material resources identified and allocated to program planning, implementation, and evaluation?
6. Has the program identified how to overcome human resource deficiencies?
7. Has the program anticipated possible obstacles and identified methods for overcoming them?
8. Does the intervention allow for local-level flexibility?
9. Has the program considered cultural differences that will need to be addressed in program design and implementation?

Pilot Implementation

10. Will the intervention be tested on a small scale before full operation?
11. Are there specified methods to assess program performance?
12. Does the program articulate how coordination between levels will occur?

Full Implementation

13. Are measures to ensure quality of program delivery in place?
14. Is regular feedback from program users part of program operations?

TABLE 33.1 *(Continued)*

Adjustment

15. Have adjustments to the program been made in light of program evaluation?
16. Are stakeholders involved in the updating of the program?
17. Has the program team considered how the political, social, or economic context has changed since the program was designed? Has the team identified ways to adjust the program to the new context?

Sustainability

18. Is regular monitoring of the program taking place?
19. Are decision makers made aware of program performance?
20. Are resources allocated to the program on a periodic basis?

is a checklist that takes into account factors that influence implementation performance and that are too often overlooked or given minimal attention. Practitioners can visit the checklist throughout the implementation process as a reminder of key elements.

Implementation is the most neglected aspect of public health intervention. Paying it more attention will yield handsome global health dividends.

References

Bartholomew, L. K., Parcel, G. S., Kok, G., & Gottlieb, N. (2006). *Planning health promotion programs: An intervention mapping approach.* San Francisco: Jossey-Bass.

Beaulieu, L. J. (2002). *Mapping the assets of your community: A key component for building local capacity.* Mississippi State, MS: Southern Rural Development Center.

Boyd, N. R., & Windsor, R. A. (2003). A formative evaluation in maternal and child health practice: The Partners for Life nutrition education program for pregnant women. *Maternal and Child Health Journal, 7*(2), 137–143.

Guldbrandsson, K. (2008–2009). *From news to everyday use: The difficult art of implementation.* Ostersund, Swedan: Swedish National Institute of Public Health.

Huber, D., Saeedi, N., & Samadi, A. K. (2008). Achieving success with family planning in rural Afghanistan. *Bulletin of the World Health Organization, 88*(3), 227–231.

Levine, R., & The What Works Working Group. (2007). *Case studies in global health: Millions saved.* Sudbury, MA: Jones and Bartlett.

Mora, J. O., Dary, O., Chinchilla, D., & Arroyave, G. (2000). *Vitamin A sugar fortification in Central America: Experience and lessons learned.* Arlington, VA: MOST, The USAID Micronutrient Program.

Prinja, S., Gupta, M., Singh, A., & Jumar, R. (2010). Effectiveness of planning and management interventions for improving age-appropriate immunization in rural India. *Bulletin of the World Health Organization, 88*(2), 97–103.

Sato, M. (2007). *Challenges and successes in family planning in Afghanistan.* MSH Occasional Papers 6. Management Sciences for Health: Cambridge, MA.

Smylie, J., Martin, C. M., Kaplan-Myrth, N., Steele, L., Tait, C., & Hogg, W. (2004). Knowledge translation and indigenous knowledge. *The International Journal of Circumpolar Health, 63*(Suppl. 2), 139–143.

Taegtmeyer, M., & Chebet, K. (2002). Overcoming challenges to the implementation of antiretroviral therapy in Kenya. *The Lancet Infectious Diseases, 2,* 51–53.

United Nations Department of Economic and Social Affairs Population Division. (2009). *World Population Prospects: The 2008 Revision* (CD-Rom Edition—Extended Data Set in Excel and ASCII Formats). New York: United Nations.

United Nations Development Programme. (2007). *MDG monitor.* Retrieved February 2, 2010, from http://www.mdgmonitor.org/map.cfm?goal=4&indicator=0&cd=.

van Teijlingen, E. R., & Hundley, V. (2001). The importance of pilot studies. *Social Research Update, 35,* 1–7.

34

Corporate Social Responsibility and Global Health

Roy Ahn and Lynda Tyer-Viola

In November 2008, against the backdrop of massive economic woes, the Director-General of the World Health Organization (WHO) issued a statement urging governments to support global health-related activities (Chan, 2008). The Director-General noted the irony of the timing of the world's recent economic downturn: "It comes in the midst of the most ambitious drive in history to reduce poverty and distribute the benefits of our modern society, including those related to health, more evenly and fairly in this world—the Millennium Development Goals" (Chan, 2008). The achievement of these goals, known as the MDGs, would require significant financial resources; the World Bank (n.d.) asserted a price tag of "between $20 and $25 billion per year for all the [MDG] health-related goals" (p. 7). The push to attain the MDGs is just one illustration of today's intense interest in the topic of global health.

This interest has sparked discussion about the means required to achieve significant improvements in health. In addition to government, other sectors have also played important roles in advancing global health. For example, large philanthropic foundations, such as the Bill & Melinda Gates Foundation, have infused billions of dollars into global health programs during the past decade (Bill & Melinda Gates Foundation, n.d.). Civil society organizations have also contributed to global health, especially through research, as well as the use of such research to inform public policy (Bhan, Singh, Upshur, Singer, & Daar, 2007). The identification of multiple stakeholder groups underscores the extraordinary complexity and magnitude of global health problems and the solutions required to address these problems (e.g., Reich, 2002).

Here we ask: "Where do multinational corporations fit into the world of global health?" Large, multinational corporations have impacts on global health, in both beneficial and deleterious ways. Corporate medical product donation programs for developing countries, for example, are one very direct way health companies contribute to global public

Roy Ahn is Associate Director of Policy and Research at the Division of Global Health & Human Rights, Department of Emergency Medicine, Massachusetts General Hospital (MGH), and an instructor in surgery at Harvard Medical School. Lynda Tyer-Viola is a senior advisor at the Division of Global Health & Human Rights and an assistant professor at the MGH Institute of Health Professions School of Nursing.

health. By contrast, companies whose products or services lead to consumer morbidity or mortality obviously harm global public health. What are the advantages as well as the pitfalls of corporate sector involvement in global health? What is the most effective role for the corporate sector in advancing global health?

The idea of engaging the corporate sector to solve global health problems may be distasteful to some in the public health arena. One needs to only review the health community's long, rancorous relationship with the global tobacco industry to understand why a mistrust of business may persist, especially toward specific corporate industries. This mistrust may also explain the pessimistic view that corporate "good deeds" represent nothing more than slick attempts to polish corporate images. However, a competing perspective casts corporations, with their significant resources and expertise, as potentially useful agents for positive social change. The mantra of "public/private partnerships," in which groups from different sectors work together on a common issue, posits that governments need help from business and civil society in order to achieve the improvements in population health to which they aspire (e.g., Reich, 2002, pp. 1–2). Key assumptions of this perspective are that corporations also stand to gain—commercially, image-wise—from these arrangements, and can bring considerable technical and/or financial resources to these issues (Brown, Khagram, Moore, & Frumkin, 2000; Elias, Gerrans, & LaForce, 2008; Mahmud & Parkhurst, 2007; Reich, 2002). Although sometimes controversial (Buse & Walt, 2002), these partnerships represent one example of corporate involvement in global health. The remainder of this chapter provides an overview of corporate social responsibility (CSR) and its relation to global health (Ahn, 2005).

What Is Known About Corporate Social Responsibility?

Engaging the private sector in global health initiatives requires a working understanding of large multinational corporations—their structures, motivations, and capabilities. According to *Fortune* magazine, the world's largest corporation in 2008, Wal-Mart, earned revenues of nearly 380 billion USD in 2007 and employed more than 2 million people. By comparison, the 500th largest global corporation, Fluor, had revenues of nearly 17 billion USD in 2007 (Global 500, 2008). The economic power of these institutions suggests that they can significantly affect public health.

A conceptual debate about what companies can and should do to advance societal goals may be fairly novel in public health circles, but the broader topic of the role of business in society has a long lineage, dating back several decades, in the academic business literature (e.g., Carroll, 1979). Some business scholars have argued that a corporation's "social responsibility" should be limited to making money, legally (Friedman, 1970), whereas others have held corporations to a higher moral standard: "The idea of social responsibilities supposes that the corporation has not only economic and legal obligations but also certain responsibilities to society which extend beyond these obligations" (McGuire, quoted in Wartick & Cochran, 1985, p. 764). For example, corporate philanthropy could be considered one form of those "certain responsibilities."

In the 1980s, business scholars posited that corporate actions were largely dictated by managements' perceptions of how a host of stakeholders might view their actions. In other words, corporate stakeholders, defined as "employees, customers, suppliers, stockholders, banks, environmentalists, government, and other groups who can help or hurt the corporation," were very influential in corporations' organizational decision making (Freeman, 1984, p. vi). In effect, the "stakeholder theory" insinuated that corporations responded not only to *stock*holders but also to a broader group of *stake*holders (Clarkson, 1995; Freeman, 1984; Wood, 1991). This theory argues that shareholders, labor unions, government regulators, and other stakeholders can influence corporate management to act in responsible ways (Freeman, 1984). The shift away from the view that only share-holders can influence corporate management decision making would prove critical in shaping contemporary opinions of corporate responsibility.

This groundbreaking work provided the platform for what is defined today as CSR and its sister term, *corporate social performance* (CSP). "Corporate social responsibility encompasses not only what companies do with their profits, but also how they make them" (Corporate Social Responsibility Initiative, John F. Kennedy School of Government, Harvard University, n.d.). CSP is broader than CSR in that it has a decided emphasis on measurement (i.e., how can corporations document and report exactly how respon-sible they are?). It entails "[a] business organization's configuration of principles of social responsibility; processes of social responsiveness; and policies, programs, and observ-able outcomes as they relate to the firm's societal relationships" (Wood, 1991, p. 693).

Philanthropy and Beyond

Philanthropy—defined here as donations of funds as well as nonmonetary resources—is the most visible expression of CSR. In global health, examples of corporate philanthropy abound, especially in terms of corporate responses to natural disasters. For example, corporations donated hundreds of millions of dollars for relief efforts in the aftermath of the catastrophic South Asian tsunami of 2004 (Thiede, 2005) and more than 500 million USD for Hurricane Katrina–related efforts (Jones, 2005). Two prominent business schol-ars coined a phrase to describe the degree of reliance on corporations in humanitarian relief: "Misery loves companies" (Margolis & Walsh, 2003, p. 268).

During nondisaster periods, corporate philanthropy in global health can be creative and impactful. Pharmaceutical companies, in particular, have been adept at working with government and civil society in "partnerships," such as drug donation programs for developing countries (Mahmud & Parkhurst, 2007; Reich, 2002). In fact, some scholars have argued for health product companies' "special responsibilities to the sick poor" precisely because their business activities are so tightly aligned with health impact: "These companies have the competence, resources, and expertise to actually make a dif-ference" (Roberts, Breitenstein, & Roberts, 2002, pp. 77–78). However, not all pharma-ceutical corporate philanthropy involves drugs; some efforts aim to strengthen health systems. GlaxoSmithKline has invested in local partnerships in health education via its Thai Nursing program, which has "trained 500 nurses over a five-year period in sub-jects including primary care, healthcare prevention and promotion, patient home visita-tion, disease management and control, and health promotion campaigns" (Mahmud & Parkhurst, 2007, p. 31). Among nonhealthcare companies, Nike, through its foundation, directs significant funding toward "empowerment" programs in developing countries that are designed to provide opportunities for girls to become entrepreneurs in their communities (Nike Foundation, 2008). By reducing poverty, these programs can lead to improved health outcomes for girls and their families in these communities.

Philanthropy, however, represents only one piece of the CSR puzzle: "Corporate social responsibility encompasses not only what companies do with their profits, but also how they make them" (CSR Initiative, n.d.). Beyond philanthropy, a corporation's day-to-day actions could potentially have substantial effects on global health. For instance, the 200-plus member Global Business Coalition on HIV/AIDS, Tuberculosis, and Malaria (2008) described how company policies on HIV/AIDS have changed and improved over time, "moving past nondiscrimination clauses to encompass total health policies, including the provision of treatment and care to employees, and occasionally, their families." This policy shift alone could improve health for thousands of workers and their families around the world.

Considerations for the Future

CSR and related business ethics concepts such as CSP are not solely exercises in navel-gazing; corporate managers have also expressed concerns about CSR-related issues. A 2007 McKinsey & Company survey of corporate managers around the world noted that "Eighty four percent [of corporate managers] … agree that making broader contributions to the public good should accompany generating high returns to investors; only 16% believe that high returns to investors should be a corporation's sole focus" (Bonini, Greeney, & Mendonca, 2007, p. 2). The respondents cited "Environmental issues, including climate change," "political influence and/or political involvement of companies," and "healthcare benefits and other employee benefits" at the top of the list of topics "likely to have the most impact, positive or negative, on shareholder value over the next 5 years" (Bonini et al., 2007, p. 4). Hence, there is good reason to believe that corporations intend to engage in CSR in the future.

What can the global health sector learn from the business management literature? First, *all* corporations, not just health-focused corporations, have the ability to contribute to improvements in global health. Corporate health philanthropy, in particular, has leveraged corporate resources to effect, in a very direct way, improved health outcomes for large numbers of people, including vulnerable populations.

However, the CSR literature highlights many day-to-day corporate attributes besides philanthropy that have the potential to improve the health of multiple stakeholder groups: how a corporation manufactures, distributes, markets, and prices its products; how a corporation treats workers and their families via its workplace policies; and so on (Ahn, 2005). Corporate workplace policies represent an excellent area where corporations can materially benefit global health. Three *Fortune* Global 500 corporations employ more than 1 million workers apiece, and 32 of them employ more than 300,000 workers each (Global 500: Top Companies, 2008). A single change in human resource policy (e.g., providing health benefits to all workers) in these behemoth organizations has the potential to improve the health of millions of workers and their families.

Corporations can make the greatest positive impacts on global health if they maximize activities that promote health *and* minimize those activities that harm health. The occupational safety and health community has long understood the health-promoting and health-harming activities of corporations (Levy & Wegman, 2000). In addition, a new, albeit controversial, literature on the effects of nonhealth factors on health is emerging. For example, climate change may lead to changes in disease patterns that ultimately harm human health (Campbell-Lendrum, Corvalan, & Neira, 2007; Epstein, 2005). The field of social epidemiology has examined potential associations between social factors (e.g., poverty, discrimination) and adverse population-health outcomes (Berkman & Kawachi, 2000; Marmot, 2005). Many corporate activities, such as industrial emissions and workplace policies, could affect these nonhealth outcomes and may, therefore, indirectly contribute to changes in population health.

Whether through philanthropy, workplace policies, or products and services that improve health, the corporate sector is well positioned to make significant contributions to global health. Ultimately, the challenge for each corporation is to recognize the consequences—good and bad—of its own actions on the myriad stakeholders it affects and to make modifications in its behavior accordingly.

References

Ahn, R. (2005). *Corporate social performance and global health*. Unpublished doctoral dissertation, Harvard School of Public Health, Harvard University.

Berkman, L. F., & Kawachi, I. (Eds.). (2000). *Social epidemiology*. New York: Oxford University Press.

Bhan, A., Singh, J. A., Upshur, R. E. G., Singer, P. A., & Daar, A. S. (2007). Grand challenges in global health: Engaging civil society organizations in biomedical research in developing countries. *PLoS Medicine, 4*(9), e272.

Bill & Melinda Gates Foundation. (n.d.). *Grants*. Retrieved November 30, 2008, from http://www.gates-foundation.org/grants/Pages/overview.aspx

Bonini, S., Greeney, J., & Mendonca, L. (2007). Assessing the impact of societal issues: A McKinsey global survey. *The McKinsey Quarterly*, 1–9. Retrieved November 28, 2008, from http://www.mckinseyquarterly.com/Assessing_the_impact_of_societal_issues_A_McKinsey_Global_Survey_2077

Brown, L. D., Khagram, S., Moore, M. H., & Frumkin P. (2000). *Globalization, NGOs, and multi-sectoral relations*. Hauser Center for Nonprofit Organizations and the John F. Kennedy School of Government, Harvard University.

Buse, K., & Walt, G. (2002). The World Health Organization and global public–private health partnerships: In search of "good" global health governance. In M. Reich (Ed.), *Public–private partnerships for public health* (pp. 169–195). Boston, MA: Harvard University Press.

Campbell-Lendrum, D., Corvalan, C., & Neira, M. (2007). Global climate change: Implications for international public health policy. *Bulletin of the World Health Organization, 85*(3), 235–237.

Carroll, A. (1979). A three-dimensional conceptual model of corporate social performance. *Academy of Management Review, 4*(4), 497–505.

Chan, M. (2008). *Impact of the global financial and economic crisis on health*. World Health Organization. Press statement, 11/12/08. Retrieved November 21, 2008, from http://www.who.int/mediacentre/news/statements/2008/s12/en/index.html

Clarkson, M. (1995). A stakeholder framework for analyzing and evaluating corporate social performance. *Academy of Management Review, 20*(1), 92–117.

Corporate Social Responsibility Initiative, John F. Kennedy School of Government, Harvard University. (n.d.) *Initiative: Our approach*. Retrieved November 25, 2008, from http://www.hks.harvard.edu/m-rcbg/CSRI/init_approach.html

Elias, C. J., Gerrans, Y., & LaForce, F. M. (2008). Public–private partnerships drive innovation to improve the health of poor populations. In *Global forum update on research for health* (pp. 157–160). Woodbridge, UK: Pro-Book Publishing Limited.

Epstein, P. R. (2005). Climate change and human health. *New England Journal of Medicine, 353*, 1433–1436.

Freeman, R. E. (1984). *Strategic management: A stakeholder approach*. New York: Basic Books.

Friedman, M. (1970, September 13). The social responsibility of business is to increase its profits. *The New York Times Magazine*, 124–126.

Global Business Coalition on HIV/AIDS, Tuberculosis and Malaria. (2008). *The maturing of business action*. New York: Global Business Coalition on HIV/AIDS, Tuberculosis and Malaria.

Global 500. (2008, July 21). Retrieved November 27, 2008, from http://money.cnn.com/magazines/fortune/global500/2008/full_list/

Global 500 Top Companies: Biggest employers. (2008, July 21). Retrieved December 1, 2008, from http://money.cnn.com/magazines/fortune/global500/2008/performers/companies/biggest/

Jones, D. (2005, December 9). Corporate giving for Katrina reaches $547 million. *USA Today.* Retrieved November 30, 2008, from http://www.usatoday.com/money/companies/2005-09-12-katrina-corporate-giving_x.htm

Levy, B., & Wegman, D. (2000). *Occupational health: Recognizing and preventing work-related disease and injury* (4th ed.). Philadelphia: Lippincott Williams & Wilkins.

Mahmud, A., & Parkhurst, M. (2007). *The role of the health care sector in expanding economic opportunity.* Corporate Social Responsibility Initiative, Harvard Kennedy School of Government. FSG Social Impact Advisors and the Fellows of Harvard College.

Margolis, J. D., & Walsh, J. P. (2003). Misery loves companies: Rethinking social initiatives by business. *Administrative Science Quarterly, 48*(2), 268–305.

Marmot, M. (2005). Social determinants of health inequalities. *The Lancet, 365,* 1099–1104.

Nike Foundation. (2008, May 27). *Nike Foundation and Buffetts join to invest $100 million in girls.* Retrieved November 30, 2008, from http://www.nikefoundation.org/files/The_Girl_Effect_News_Release.pdf

Reich, M. R. (Ed.). (2002). *Public–private partnerships for public health.* Cambridge, MA: Harvard University Press.

Roberts, M., Breitenstein, A. G., & Roberts, C. S. (2002). The ethics of public–private partnerships. In M. R. Reich (Ed.), *Public-private partnerships for public health* (pp. 67–85). Cambridge, MA: Harvard University Press.

Thiede, B. (2005, February 11). Tsunami relief marks shift in corporate efforts. *Charlotte Business Journal.* Retrieved November 30, 2008, from http://charlotte.bizjournals.com/charlotte/stories/2005/02/14/focus3.html?surround=etf

Wartick, S. L., & Cochran, P. L. (1985). The evolution of the corporate social performance model. *Academy of Management Review, 10*(4), 758–769.

Wood, D. J. (1991). Corporate social performance revisited. *Academy of Management Review, 16*(4), 691–718.

World Bank. (n.d.) *The costs of attaining the Millenium Development Goals.* Retrieved November 29, 2008, from http://www.worldbank.org/html/extdr/mdgassessment.pdf

IV

Recommendations for the Future

Introduction

Joyce J. Fitzpatrick

Beyond the individual projects, countries, and models, health professionals have a collective responsibility to address global health issues at the broadest level. In this section there are two examples of how to move the dialogue and debate to the policy level. In Chapter 35, Garson describes ways in which the Problem Solving for Better Health® (PSBH®) model can be moved from the individual project level to informing and influencing policy development and analysis. He provides specific recommendations that could be implemented and outlines next steps in the movement to the policy level. He identifies models for change that have been implemented in relation to other topics, for example institutes, conferences, student placements, etc. Garson concludes that we should link the "thinkers" with the "doers" so as to maximize resources and progress toward achieving our healthcare goals more quickly.

In the final chapter, Smith calls all citizens to action to create a better world and global health for all. He highlights the problems inherent in many of the current approaches to solving health problems, some of which create additional problems for those they are intended to serve. Very often the approaches initiated by health professionals are distancing, particulate, and biased, rather than humanistic and holistic. Smith calls for a grand plan for global health that incorporates vision, passion, commitment, and persistence, but at the same time includes a practical, flexible dimension. According to Smith, all individuals should be engaged in planning for their own health and empowered to make a difference in their own lives and the lives of their fellow citizens. While Smith's vision of health and a healthy world presents a challenge, the PSBH model, and the other partnership models described in this book, provide evidence of both the vision and the practical approaches that have made a difference. Smith challenges us further to succeed in our individual and collective work, and importantly, he provides the structure and the tools for implementing change.

35

From Individual Problem Solving to Evidence-Based Policy

Arthur Garson, Jr.

Across the world, countries face challenges in improving the health of their societies. Although their circumstances may differ, all countries, whether developed or developing, can benefit from the experiences of one another. The diseases of underdeveloped countries, including HIV/AIDS, malnutrition, chronic diarrhea, tuberculosis (TB), and malaria, all have similar roots in poverty. Meanwhile, developed countries "export" diseases such as obesity and hypertension that are now on the rise in developing economies. Developed parts of the world can share lessons on how to organize care, providing coverage and access. Underdeveloped countries can certainly learn from developed countries how to provide advanced medicine, although advanced medicine does not always facilitate the greatest good for the greatest number. Finally, underdeveloped countries can teach developed countries how to provide, in some cases, the most efficient care with the most limited resources.

Improvements in health can be made by various actors at all points along a continuum—from individuals to foundations to governments. The majority of effective improvements occur when all levels are involved: identifying problems and solving them locally and then applying these local solutions more broadly to collect data and solve problems at the level of a state or country. These "bottom-up" approaches, when individual project data are appropriately aggregated, can provide important information to governments; similarly, "top-down" approaches from policymakers who are aware of the major issues of the country can be aided by utilizing individuals to introduce new programs and collect data. Each approach informs the other.

Bottom Up: Individuals to Policymakers

A prototype of the bottom-up approach has been in operation for decades in the form of Problem Solving for Better Health® (PSBH®), Problem Solving for Better Health Initiative™ (PSBHI™), and Problem Solving for Better Health-Nursing™ (PSBHN™), all pioneered

Arthur Garson, Jr., is the Executive Vice President and Provost of the University of Virginia.

by the Dreyfus Health Foundation (DHF, 2007; The Health Foundation [THF], 1992; Hoyt, 2007;). As this book describes, the programs involve grassroots "small-scale problem-solving projects that … directly benefit many people" (THF, 1992). This approach is locally defined and may involve taxi drivers, bureaucrats, farmers, health professionals, and others. Interestingly, the PSBH paradigm can also be taught in professional schools, specifically medical and nursing schools. The program has been highly successful in India and China, training students in the essentials of clinical research and demonstrating how small projects can be accomplished with important results in a limited period of time. In all of its incarnations, the PSBH process has been tremendously successful in more than 30 countries (including the United States), with more than 30,000 people generating over 20,000 projects (DHF, 2007; Hoyt, 2007; THF, 1992).

The advantages of bottom-up projects are several. They have the potential to solve the problems relevant to people in communities. They suggest possible comprehensive solutions when aggregated (i.e., when data from several small studies collected with identical methodology are combined for analysis). They can grow from a single local program to become more widespread, demonstrating the depth of the problem as well as potential solutions that can lead to policy change. As has been said, "the plural of anecdote is policy;" the bottom-up approach generates a large number of "anecdotes" that can be combined with applicable data to attract the attention of policymakers. The bottom-up approach can also identify and promote leaders who are capable of solving important problems. Finally, such local bottom-up approaches can generate further questions in a community, which can then be answered with more local solutions.

Disadvantages of the bottom-up approach must also be considered, however. Such an approach requires local application of practical ways to solve a problem. It is important for individuals to understand how previous problems have been solved—or not solved. Innovation is required if new methods of problem solving are needed. The individual who is proposing the program also must be able to implement, and, therefore, to lead and to marshal human resources (whether laypeople, physicians, or nurses), as well as find financing. Such bottom-up approaches also rely on questions developed by individuals, which may not be the most crucial in solving the country's health problems, or even the community's health problems. Finally, a methodology is required to move from collected data to policy; it is not likely that seminars and journal articles will suffice. It is important to have access to policymakers who are willing to receive such data and consider policy implementation based upon the data.

Innovation and aggregation seem to be at odds: to stimulate innovation means approving some projects with low probabilities of success. Nevertheless, virtually every project (except those with a truly local problem and local solution) should be carried out with an eye on "aggregation," meaning that if the pilot study is successful, it can be reproduced in other larger samples either in the same area or beyond. This implies the need for two types of projects for PSBH/PSBHI/PSBHN: (1) the typical pilot project and (2) the follow-up or aggregation type study. In the latter, an individual would find a methodology in the DHF database that had already been demonstrated to be effective, and then would use this methodology in an aggregation study.

To facilitate this, a database could be available to participants before and during the workshop. During the PSBH workshop, participants could reference the database for prior approaches and prior outcomes (either positive or negative) to determine the applicability of prior approaches to the current identified problem. The database would be searchable (coded) and provide enough specific information to determine whether a similar problem has been targeted elsewhere, the method (in sufficient detail to be reproduced in future studies allowing for data aggregation), the number of subjects, and the results. The database would also include "lessons learned"—ways to approach the problem in a different manner the next time others attempt a similar project, as well as possible applicability to larger studies. In addition, the database might include fields for possible policymaker contacts and possible funding mechanisms.

The PSBH process could potentially be enhanced by adding a sixth step, entitled "move forward together." The intent of this step would be to discuss how to move from the individual study to groups of studies that could have aggregated data. In this way, projects could be sustained and ultimately move from lay community members to health professionals, foundations, and governments. Step 6 would not be applicable to projects that solve unique local problems in unique ways but, if possible, projects should answer this final question. This would lead to "think small ... but prepare to take the next step" (DHF, 2007; Hoyt, 2007; THF, 1992). The "next step" might not necessarily involve the aggregation of data leading directly to policy but could involve aggregation of *some* data that then generate questions that can serve as suggested further projects.

To learn as much as possible from all of the PSBH/PSBHI/PSBHN projects, a formal worldwide learning consortium could be created so that not only problems and methodology, but also approaches to health policy around the world, can be shared. This consortium would mainly communicate online, but such online consortia benefit from face-to-face meetings, organized around individual problems. Annual meetings would be attended by representatives of as many countries as possible.

Top Down: Policymakers to Individuals

A proposed Institute for Health Systems and Policy would assess and improve the healthcare delivery systems in the United States and other countries. The institute would have a tripartite mission of service to the public, research, and education. It would combine original research on public health with a number of sources, such as multiple studies based upon grassroots primary care data collection. The research activities could be shared through new Web-based tools, bringing experts together to develop novel insights and strategies regarding common challenges facing the world's health systems. With access to these suggested strategies, decision makers could develop evidence-based policies that lead to improvements in health systems.

The initial focus of the institute would be in the intertwined policy areas that are essential to providing better health to the world's population: access and coverage. Evidence-based policy and implementation strategies would suggest the changes necessary in health systems so that ultimately every member of the public will have timely and appropriate access to healthcare practitioners. This would require studies of the healthcare workforce—planning, training, and models of care that can then be translated into delivery models for underserved regions. These larger societal studies should include topics such as improvements in transportation, education, and job creation, all of which improve the health of communities as well as the individuals that reside within them. One example, discussed earlier in this book, is the use of community health workers (e.g., grandparents) functioning in a team model linked by innovative electronic media that allow supervision, data collection, and continuous learning. After initial pilot programs demonstrate a working model of improved access, major grant funding could be sought to implement these models, where appropriate, throughout the world.

Given that access and coverage are intertwined and inextricably related to quality and cost in every healthcare system, the institute would bridge and amplify the interconnections with targeted studies. These would include developing new ways to incent personal responsibility in patients and the practice of care determined to be of high value by practitioners and healthcare facilities, implementing information technology and other methods to improve quality and reduce the cost of care, developing a consistent measure of the value of treatments and tracking its application throughout the system, developing financial relationships within healthcare systems that strengthen the business case for quality improvement, designing systematic strategies to address public health problems in different parts of the world (e.g., obesity or diarrhea) that damage health and drive up costs, and applying ethical ways to allocate limited resources.

The institute faculty would teach undergraduates, students in health professions, and graduate students, either in person or using distance education around the world. In addition, the institute would sponsor and provide mentorship for research fellows from within and outside the institute, and provide targeted grants to researchers studying innovations in health systems. The institute would offer certificates in health systems and public policy to students around the world.

As a national and international leader in the study and improvement of health system performance, the institute for Health Systems and Policy would apply Web-based technology to teach, to develop empirical research, and to use this evidence to shape the evolution of public policies and improve health worldwide. In maximizing the advantages of a small institute, it would be important to demonstrate results: work done by the institute should result in improved health systems, and the work should be recognized both by the health system itself as well as by others through publications and seminars. Such a small institute would also become a specialist in partnering with academic institutions, foundations, nongovernmental organizations, and governments to address larger problems, with the institute providing a unique niche. For example, the institute may have greater access to "on the ground" data collection than others; alternatively, the institute may have experts in particular areas, such as those providing access to care in underserved regions.

The advantage of a top-down approach is clear/simple: The questions would have the attention of the policymakers, foundations, or governments that are issuing the questions. Presumably these are crucial questions whose answers will lead to improved health.

The disadvantages of a purely top-down approach are also important to acknowledge. For one thing, the question may be the wrong question. It may be too narrow, important only to a single or a few policymakers driven more by local politics than overall urgent needs. A question might ask for a politically expedient solution rather than requiring an answer to a fundamental policy issue. This is one of the gray areas in practical policy: whether to "move the ball down the field" incrementally or to "throw the long ball" of substantive change. The United States generally moves the ball down the field incrementally, due at least partially to a political process that requires agreement by numerous committees and separate parties; broad social policy changes are generally unacceptable to a sufficient majority. Other countries, however, have been somewhat more successful in large-scale policy change.

While not "wrong," certain questions issued by policymakers tend to deal more with process than with outcome, and although they are required for system improvement they seem distant to actual improvement in the health of the local community (e.g., how to improve the efficiency of billing is an important question that could save money, and this money could be used to pay for care for the uninsured—but these two may not be clearly linked). In many cases the connection cannot be made, and process improvement questions are difficult to translate to improvement in health at the local level. Policymakers also tend to ask questions that available data can already answer rather than asking a more generalizable question. For example, the data are available on every Medicare patient. But because Medicare patients are generally older than the 65 years, and consistent and comprehensive information on those younger than 65 is lacking, Medicare studies are not generalizable to the greater population.

An extension of this problem is that policymakers tend to ask smaller questions because funding and timeframes are generally short. Therefore, even large studies require further aggregation to be applicable to overall policy. Finally, as noted with bottom-up approaches, once a policy is developed the actual implementation requires leaders and the devotion of appropriate people whether in the health system or the local community. Such implementation may fail if the local implementation was not considered thoroughly.

The Ideal: The Circle

The ideal prototype is a circle, moving from PSBH problem identification, data collection, and aggregation to information that influences policy and improves health—or, to begin at another part of the circle, if a system has set priorities and targets for improved health, the grassroots network can be activated to collect data, testing different hypotheses of how to improve health at the local level. Specifically, there are four ways this integration could proceed:

1. A joint advisory council for DHF and the institute could be created with the leadership of both entities, including advisory board members of both, as well as several national and international outside policy experts. This joint advisory council would discuss, among other issues, projects that appear the most promising for aggregation from PSBH (the bottom-up approach) as well as those potential projects of the institute for which an aggregated approach to data collection by PSBH (the top-down approach) would be worthwhile.
2. Joint DHF/institute conferences could be held on how to move from data to evidence-based policy and "around the circle." Sessions on specific projects would also be held. These conferences would occur at least yearly, but could occur more frequently within certain regions or related to certain projects/problems. Follow-up to any of these meetings would be through an online worldwide learning consortium.
3. Institute students could learn how to identify and access health system challenges during a 1-year intense program in research and service learning that identifies and solves limited problems (based upon PSBH); the aggregated data from these projects would inform evidence-based policy.
4. The PSBH methodology could be taught to Ministries of Health in key countries. Yearly workshops would be developed, with ministry personnel helping to solve

local problems. This would not only involve individuals in problem solving but also sensitize ministry personnel to use the aggregated data in their own country as a basis for evidence-based policy.

5. This "ideal" circle where data inform policy and policy generates further questions to be answered by more data is best served with an integrated approach. Many organizations do each of these functions quite well, from individual data gathering to community-based service interventions and policy development. The proposed plan is to combine a "think tank" with a "do tank," to produce evidence-based policy for the benefit of the world's health.

The major advantages to integration are the production of evidence-based policy based upon data either originating from individuals and systems or from the policymakers asking questions that can be answered by data collection at the local level. In any new entity, maximizing the advantages and minimizing the disadvantages requires planning, execution, and integration. The goal is better health for all, in this instance through the development of policy, whether from individual ideas or collective thinking.

References

Dreyfus Health Foundation. (2007). *Problem Solving for Better Health (PSBH) participant's handbook*. New York: Author.

The Health Foundation. (1992). *Problem-Solving for Better Health*. New York: Author.

Hoyt, P. (2007). An international approach to Problem Solving for Health-Nursing™ (PSBHN). *International Nursing Review, 54,* 100–106.

36

The Call to Action

Barry H. Smith

This book began with the statement that we live in a broken world. The evidence of this is overwhelming and reinforced every day. There is far too much disease, suffering, death, and lost human potential for far too much of the world's population. Add to that man's inhumanity to man, with hate and violence, as well as our tendency to indulge in activities that harm us (e.g., poor eating habits, tobacco use, risky behaviors), and the picture is discouraging. The negative statistics are often staggering. I do not need to repeat them here.

The problem of brokenness is global. Although the developing countries bear the largest part of this burden, the fact is there are serious problems across the entire world. One can be disenfranchised, isolated, and powerless anywhere. The effects of globalization have led to infectious disease problems in even the most remote corners of the world, threatening the health of everyone, rich and poor. Some communicable diseases, such as smallpox and polio, have come under increasingly better control, whereas chronic diseases such as diabetes, cancer, hypertension, cardiovascular disease, and mental illness have come to the fore in every country. Because of their complexity and frequent collateral damage to organ systems, these diseases are often less amenable to more straightforward solutions, such as clean water and antiparasitic or antibacterial agents. Furthermore, because many of these problems occur most frequently in people more than 65 years of age, these diseases have enormous implications for families and the economic burdens of any society.

Although it remains the overwhelming tendency to think of health and disease in biological terms that involve physiology, genes, parasites, bacteria, and viruses, a major point in this book is that health should be seen more broadly. Health is not only a total state of well-being but also a product of the functioning of one's society, and the individual within society. A human being is not defined by one or more disease states but rather as an integrated whole that includes his or her biological, social, cognitive, emotional, and spiritual dimensions.

The preceding chapters are based on the above conception of health and the recognition that we must deal with individuals, families, communities, and societies that are integrated wholes (even better, the products of complex multisystem interactions) to change the situation—to heal our world (Resnicow & Page, 2008; Scotch, Parmanto, Gadd, & Sharma, 2006). Most of the efforts that have been described here are products of the Dreyfus Health Foundation's (DHF) Problem Solving for Better Health® (PSBH®) program. This is not the only model; other examples are included in Section III and there are certainly many more. It is clear that multiple approaches (e.g., medical, biological, economic, and educational) are necessary to address the brokenness that we see around us everyday. Grassroots as well as top-down components must be integrated; the keys to the ultimate success of better health and quality of life for humanity lie in the obligatory complementarity of these different components. There is no such thing as one approach to deal with the whole problem. To insist that there is a single approach is a big mistake, just as not trying to bring the approaches together in an integrated fashion is a grave error. Sadly, we seem to persist in making both of these mistakes.

Granting that multiple approaches are needed, it is also crucial to stress the importance of bringing "the people" into the processes. People are an absolutely necessary element. If this is not done, programmatic failure, in the strictest sense of being measured against what needs to be accomplished, is a certainty. One of the major strengths of PSBH is that bringing "the people" into the process is exactly what the program is designed to do. In some countries or regions this has been done by working directly at the community, family, and individual levels. In other countries, most specifically China and India, because of the large numbers of people to be reached, the initial efforts have been with health workers, involving them so that they become the ones to spread the model of responsibility, capability, and action to everyone in the country as quickly as possible. In most places there is likely to be a mix of both approaches. This is desirable because it speaks to the necessary integration of the different levels and modes of solving the region's problems.

The PSBH results and the positive outcomes from the other models reported here demonstrate that measurable differences in health and quality of life can be achieved, yet, we must recognize that these successes are not nearly enough. Despite what has been accomplished, we have not made much of a dent in the problems from which hundreds of millions, even billions, of people are suffering. We are all guilty when we become comfortable with the statistics of death, morbidity, and lost human potential; when we do not regard people with true respect; when we forget or ignore that people are integrated wholes and we implement programs that ultimately will fail; when we wait for prerequisites or make other excuses for our own failures; or when we insist that our own approach is the only right one.

So, what is to be done? This book serves as a clarion call to action—a call for a revolution of and by the people. First we need to define "the people." Who exactly are they? In philanthropy, they are generally the "disadvantaged," the people who have been or are the targets or recipients of present efforts for better health around the world. They are the ones who suffer most from the problems that we have been discussing. They are most often those living in poverty. They lack education and either do not have jobs or are working at the most menial and most physically demanding of tasks. They may live in slums, like those of Mumbai or Chennai in India, or the favelas of Brazil, where the homes are simple, often made of discarded metal, pipes, or even cardboard and mud. They may live in rural areas and work their own small plots of land or the farms of others. They work hard. They are subject to injury and disease with little or no access to healthcare. Their life expectancy is short compared to that of the better-off citizens of their countries. They do not have the opportunities to make changes in their own lives or to make life better for their families.

That is the usual description of the common people, and most especially, those who are poor. However, the picture presented in the preceding paragraph is not a true representation. First of all, there is a kind of bias, albeit often unintended, that "the people" are second-class citizens. There is a subtle condescension hidden in words that appear simply to be factual. Second, and far more important, the earlier description leaves out the humanity and enormous capabilities of these people. They are the missing pieces. Despite their disadvantages, they are in essence the equals of those of us who are more fortunate.

A revolution for the good of all can only begin, grow, and ultimately succeed in making changes for the better if "the people" are made central to it. They must be the drivers and leaders. In other words, they must be seen as full and equal partners. Their experience, wisdom, and abilities must be the foundation on which the revolution is built.

It is one thing to talk about a revolution for the good and quite another to see it through to making the changes that are needed. Fortunately, as the chapters in this book make clear, a transformation is already underway. It is also important to realize that truly successful revolutions do not just happen. History teaches us that for a revolution to be successful there must be several ingredients: a grand or strategic vision, passion, commitment, persistence, and a practical but flexible tactical plan that includes the mobilization of the people on a large scale. Without all these elements, one ends up with an insurgency or some lesser societal turmoil.

Our revolution is just beginning. The PSBH program has reached more than 30 countries. Other programs, such as those of Ashoka, The Carter Center, and the Clinton Global Initiative; foundation efforts, such as those of the Bill & Melinda Gates Foundation, the Rockefeller Foundation, and the W. K. Kellogg Foundation; government aid efforts, such as those of Irish AID, the United Kingdom's Department For International Development, Australia's AusAid, Japan's Official Development Assistances, Sweden's Sida (International Development Agency), the Czech Republic's Development Cooperation and Humanitarian Aid, and the United States Agency for International Development; and the rapidly increasing aid efforts from countries such as China, Brazil, and India, are reaching even larger numbers of people around the world. In a very real sense, there is no country that is not experiencing an ongoing development process.

Unfortunately, the benefit of much of the aid from a variety of sources fails to impact the lives of "the people." Tremendous amounts of resources are available. They need to be leveraged to achieve far more than they are achieving now. Bringing the people into the systems as active participants and leaders is critical.

It is also worth noting the fact that according to figures from the Progressive Policy Institute (2007), "The world's truly generous people are migrant workers—Indonesian maids in Hong Kong, Filipina nurses in California, Haitian farmworkers in Florida, Beninois and Malians in France, Turks in Germany—whose 286 billion USD in remittance payments for 2006 is easily more than twice all the aid provided by governments and multilateral financial institutions." That fact is rather humbling, but it also suggests a tremendous opportunity for a revolution for the good. The leadership of the people already exists and is thriving, but its potential has only barely begun to be unleashed.

The following are some specific elements of our call to action:

(a) Formation of a central but global steering group. Members need not be in one location but can be linked by technology. Diversity in every respect is essential. All must be totally committed and passionate. Taking action is paramount. No excuses!

(b) Commitment to the viewpoint that every death that occurs each day, that every bit of human suffering, that every unnecessary disease, that every bit of diminished human potential, is unacceptable. Every day there must be a measurable reduction in each of these elements.

(c) Commitment by all involved that this revolution is not about individual countries, institutions, specific programs, or people, but rather about measurable change in people's lives and quality of life. Everything is to be subsumed toward the goal of measurable, sustainable, and replicable change for the good. It is important to note that it is not about who is to get what resources, but rather how the resources that are available might be used to maximum effect.

(d) Mapping and evaluation of current global assets available. This asset map is to include as many projects and ongoing programs as possible, with analysis as to how they might be evaluated and leveraged. Garson, in Chapter 35, has specific suggestions for moving from individual problem solving to evidence-based policy, which creates an environment in which the revolution can thrive.

(e) Creation of an international core group of experts in complex system analysis, model building, and outcome prediction (Resnicow & Page, 2008; Scotch et al, 2006). These experts will provide the evidence base for the activities identified previously and also help build the broader vision.

(f) Ongoing global mobilization of "the people" through a multilevel set of processes that includes face-to-face or one-on-one encounters, mass rallies that take lessons from successful political movements, and technological connectivity. The Internet will be used to disseminate information quickly. Data on the success or failure of efforts around the world will be collected on an ongoing basis to evaluate progress or lack of it and provide feedback and encouragement to the members of the global revolutionary force. The media will be recruited to be part of, as well as report on, the progress of the revolution.

(g) Continued spreading of tools, such as PSBH, that need to reach every corner of the world and each and every person to convey the message of personal and collective responsibility, innate capability, and individual and collective progress in the revolution. The ongoing and continuous feedback provided by the data collection and evaluation system described will be a critical piece of this effort.

(h) Victory—of, by, and for all people everywhere!

Is this a dream? Can we achieve the goal of changing the world for the better? Not only *can* this revolution for the good succeed, it *must*. The key to making it happen is us—all of us. Start making a difference today!

References

Progressive Policy Institute. (2007, November 7). *Developing countries' foreign aid programs have tripled since 2001.* Retrieved August 14, 2009, from http://www.ppionline.org

Resnicow, K., & Page, S. E. (2008). Embracing chaos and complexity: A quantum change for public health. *American Journal of Public Health, 98*(8), 1382–1389.

Scotch, M., Parmanto, B., Gadd, C. S., & Sharma, R. K. (2006). Exploring the role of GIS during community health assessment problem solving: Experiences of public health professionals. *International Journal of Health Geographics, 5,* 39–49.

Appendix

Dreyfus Health Foundation

National Coordinators

Belarus: Dr. Vladimir Gordeiko
Brazil: Dr. Daniel Becker
Bulgaria: Mrs. Yanka Tzvetanova
Cameroon: Dr. Paul Tan
China: Madame On Ning and Ms. Hsin-Ling Tsai
Dominican Republic: Dr. Adelaida Oreste
El Salvador: Dr. Ignacio Paniagua Castro and Dr. Mauricio Lozano
Ghana: Mrs. Lynda Arthur
Guyana: Ms. Ismay Murray and Dr. Wallis Best Plummer
India: Dr. V. Raman Kutty
Indonesia: Dr. Alex Papilaya
Jordan: Mr. Mahmoud M. Alkam and Dr. Darwish Badran
Kenya: Ms. Mary Muyoka
Kyrgyzstan: Dr. Aibek Mukambetov
Latvia: Dr. Velta Lubkina
Lesotho: Dr. William J. Bicknell
Lithuania: Ms. Giedre Donauskaite-Tang
Malawi: Dr. Maureen L. Chirwa
Mexico: Dr. Héctor Marroquín Segura
Peru: Ms. Anna Zucchetti
Poland: Dr. Jan Sobotka and Dr. Katarzyna Broczek
Romania: Mr. Paul Florea and Mrs. Ana Florea
Ukraine: Dr. Oleksandra Sluzhynska
United States: Ms. Marsha Johnson Copeland
Vietnam: Dr. Tran Duc Thai
Zambia: Mrs. Ruth Chikasa

Regional Coordinators

Africa: Mrs. Ruth Chikasa
Asia: Madame On Ning
Eastern Europe, Middle East, and Central Asia: Dr. Jan Sobotka
Latin America: Dr. Daniel Becker
United States of America: Ms. Marsha Johnson Copeland

Index

Note: Page references followed by "*f*" and "*t*" denote figures and tables, respectively.